Drug Delivery: Evaluation, Formulation and Mechanisms

Drug Delivery: Evaluation, Formulation and Mechanisms

Editor: Lyda Zhang

AMERICAN
MEDICAL PUBLISHERS
www.americanmedicalpublishers.com

AMERICAN
MEDICAL PUBLISHERS
www.americanmedicalpublishers.com

Cataloging-in-Publication Data

Drug delivery : evaluation, formulation and mechanisms / edited by Lyda Zhang.
p. cm.
Includes bibliographical references and index.
ISBN 979-8-88740-071-6
1. Drug delivery systems. 2. Drugs--Administration. 3. Drugs--Dosage forms.
4. Pharmaceutical technology. 5. Biomedical engineering. 6. Pharmaceutical chemistry.
I. Zhang, Lyda.
RS199.5 .D78 2023
615.6--dc23

American Medical Publishers,
41 Flatbush Avenue,
1st Floor, New York,
NY 11217, USA

ISBN 979-8-88740-071-6 (Hardback)

Contents

Preface

Drug delivery encompasses the methods, manufacturing processes, technologies, formulations and storage systems used to transport a pharmaceutical compound to its target site in order to produce the intended therapeutic effect. Its goal is to modify a drug's specificity and pharmacokinetics by formulating it with various medical devices, excipients and drug carriers. Drug delivery techniques that are frequently utilized include controlled, targeted and steady drug delivery. Since the introduction of systems of medical applications, a variety of drugs are being used to treat a number of diseases through the administration of various conventional forms of drug delivery, including lotions, ointments, suppositories, solutions, pills, mixtures, pastes, powders, tablets, etc. The three main mechanisms of drug delivery are swelling, diffusion and erosion. This book aims to understand the evaluation, formulation and mechanisms of drug delivery. It covers in detail some existent theories and innovative concepts revolving around this domain. Those with an interest in this field of study would find this book helpful.

The information contained in this book is the result of intensive hard work done by researchers in this field. All due efforts have been made to make this book serve as a complete guiding source for students and researchers. The topics in this book have been comprehensively explained to help readers understand the growing trends in the field.

I would like to thank the entire group of writers who made sincere efforts in this book and my family who supported me in my efforts of working on this book. I take this opportunity to thank all those who have been a guiding force throughout my life.

Editor

1

Intracellular Delivery of siRNAs Targeting AKT and ERBB2 Genes Enhances Chemosensitization of Breast Cancer Cells in a Culture and Animal Model

Tahereh Fatemian [1], Hamid Reza Moghimi [2] and Ezharul Hoque Chowdhury [1,*]

[1] Jeffry Cheah School of Medicine and Health Sciences, Monash University Malaysia, Jalan Lagoon Selatan, 46150 Bandar Sunway, Malaysia

[2] School of Pharmacy, Shahid Beheshti University of Medical Sciences, 19839-63113 Tehran, Iran

* Correspondence: md.ezharul.hoque@monash.edu

Abstract: Pharmacotherapy as the mainstay in the management of breast cancer suffers from various drawbacks, including non-targeted biodistribution, narrow therapeutic and safety windows, and also resistance to treatment. Thus, alleviation of the constraints from the pharmacodynamic and pharmacokinetic profile of classical anti-cancer drugs could lead to improvements in efficacy and patient survival in malignancies. Moreover, modifications in the genetic pathophysiology of cancer via administration of small nucleic acids might pave the way towards higher response rates to chemotherapeutics. Inorganic pH-dependent carbonate apatite (CA) nanoparticles were utilized in this study to efficiently deliver various classes of therapeutics into cancer cells. Co-delivery of drugs and genetic materials was successfully attained through a carbonate apatite delivery device. On 4T1 cells, siRNAs against AKT and ERBB2 plus paclitaxel or docetaxel resulted in the largest increase in anti-cancer effects compared to CA/paclitaxel or CA/docetaxel. Therefore, these ingredients were selected for further in vivo investigations. Animals receiving injections of CA/paclitaxel or CA/docetaxel loaded with siRNAs against AKT and ERBB2 possessed significantly smaller tumors compared to CA/drug-treated mice. Interestingly, synergistic interactions in target protein knock down with combinations of CA/AKT/paclitaxel, CA/ERBB2/docetaxel were documented via western blotting.

Keywords: siRNA; drug delivery; nanoparticle; carbonate apatite; ERBB2; AKT; breast cancer

1. Introduction

Combinations of individual therapeutics indicated against malignancies might result in superior outcomes in resolving the complexity of cancer cells. Among the tackled complexities is an acquired or intrinsic resistance of the cancer cells to treatment. In fact, combining different therapeutic strategies might provide various benefits as follows: (a) Maximized therapeutic efficacy without increased overall toxicity to the host due to different mechanisms of action; (b) prevention of the development of resistance to single agents; (c) covering the heterogeneous tumor cell population with different drug sensitivity profiles; and (d) possible synergy between therapeutics, resulting in increased anticancer efficacy [1].

The underlying mechanisms of resistance might involve genetic alterations, which could be depleted via RNA interference technologies, such as small interfering RNAs (siRNAs). Phenotype modifications through suppression of mRNA transcripts by the usage of siRNA, might render the cancer cells more responsive to the accompanying chemotherapeutic agents. In the co-delivery of nucleic acids and small molecule drugs, protective vectors would assist in boosted cellular uptake, lysosomal escape, and protection against serum nucleases together with limited off-target effects.

Nano-based formulations have the potential to be versatile and multifunctional, enabling the co-delivery of multiple agents entrapped in the nanoparticles' structure to gain synergistic anticancer effects or multi-functions.

Co-delivery of drugs and siRNAs has been documented via application of different carrier systems [2–4]. In one study, doxorubicin and Bcl-2-targeted siRNA were applied via a polyethylenimine-coated graphene oxide (PEI-GO) vehicle. Here, the GO moiety adsorbs the therapeutics while PEI enhances cell membrane penetration [2]. In another example, a triblock polymer loaded with VEGF siRNA and paclitaxel delivered augmented efficacy against paclitaxel [3]. *N*-succinyl chitosan-poly-L-lysine-palmitic acid (NSC-PLL-PA) has been utilized in the synthesis of a triblock copolymer for co-delivery of P-glycoprotein-targeted siRNA and doxorubicin at pH 7.4. These therapeutics are released upon degradation of the carrier in the acidic pH of lysosomes [4].

In fact, numerous examples of synthetic dual siRNA and drug-delivery vehicles have been reported in the literature, with varying formulations and results [5–8]. However, carriers consisting of protein or peptide origins have demonstrated superiority due to biodegradability, complex structure details and functional groups, feasible adjustments in the synthesis process, and also compatibility in the construction of multifunctional hybrid materials [9].

As published data demonstrate, a lipoproteoplex has been developed for the purpose of dual delivery of siRNA and doxorubicin, with the ability to condense siRNA and encapsulate the small-molecule chemotherapeutic, doxorubicin. The lipoproteoplex demonstrates improved doxorubicin loading, resulting in a substantial decrease in MCF-7 cell viability, plus effective transfection of GAPDH (60% knockdown) in MCF-7 breast cancer cells [9].

Inorganic carbonate apatite is a recently developed nanocarrier synthesized via calcium phosphate precipitation in the presence of bicarbonate. The controlled crystal growth dynamic leads to the formation of particles with a size ranging between 50 and 300 nm. These carriers encompass optimal features of efficient endocytosis, fast dissolution rate in endosomal acidic pH, and effective release of loaded therapeutics. In more detail, addition of 3 mM of Ca in the synthesis of carbonate apatite results in the formation of nanoparticles with a size less than 50 nM. In presence of 10 nM of paclitaxel, NPs reach a maximum size of around 170 nm. Markedly, paclitaxel-loaded carbonate apatite demonstrates a $20.71 \pm 4.34\%$ loading efficiency [10]. Carbonate apatite nanoparticles have been utilized for co-delivery of anti-cancer drugs and various siRNAs, resulting in improved outcomes [11,12].

Members of the human epidermal growth factor receptor (HER) family are among the key factors in regulating the response of breast cancer cells to chemotherapy. As another mediator in the complex pathway of oncogenesis, AKT, a serine–threonine protein kinase, has been heavily studied.

AKT signaling has been shown to be regulated by enhanced HER signals, mutational activation of Ras leading to AKT activation via the PI3K pathway, or the mutational inactivation of the PTEN phosphatase resulting in diminished AKT activity. Secondary to these alterations, AKT kinase activity would be augmented. Thereafter, increased AKT kinase activity on its own and in the absence of any upregulation in AKT protein concentrations may have a broader effect on oncogenesis as well as the cellular response to cancer therapy [13].

Thus, various components of these inter-related signaling cascades have been targeted via siRNA application in this study to obtain an accurate assessment of their role in the response of the cancer cells to chemotherapy agents.

2. Materials and Methods

2.1. Materials

Dulbecco's modified eagle medium (DMEM), calcium chloride dehydrate ($CaCl_2.2H_2O$), sodium bicarbonate ($NaHCO_3$), dimethyl sulphoxide (DMSO), 3-(4,5-dimethylthiazol-2-yl)-2,5-diphenyl tetrazolium bromide (MTT), phosphoric acid solution (H_3PO_4), trifluroacetice acid (TFA; CF_3COOH), Ethylene Diamine Tetraacetic Acid (EDTA), and anti-cancer drugs docetaxel (Doc) and paclitaxel (Pac) were purchased from Sigma-Aldrich (St Louis, MO, USA). DMEM powder, fetal bovine serum (FBS), trypsin ethylene diamine tetraacetate (trypsin-EDTA), 4-(2-hydroxyethyl)-1-piperazineethanesulfonic acid (HEPES), and penicillin-streptomycin were obtained from Gibco BRL (Carlsbad, CA, USA). All functionally validated siRNAs used in this study (listed in Table 1) were obtained from Qiagen and dissolved in RNase-free water provided by the company to obtain 10-μM stock solution. MCF-7, 4T1 and MDA-MB-231 cells were originally from ATCC.

Table 1. List of validated siRNAs (Qiagen, MD, USA) that were used in this study.

siRNA	Target Sequence	Targeted Gene	Validation Cell Line	% knockdown
Hs-AKT1-5	AATCACACCACCTGACCAAGA	AKT (protein kinase B)	HeLa S3	90
Hs_MAPK1_10	AAGTTCGAGTAGCTATCAAGA	Mitogen-activated protein kinase	HeLa S3	90
Hs-ROS1-5	AAGGTAATTGCTCTAACTTTA	ROS Proto-Oncogene 1, Receptor tyrosine kinase	HeLa	87
Hs-ERBB2-14	AACAAAGAAATCTTAGACGAA	Receptor tyrosine-protein kinase ERBB-2 or human epidermal growth factor receptor 2 (HER2)	MCF-7	92

2.2. *Cell Culture*

MCF-7 and MDA-MB-231 as human breast cancer cell lines and 4T1 as a mouse breast cancer cell line were cultured in 75-cm^2 tissue culture flasks (Nunc, Orlando, FL, USA) using DMEM supplemented with 10% FBS, 1% penicillin and streptomycin, and 1% HEPES at 37 °C in a humidified 5% CO_2-containing atmosphere.

2.3. *Generation and Characterization of Carbonate Apatite*

Carbonate apatite nanoparticles were manufactured via addition of Ca^{2+} from 1 M $CaCl_2$ stock solution to the bicarbonate-buffered cell culture medium (DMEM, pH adjusted to 7.5, containing 44 mM HCO^{3-}), which already contained the third reactant (0.9 mM phosphate), followed by incubation at 37 °C for 30 min. As a result, microscopically visible carbonate apatite particles were formed through precipitation following nucleation in a supersaturated solution. Turbidity determination and size and zeta potential measurement of the variously formulated nanoparticles were employed for characterization of the resulting products [10].

2.4. *Complexation of Drugs and siRNAs with Carbonate Apatite*

Various concentrations of drugs and siRNAs (Table 1) were added in DMEM media (44 mM bicarbonate, pH 7.5) containing particular concentrations of $CaCl_2$ and subjected to a 30-min incubation at 37 °C to allow formation of complexes.

2.5. *In Vitro Viability Assay*

Cytotoxicity of carbonate apatite nanoparticles alone and also differently loaded NPs on human and murine breast cancer cell lines was assessed by MTT assay. Briefly, the cells from the exponential growth phase were seeded in 24-well plates (Griener, Frickenhausen, Germany) (approximately 50,000 cells/well) in DMEM with 10% FBS at 37 °C with 5% CO_2. After 24 h, cells were exposed to various treatments for a consecutive period of 48 h. Two days later the viability was assessed by adding 50 μL MTT solution (5 mg/mL in phosphate buffered solution (PBS)) to each well and incubating for 4 h in dark. Then, the medium was removed and 300 μL DMSO was added to each well to dissolve the purple formazan crystals. Formazan quantification in the form of optical density (OD) was performed at test and reference wavelengths of 595 nm and 630 nm by a plate reader (benchmark plus, Bio Rad).

Cell viability was determined using the following formula:

$$\text{Cell viability (\%) (CV)} = \frac{OD_{(treated)} - OD_{(reference)}}{OD_{(untreated)} - OD_{(reference)}} \times 100.$$

The reference was the optical density of DMSO only in the applied wavelengths.

Each experiment was done in triplicate and results are expressed as mean ± SD of % of cell viability. Subsequently, an increase in cytotoxic effect of the loaded NPs was calculated as follows:

$$\text{Increase in toxicity (\%)} = CV_{\text{baseline treatment}} - CV_{\text{complete treatment}},$$

where $CV_{\text{baseline treatment}}$ and $CV_{\text{complete treatment}}$ represent the cell viability resulting from the baseline treatment and complete treatment, respectively. In all bar charts (Supplementary Figures) displaying cell viability values, each two adjacent bars were compared together and an increase in toxicity was calculated for all different concentrations and expressed as mean ± SD.

2.6. *Sodium Dodecyl Sulfate Polyacrylamide Gel Electrophoresis (Sds-Page) and Western Blot*

Treated cells in each well of a 24-well plate were lysed by addition of 200 μL of whole cell IP-lysis buffer and protein sample was collected. Then, 5 μL solution was used for estimation of total protein content using the BSA assay kit according to instruction provided by the manufacturer (Quick-start Bradford protein assay kit, Bio Rad, Hercules, CA, USA).

Samples of the cell lysate containing equal amounts of total protein (e.g., 10 μg) were mixed with 10 μL of 10× loading dye and heated for 5 min at 95 °C and then resolved by SDS-PAGE using stain free mini protean SFX gels (10 wells) in 1X running buffer. In total, 7 μL of precision plus protein standards-dual color were used as a molecular weight marker to confirm the molecular weight of the proteins in the samples. The protein samples were transferred from gel to the 0.2-μm polyvinylidene difluoride (PVDF) membranes and attached using a trans-blot turbo transfer system (Bio Rad). Membranes were blocked in 5% skimmed milk in 1X TBST for an hour at room temperature.

The membrane was probed with indicated primary antibody (Table 2) overnight at 4 °C. Unbound primary antibodies were washed using 1X TBST buffer for 5 times, 5 min each, with gentle agitation. Blots were probed with horseradish peroxide conjugated secondary antibody (anti-rabbit IgG, 1:3000) for 1 h at room temperature. TBST was again used to remove excess secondary antibody by 5 wash cycles each 5 min long with gentle agitation. Clarity Western Enhanced Chemiluminescence (ECL) substrate (Bio-Rad) was applied onto the membrane in the dark for 5 min and the signals on the membrane were visualized via a Bio-Rad Gel documentation system.

Table 2. Information for the primary antibodies used for western blot in this study.

Name	Manufacturer	Molecular Weight	Clonality	Used Dilution
AKT (pan) (C67E7) Rabbit mAb	Cell signaling (Danvers, MA, USA)	60 KDa	Monoclonal	1:1000
p 44/42 MAPK (Erk 1/2) (137F5) Rabbit mAb	Cell signaling (Danvers, MA, USA)	42/44 KDa	Monoclonal	1:1000
ERBB2 (HER2)	Thermo Fisher scientific (Waltham, MA, USA)	200 KDa	Polyclonal	1:1000
GAPDH (glyceraldehyde-3-phosphate dehydrogenase)	Cell signaling (Danvers, MA, USA)	37 KDa	Monoclonal	1:3000

2.7. *Formulation of Particles for In Vivo Study*

The injectable nanoparticles were formulated in 100 μL of freshly prepared bicarbonated (44 mM) DMEM media to which $CaCl_2$ was added. Samples were then incubated at 37 °C for 30 min followed by maintenance on ice to prevent aggregation during injection. In drugcontaining samples, 1.25 mg/kg of Pac and 1 mg/kg of Doc were used prior to incubation. In case of using siRNAs, 50 nM of each siRNA was added to the media prior to incubation. The resulting therapeutics were used for iv treatment of animals.

2.8. 4T1-Induced Breast Cancer Murine Model

Female Balb/c mice with the age of 6 to 8 weeks and body weight of 15 to 20 g were used in this study.

Animals were maintained in a 12:12 light:dark condition and provided with food ab libitum and water. All experiments were performed in complete adherence to the regulations of Monash University Animal Welfare Committee. The details of the animal study were approved by Monash Animal Ethics Committee on 3 August 2012 with the project identification code of MARP/2012/087 under the title of "Delivery of anti-cancer drugs to breast cancer cells using nanoparticles". Tumor induction was performed via subcutaneous injection of 4T1 cells (in 100 μL PBS) on the mammary fat pad of mice. Injection day was considered as day 1 of the animal study. The development of tumor was regularly assessed through manual examination of the injection site. Randomization and treatment were carried out when the volume of the tumor reached an average of 13.20 ± 2.51 mm^3 (Table 3). Treatment was administered via intravenous injection through the right or left caudal vein. Duration of study was 30 days, which involved close monitoring of the animals together with recording their body weights and tumor outgrowth every other day. The following formula was used for calculation of the tumor volume:

$$\text{Tumor volume } (\text{mm}^3) = \frac{(\text{Length} \times \text{Width}^2)}{2}$$

Table 3. Treatment groups used for in vivo study.

Group	Regimen
Untreated	-
CA	7 μL of 1 M $CaCl_2$ in DMEM
CA	4 μL of 1 M $CaCl_2$ in DMEM
Pac	1.25 mg/kg paclitaxel in DMEM
Doc	1 mg/kg docetaxel in DMEM
CA/Pac	1.25 mg/kg paclitaxel and 7 μL of 1 M $CaCl_2$ in DMEM
CA/Pac	1.25 mg/kg paclitaxel and 4 μL of 1 M $CaCl_2$ in DMEM
CA/Doc	1 mg/kg docetaxel and 4 μL of 1 M $CaCl_2$ in DMEM
CA/AKT	50 nM of AKT siRNA and 4 μL of 1 M $CaCl_2$ in DMEM
CA/ERBB2	50 nM of ERBB2 siRNA and 4 μL of 1 M $CaCl_2$ in DMEM
CA/AKT/ERBB2/Pac	1.25 mg/kg paclitaxel and 50 nM of ERBB2 and AKT siRNA and 4 μL of 1 M $CaCl_2$ in DMEM
CA/AKT/ERBB2/Doc	1 mg/kg docetaxel and 50 nM of ERBB2 and AKT siRNA and 4 μL of 1 M $CaCl_2$ in DMEM

2.9. Statistics

For determining statistical significance of quantifications, student's *t*-test was used; all data are presented as mean ± SD. Data was considered significant for p values < 0.05.

3. Results and Discussion

3.1. Cytotoxicity of siRNA-Loaded NPs on MCF-7 and 4T1 Cells

To explore the efficacy of carbonate apatite in the delivery of siRNAs into the cells and also evaluate the effect of single gene knock down on the viability of cancer cells, carbonate apatite nanoparticles harboring single siRNA were tested on MCF-7 and 4T1 cells. Here, 4 mM of $CaCl_2$ was applied in the presence of various amounts of single siRNAs to produce treatment formulations.

Binding of siRNA to NPs, in the presence of increasing concentrations of calcium and fixed siRNA amounts, is saturable and reaches a plateau level, in spite of the escalating pattern of particle size. Higher amounts of calcium together with limited endogenous phosphate (0.9 mM) accounts for an increased particle size due to aggregation and not larger individual particles. Limited surface area of the particles secondary to aggregation results in restricted siRNA binding [14].

Remarkably, CA capacity in the efficient delivery of siRNAs into their action site is displayed by the considerable enhancement in the cytotoxic effects for almost all amounts of siRNAs complexed with CA compared to free siRNA. The most killing effect on MCF-7 and 4T1 seems to be achieved by muting the HER2 or ROS1 cascade (Table 4) (Supplementary Figures S1 and S2), indicating the strong impact of ERBB2 or ROS signaling on the survival of both cell lines.

Table 4. Cytotoxicity (%) enhancement on 4T1 and MCF-7 cells treated with various siRNAs (1 pM, 10 pM, 100 pM, 1 nM, and 10 nM) incorporated into an apatite structure formed with 3 mM of $CaCl_2$. The data is presented as mean ± SD compared to free siRNA.

Cell line	Treatment	siRNA Concentration				
		1 pM	10 pM	100 pM	1 nM	10 nM
4T1	CA/ERBB2	16.44 ± 5.77	33.24 ± 9.14	26.70 ± 3.93	28.09 ± 6.28	19.80 ± 1.13
	CA/AKT	14.11 ± 5.41	−4.58 ± 5.01	3.42 ± 1.23	−3.27 ± 4.48	−3.96 ± 2.98
	CA/MAPK	10.68 ± 3.69	−0.72 ± 0.87	17.59 ± 1.04	5.36 ± 1.15	25.45 ± 4.64
	CA/ROS1	13.85 ± 6.99	14.68 ± 3.87	27.46 ± 1.17	16.65 ± 1.44	35.56 ± 2.81
MCF-7	CA/ERBB2	07.49 ± 8.01	24.56 ± 3.19	13.82 ± 3.34	19.29 ± 3.91	8.63 ± 1.67
	CA/ROS1	12.52 ± 2.79	13.69 ± 3.07	23.97 ± 2.13	28.88 ± 2.29	29.70 ± 3.96

In another research, carbonate apatite nanoparticles have been confirmed as efficient carriers for electrostatically associated siRNA inside the cells, releasing bound siRNA from endosomes to the cytosol through pH-responsive self-dissolution. This was concluded based on the significant increase in the fluorescence intensity of the intracellular components from the cells treated with CA/fluorescent siRNA compared to untreated and CA-treated cells [14].

Moreover, application of different concentrations of 'Allstars Negative Control siRNA' (1 pM to 10 nM) loaded into a carbonate apatite structure resulted in no alteration of breast cancer cells' viability [11].

However, the duration of response of the cancer cells to single-oncogene inhibitors, even the most potent oncogenes, is mostly short due to the development of resistance or upregulation of compensatory mechanisms in survival and proliferation signaling. Therefore, sustained and significant outcomes are mainly achieved with combinations of various classes of anti-cancer therapies. In case of no initial response to treatment or development of drug resistance, combinatory regimens are of great benefit to induce therapeutic response. In fact, putting off the causal cascades of resistance by one agent might result in re-sensitization of the cells to other therapeutics in the combination.

Markedly, pharmacokinetics and pharmacodynamics interactions between the agents in combination therapy might develop in case of a shared action site, uptake, and metabolism or elimination routes.

Delivery of drugs and siRNAs by means of carbonate apatite nanoparticles into cells was further studied. The aim was to evaluate the impact of silencing different signaling pathways on the response of cancer cells to the cytotoxic effects of drugs. Different concentrations of paclitaxel, docetaxel, mitomycin C, and topotecan (10 pM, 100 pM, and 1 nM) were used together with 1 pM of siRNAs against AKT, ERBB2, MAPK, and ROS1 and 3 mM Ca. Based on extensive experiments and with the aim of exploring possible synergistic effects, the lowest effective doses of therapeutics were applied. This was to perhaps achieve a therapeutic effect with lower doses and hence less side effects.

Notably, application of anti HER2 siRNA together with any of the four drugs caused positive changes in cytotoxicity against 4T1 cells (Supplementary Figures S3–S6). Additionally, co-delivery of Pac and ROS1 siRNA or Doc and MAPK siRNA seemed to sensitize 4T1 cells to the drug to a great extent.

Response of MDA-MB-231 cells to chemotherapy in case of single pathway silencing was also explored. Paclitaxel and docetaxel were used in complexes of carbonate apatite using 3 mM Ca and 10 pM, 100 pM, and 1 nM of the drug together with 1 nM of each siRNA. As the cell viability data reveals, Pac efficacy benefits from silencing ERBB2 or ROS1 pathways in terms of a highest increase in cytotoxicity on MDA-MB-231 cells (Supplementary Figure S7). Whereas, AKT or ERBB2 pathways display a significant role in response to docetaxel in MDA-MB-231 cells, as with knock down of these two oncogenes, all concentrations of Doc exert a substantial higher cytotoxicity (Supplementary Figure S8).

As the next step, simultaneous silencing of AKT and ERBB2 oncogenes was implemented to check if these pathways have any impact on the response to classical anti-cancer drugs.

Carbonate apatite was formed with 3 mM of $CaCl_2$ and 1 pM of AKT and ERBB2 siRNA together with 10 pM, 100 pM, and 1 nM of paclitaxel, docetaxel, mitomycin C, and topotecan. Based on cell viability results (Supplementary Figure S9), knock down of AKT and ERBB2 seems to have the greatest impact on the response to paclitaxel or docetaxel in 4T1 cells. The highest enhancement in cytotoxicity on 4T1 is equal to 19.97 ± 1.73% for Pac and 15.16 ± 3.55% for Doc, resulting from simultaneous blockade of AKT and ERBB2 signaling. Thus, these combinations were applied for in vivo studies since the animal tumor model was developed by local injection of 4T1 cells in mice.

On MDA-MB-231 cells, application of siRNAs for simultaneous silencing of two pathways led to augmented cytotoxicity of paclitaxel as well. This effect was higher with usage of AKT and ROS1 siRNA or co-delivery of AKT and MAPK siRNAs in the presence of Pac (Supplementary Figure S10).

Tables 5–7 demonstrate the enhancement of the cytotoxic effect of classical anti-cancer drugs resulting from the silencing of various pathways in MCF-7, 4T1, and MDA-MB-231 cells, respectively.

Table 5. Effect of silencing various pathways on cytotoxicity of classical anti-cancer drugs in MCF-7 cells. Data is presented as mean ± SD compared to CA/drug.

Treatment on MCF-7 Cells	Drug Concentration		
	10 pM	**100 pM**	**1 nM**
CA/Pac/AKT	10.93 ± 1.05	8.33 ± 0.84	3.31 ± 0.45
CA/Pac/ERBB2	7.25 ± 1.91	4.11 ± 0.35	3.40 ± 1.81
CA/Pac/MAPK	−10.79 ± 2.12	1.53 ± 0.55	2.06 ± 0.35
CA/Pac/ROS1	4.19 ± 1.41	3.14 ± 0.74	3.64 ± 0.19
CA/Doc/AKT	5.14 ± 1.22	10.45 ± 1.33	11.69 ± 2.18
CA/Doc/ERBB2	8.95 ± 2.28	10.25 ± 0.99	14.28 ± 1.04
CA/Doc/MAPK	3.22 ± 0.91	4.27 ± 0.08	3.67 ± 1.72
CA/Doc/ROS1	1.06 ± 0.59	2.83 ± 0.71	1.25 ± 0.53

Table 6. Effect of silencing various pathways on cytotoxicity of classical anti-cancer drugs in 4T1 cells. Data is presented as mean ± SD compared to CA/drug.

Treatment on 4T1 Cells	Drug Concentration		
	10 pM	**100 pM**	**1 nM**
CA/Pac/AKT	−15.93 ± 0.95	8.70 ± 2.14	−2.68 ± 0.54
CA/Pac/ERBB2	12.93 ± 0.36	9.15 ± 0.14	2.42 ± 2.84
CA/Pac/MAPK	−13.79 ± 1.18	2.53 ± 0.20	2.16 ± 0.11
CA/Pac/ROS1	10.09 ± 1.03	2.04 ± 0.85	7.24 ± 0.07
CA/Doc/AKT	−5.04 ± 0.77	−9.43 ± 0.51	1.30 ± 0.62
CA/Doc/ERBB2	5.85 ± 1.08	7.21 ± 1.17	2.20 ± 1.95
CA/Doc/MAPK	3.16 ± 0.21	5.07 ± 0.98	2.67 ± 0.76
CA/Doc/ROS1	2.76 ± 0.58	1.81 ± 0.97	0.05 ± 0.42

Table 6. *Cont.*

Treatment on 4T1 Cells	Drug Concentration		
	10 pM	100 pM	1 nM
CA/Mito/AKT	0.20 ± 0.71	4.97 ± 1.15	1.92 ± 0.28
CA/Mito/ERBB2	2.13 ± 3.64	5.11 ± 0.85	1.71 ± 0.38
CA/Mito/MAPK	1.26 ± 1.23	0.23 ± 1.45	7.77 ± 0.95
CA/Mito/ROS1	0.72 ± 0.92	0.52 ± 0.16	4.20 ± 1.12
CA/Topo/AKT	0.02 ± 1.64	3.09 ± 0.42	5.28 ± 3.07
CA/Topo/ERBB2	4.54 ± 2.27	5.85 ± 0.47	0.86 ± 2.51
CA/Topo/MAPK	6.54 ± 0.55	0.55 ± 0.51	4.74 ± 0.88
CA/Topo/ROS1	0.58 ± 0.25	0.03 ± 0.36	0.52 ± 0.81
CA/Pac/AKT/ERBB2	19.97 ± 1.73	5.48 ± 2.09	11.63 ± 2.23
CA/Doc/AKT/ERBB2	7.87 ± 1.82	1.45 ± 0.37	15.16 ± 3.55
CA/Mito/AKT/ERBB2	6.04 ± 0.28	0.59 ± 0.47	4.60 ± 0.82
CA/Topo/AKT/ERBB2	−10.41 ± 0.66	−4.73 ± 1.52	−10.77 ± 0.71

Table 7. Effect of silencing various pathways on cytotoxicity of classical anti-cancer drugs in MDA-MB-231 cells. Data is presented as mean ± SD compared to CA/drug.

Treatment on MDA-MB-231 Cells	Drug Concentration		
	10 pM	100 pM	1 nM
CA/Pac/AKT	4.60 ± 1.53	−8.84 ± 0.92	7.55 ± 1.43
CA/Pac/ERBB2	12.03 ± 2.44	0.59 ± 1.32	12.03 ± 3.57
CA/Pac/MAPK	8.96 ± 2.16	0.35 ± 0.36	8.25 ± 1.28
CA/Pac/ROS1	11.08 ± 2.09	0.35 ± 0.09	7.90 ± 1.83
CA/Doc/AKT	3.66 ± 0.24	8.97 ± 2.94	16.16 ± 4.52
CA/Doc/ERBB2	20.05 ± 4.61	7.97 ± 3.06	8.02 ± 1.49
CA/Doc/MAPK	−1.06 ± 0.58	6.14 ± 2.73	6.49 ± 1.91
CA/Doc/ROS1	0.59 ± 0.34	10.74 ± 3.16	7.90 ± 1.52
CA/Pac/AKT/ERBB2	7.07 ± 2.22	3.71 ± 0.85	13.29 ± 1.12
CA/Pac/AKT/MAPK	18.62 ± 3.64	14.42 ± 2.14	3.37 ± 3.47
CA/Pac/AKT/ROS1	11.26 ± 1.05	−0.12 ± 0.93	22.40 ± 3.44
CA/Pac/ERBB2/MAPK	1.32 ± 0.07	−1.44 ± 0.12	12.22 ± 2.33
CA/Pac/ERBB2/ROS1	−0.48 ± 0.52	−9.70 ± 0.49	5.51 ± 1.86
CA/Pac/MAPK/ROS1	9.58 ± 1.24	−4.79 ± 0.93	6.23 ± 2.22

According to the cell viability data displayed in Table 5, silencing AKT or ERBB2 regulates the response of MCF-7 cells to paclitaxel or docetaxel substantially. Thus, the effect of these therapeutic agents on the protein expression was further evaluated via Western blotting.

Induction of cell death followed by application of therapeutically loaded carbonate apatite could be associated with involvement of the apoptotic pathway, based on escalation of caspase-7-mediated signaling [12].

Silencing of AKT or HER2 signaling to expedite treatment outcomes in cancer is backed up by a solid body of knowledge. Expression of HER2 in MCF7 cells has been shown to increase under certain conditions [15,16].

According to recent research, docetaxel induces either apoptosis accompanied by survivin upregulation or necrosis and a lower rate of survivin upregulation in various breast cancer cell lines, based on cells receptor expression profile and the molecular phenotype. Additionally, inhibition of p-AKT was shown to revert survivin upregulation and also induce docetaxel-dependent apoptosis [17].

In another study, inhibition of NRF2 in ERBB2-overexpressing ovarian carcinoma cells was shown to suppress ERBB2 expression, which led to a decrease in phospho-AKT and enhanced p27 protein together with increased sensitivity of these cells to docetaxel cytotoxicity and apoptosis [18].

There are also other published data associating increased paclitaxel-induced apoptosis with inhibition of AKT in ovarian cancer cells. While paclitaxel-resistant cells demonstrated higher levels of p-AKT compared to paclitaxel-sensitive cells, inhibition of AKT increased paclitaxel therapeutic efficacy in both cell lines [19].

Moreover, combination of shRNA against AKT1 with paclitaxel exerted synergistic anti-cancer effects, thus inhibiting the growth of human breast cancer MDA-MB-231 and MCF-7 cells, and breast cancer MDA-MB-231 cell xenografts in mice as well. The combination therapy demonstrated enhanced anti-cancer effects through inhibition of AKT1 signaling and induction of apoptosis [20].

Extensive in vitro and in vivo research has associated ERBB2 overexpression with resistance of breast cancer cells to certain chemotherapeutic agents, namely docetaxel and paclitaxel. Furthermore, in clinical studies, herceptin, the anti-ERBB2 antibody, enhanced the antitumor activity of paclitaxel and doxorubicin against ERBB2-overexpressing human breast cancer xenografts, and the paclitaxel response rate of patients with ERBB2-overexpressing breast cancers was significantly higher among patients receiving paclitaxel plus herceptin than those receiving paclitaxel alone [21]. Additionally, co-administration of a PI3K inhibitor with cytotoxic or targeted anticancer agents, such as carboplatin, paclitaxel, or erlotinib, led to increased tumor growth inhibition over the corresponding single agents [22].

Moreover, high AKT activity has been shown to be responsible for the enhanced resistance of ERBB2-overexpressing cancer cells toward chemotherapeutic agents, and inhibition of AKT activation by peptide aptamer resulted in the restoration of regular sensitivity of breast cancer MCF7 cells towards paclitaxel [23].

In another research, siRNA-based knockdown of HER-2 conferred increased sensitivity to paclitaxel in endometrial cancer cells, attenuating the induction of p-AKT on paclitaxel stimulation, which was cancelled by inactivating AKT by the introduction of a dominant-negative form [24].

3.2. *Effect of CA/siRNA/Drug at the Protein Level*

As cell viability assays revealed, silencing AKT or ERBB2 exerts the maximum effect on the enhancement of cytotoxicity of Pac or Doc on MCF-7. Thus, the underlying mechanism of reduced viability following administration of these treatments was investigated via western blotting. This was performed to confirm that the applied siRNA is effective in the knock down of the target protein synthesis and also to observe the changes in protein expression leading to enhanced chemo sensitivity.

AKT expression following treatment of MCF-7 cells with free AKT siRNA and CA-complexed AKT siRNA was assessed and compared with untreated cells. As the bands on the blot and densitometry analysis reveal (Figure 1), complexation of siRNA with carbonate apatite leads to significantly decreased expression of AKT compared to free AKT siRNA and untreated cells (p value < 0.05). This confirms the efficacy of CA in the successful delivery of siRNA and knock down of the target protein.

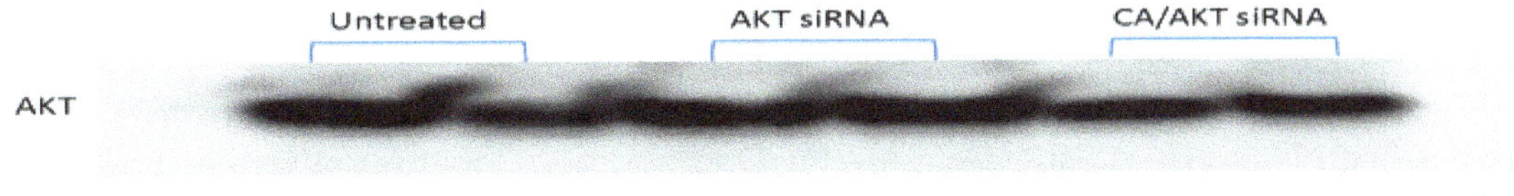

Figure 1. AKT protein expression in MCF-7 cells. Cells were treated with media (untreated), free AKT siRNA, and CA/AKT siRNA formed with 3 mM of $CaCl_2$ and 1 nM siRNA for 44 h. Cellular lysates were resolved by SDS-PAGE and transferred in PVDF membrane followed by incubation with primary antibodies raised in rabbit against AKT. HRP-conjugated goat anti-rabbit secondary antibody was used to detect the chemiluminescent signals.

The same experiment design was utilized with MAPK siRNA. According to Figure 2, free MAPK siRNA does not change the expression level of MAPK protein whereas CA/MAPK significantly knocks down production of the target protein (p value < 0.05).

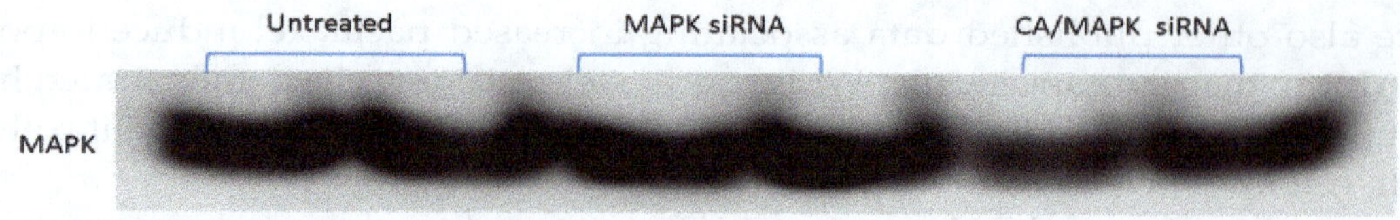

Figure 2. MAPK protein expression in MCF-7 cells. Cells were treated with media (untreated), free MAPK siRNA, and CA/MAPK siRNA formed with 3 mM of $CaCl_2$ and 1 nM siRNA for 44 h. Cellular lysates were resolved by SDS-PAGE and transferred into PVDF membrane followed by incubation with primary antibodies raised in rabbit against AKT. HRP-conjugated goat anti-rabbit secondary antibody was used to detect the chemiluminescent signals.

Next, changes in protein expression resulting from the combinations of drugs and siRNAs, as highlighted in the cell viability data, were studied. MCF-7 cell lysate treated with free and CA-bound AKT siRNA, CA/AKT/Pac and CA/Pac were loaded on the gels. According to the resulting bands (Figure 3), the lowest level of AKT protein was obtained by CA/AKT/Pac treatment versus CA/Pac or CA/AKT. This implies the development of synergistic interactions to suppress survival pathways in the presence of classical anti-cancer drugs together with genetic downregulation of survival proteins, which in turn might lead to enhanced sensitivity of the cells to the anti-cancer medication.

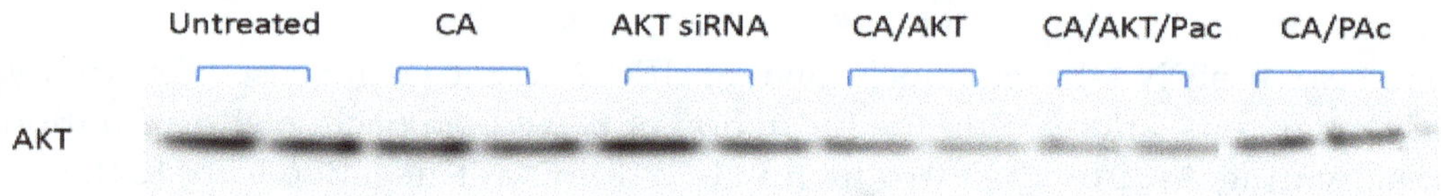

Figure 3. AKT protein expression in MCF-7 cells. Cells were treated with media (untreated), carbonate apatite, free AKT siRNA, CA/AKT siRNA, CA/AKT/Pac, and CA/Pac. Ingredients include 3 mM of $CaCl_2$, 1 nM siRNA, and 1 nM Pac. Cellular lysates were run in SDS-PAGE and transferred into PVDF membrane and incubated with primary antibodies raised in rabbit against AKT. HRP-conjugated goat anti-rabbit secondary antibody was used to detect the chemiluminescent signals.

The same synergistic pattern, but with a lower potency, was observed with application of CA/AKT/Doc in the downregulation of AKT protein against CA/AKT or CA/Doc (Figure 4).

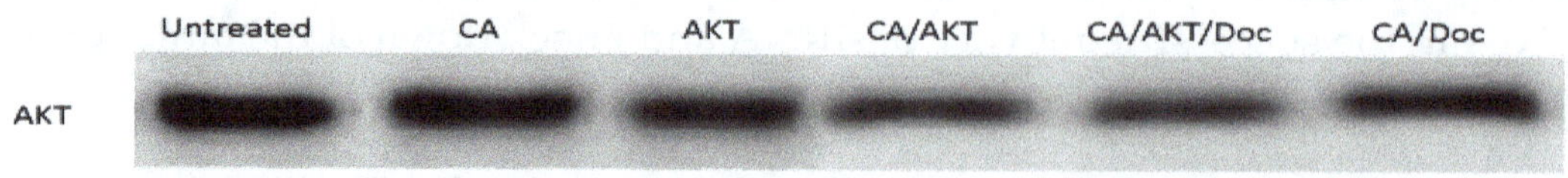

Figure 4. AKT protein expression in MCF-7 cells. Cells were treated with media (untreated), carbonate apatite, free AKT siRNA, CA/AKT siRNA, CA/AKT/Doc, and CA/Doc. Ingredients include 3 mM of $CaCl_2$, 1 nM siRNA, and 1 nM Doc. Cellular lysates were run in SDS-PAGE and transferred into PVDF membrane and incubated with primary antibodies raised in rabbit against AKT. HRP-conjugated goat anti-rabbit secondary antibody was used to detect the chemiluminescent signals.

Based on a substantial enhancement in efficacy, the impact of different combinations of ERBB2 siRNA with paclitaxel or docetaxel on the expression level of ERBB2 protein was also examined. As the blot in Figure 5 shows, the highest knock down was achieved by co-delivery of CA-bound Doc and ERBB2 siRNA followed by CA/Pac/ERBB2. Again, the synergy in the therapeutic efficacy of the drug together with siRNA is present since the impact of the drug or siRNA as a single agent is considerably weaker.

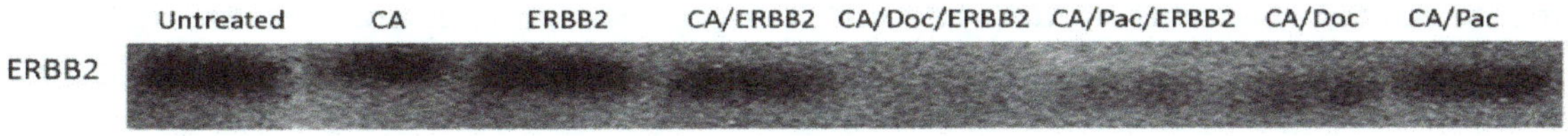

Figure 5. ERBB2 protein expression in MCF-7 cells. Cells were treated with media (untreated), carbonate apatite, free ERBB2 siRNA, CA/ERBB2 siRNA, CA/Doc/ERBB2, CA/Pac/ERBB2, CA/Doc, and CA/Pac. Ingredients include 3 mM of $CaCl_2$, 1 nM siRNA, and 1 nM drug. Cellular lysates were run in SDS-PAGE and transferred into PVDF membrane and incubated with primary antibodies raised in rabbit against ERBB2. HRP-conjugated goat anti-rabbit secondary antibody was used to detect the chemiluminescent signals.

3.3. *In Vivo Efficacy of CA/Drug/siRNA*

According to cell viability data on 4T1 cells and the enhancement in the cytotoxicity of drugs, co-delivery of AKT and ERBB2 siRNAs together with Pac or Doc resulted in the highest increase in the drug's efficacy. Thus, these two combinations were applied in animal study.

For comparison of the in vivo efficacy of the therapeutics in the first batch, animals were treated on day 8 and 11. Formulations were prepared by mixing 4 mM Ca, 1.25 mg/kg Pac, 50 nM AKT siRNA plus 50 nM ERBB2 siRNA in 100 μL of HCO_3-DMEM. There were no significant changes in the pattern of body weight change and also general signs and symptoms of the animals among different groups of the studies.

As the t-test results reveal, CA-AKT-ERBB2-Pac treatment significantly reduced the tumor volume on day 14 and 16 compared to Ca/Pac. Moreover, the group treated with CA/ERBB2 displayed significantly smaller tumors compared to the CA group on day 12 and 14. The effect of Pac complexed with CA on tumor regression was significant on day 14 versus free paclitaxel therapy (Figure 6).

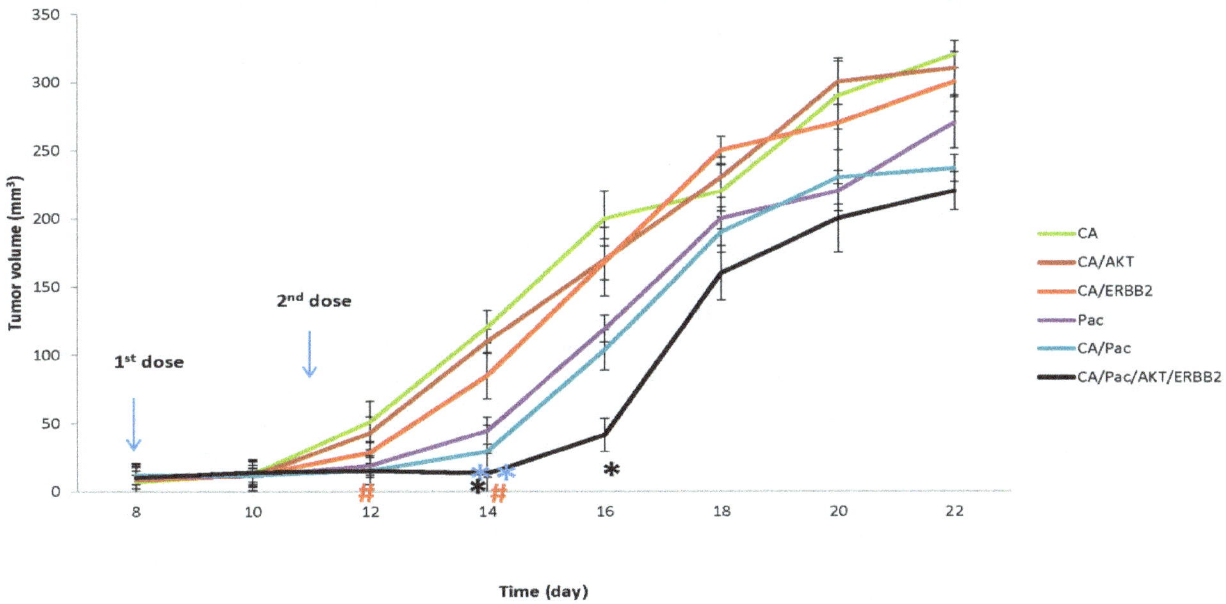

Figure 6. Effect of silencing AKT and ERBB2 pathways on in vivo efficacy of paclitaxel. Mice were purchased from Razi Research Institute, Tehran, Iran. Approximately 10^6 4T1 cells were inoculated subcutaneously on the mammary pad of mice. Based on tumor volume calculations, mice were randomized and treated intravenously through tail-vein injection on day 8 and 11. The therapeutics included 100 μL of carbonate apatite entailing 4 μL of 1M $CaCl_2$ and 50 nM of AKT and ERBB2 siRNA plus 1.25 mg/kg Pac. Body weight and tumor outgrowth were monitored every other day. Data is represented as mean ± SD, $n = 6$ and values are significant when * p value < 0.05 for CA/Pac/AKT/ERBB2 vs. CA/Pac, # p value < 0.05 for CA/ERBB2 compared to CA and ** p value < 0.05 for CA/Pac against Pac.

In another batch, injections on day 10 and 13 encompassed preparations of 4 mM Ca, 1 mg/kg Doc, 50 nM AKT siRNA, and 50 nM ERBB2 siRNA in 100 μL bicarbonated DMEM (Figure 7).

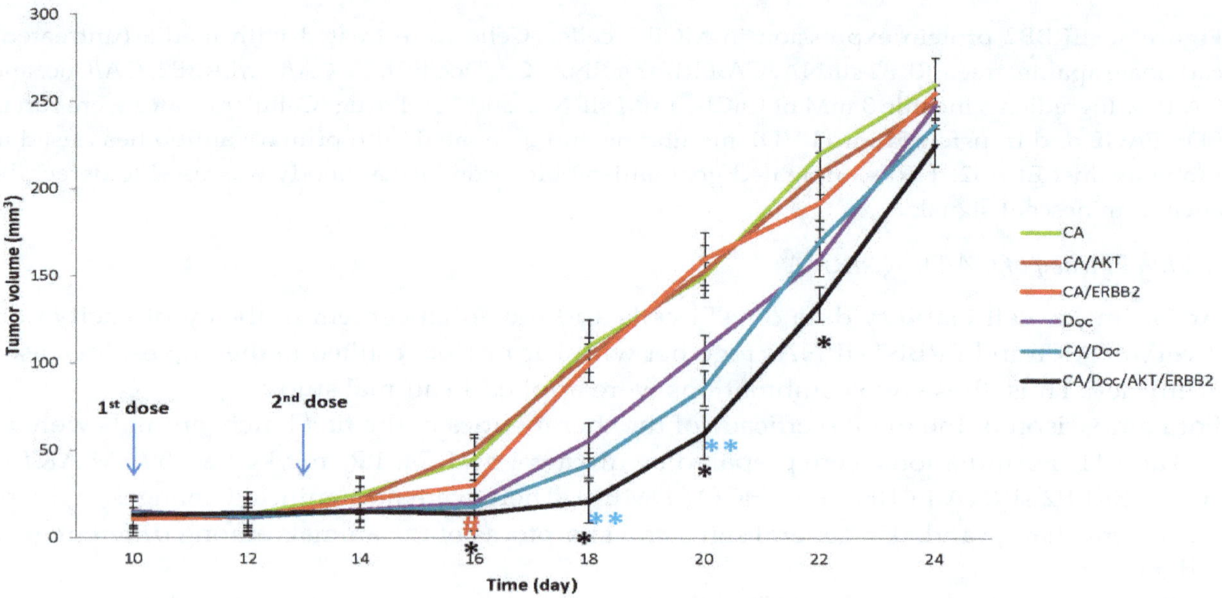

Figure 7. Effect of silencing AKT and ERBB2 pathways on in vivo efficacy of docetaxel. Mice were purchased from Razi Research Institute, Tehran, Iran. Approximately 10^6 4T1 cells were inoculated subcutaneously on the mammary pad of mice. Based on tumor volume calculations, mice were randomized and treated intravenously through tail-vein injection on day 10 and 13. The therapeutics included 100 μL of carbonate apatite entailing 4 μL of 1M $CaCl_2$ and 50 nM of AKT and ERBB2 siRNA plus 1mg/kg Doc. Body weight and tumor outgrowth were monitored every other day. Data is represented as mean ± SD, $n = 6$ and values are significant when * p value < 0.05 for CA/Doc/AKT/ERBB2 vs CA/Doc, # p value < 0.05 for CA/ERBB2 compared to CA and ** p value < 0.05 for Ca/Doc against Doc.

According to the p values calculated in the t-test, treatment of animals with CA/Doc/AKT/ERBB2 resulted in significantly smaller tumor volumes on days 16, 18, 20, and 22 compared to CA/Doc. Whereas CA/ERBB2 displayed a significant anti-tumor efficacy only on day 16 compared to CA, and CA/AKT was not effective in tumor regression. Animals treated with CA/Doc had significantly smaller tumors on day 18 and 20 compared to Doc-treated animals.

ERBB2 overexpression has been linked to elevated levels of inhibitory phosphorylation of Cdc2 and suppression of paclitaxel-induced cell death in breast cancer cells via deregulation of the G2/M cell cycle checkpoint. This provides a mechanistic rationale for the association between ERBB2 overexpression and paclitaxel resistance. Interestingly, overexpression of a subunit of PI3k in ovarian cancer cells has been shown to confer paclitaxel resistance. Additionally, selective inhibition of the PI3k pathway could restore the efficacy of paclitaxel in those cells [25]. Thus, alterations in the expression and activity levels of key components of these signaling networks regulating cellular proliferation and survival may confer paclitaxel resistance. Further, circumvention of this type of resistance might be achieved via application of selective inhibitors of these proteins to increase drug sensitivity.

Simultaneous targeting of AKT and ERBB2 to achieve improvements in eradication of oncogenesis has been brought up in various studies.

Overexpression or activation of HER members and also AKT has been linked to limited benefits of treatment in patients, leading to poor prognosis in breast cancer. In fact, functionally relevant alterations in AKT1 could be a putative mediator of tumor progression and drug resistance. Moreover, amplification or gain-of-function mutations of ERBB2 can account for hyperactivation of the AKT cascade in breast cancer cells. Crosstalk with heterologous receptors and amplification of HER2 signaling, amplifications of the PI3K/AKT pathway, and de-repression and/or activation of compensatory survival pathways through increased PI3K/AKT signaling are among the resistance mechanisms against anti-HER2 therapy. Factors associated with resistance to ERBB2-targeted agents have been invariably associated with a reactivation of the PI3K/AKT signaling cascade [26,27]. However, defects in HER2/PI3K/AKT axes and their impact on regulation of the response of cancer cells to treatment need further investigation.

In an experimental design, HER2-positive MCF7 cells showed a PI3K-dependent increase in AKT activity together with increased resistance to a panel of five chemotherapeutic agents with known different mechanisms of action (paclitaxel, doxorubicin, 5-fluorouracil, etoposide, and camptothecin). Selective inhibition of PI3K or AKT in these HER2-overexpressing MCF7 cells reduced the levels of phosphorylated (activated) AKT and sensitized the cells to the chemotherapeutic agents. It has been further confirmed that expression of a constitutively active AKT vector alone in MCF7 cells caused similarly increased resistance of the cells to the chemotherapeutic agents [13]. Therefore, the HER2/PI3K/AKT pathway is confirmed to play a causal role in the resistance of breast cancer cells against several therapeutics, and targeting components of this pathway might resolve the resistance and enhance the efficacy of the treatments. In view of that, the in vitro and in vivo results of this study are in alignment with the documented role of AKT and ERBB2 in drug resistance.

Strikingly, the efficacy of simultaneous knock down of AKT and ERBB2 in augmenting the response of cancer cells to docetaxel was reported for the first time in this study.

Markedly, the strategic location of AKT and its activation by multiple upstream signal transduction pathways makes it a better target than its upstream targets, such as HER2, Ras, or PI3K, in sensitizing cancer cells to chemotherapy or radiotherapy. Thus, there could be clinical benefits from an appropriate combination of conventional chemotherapeutic drugs with a new generation of signal transduction inhibitors that inhibit the HER/PI3K/AKT pathway for the treatment of breast cancer.

A summary of the ERBB2 and AKT signaling cascades regulating cell's proliferation, survival, and resistance to apoptosis and treatment is illustrated in Figure 8. This is for clarification of the enhanced efficacy of Pac or Doc attained by simultaneous blockade of AKT and ERBb2 cascades and the impact on the response of the cells to the drugs.

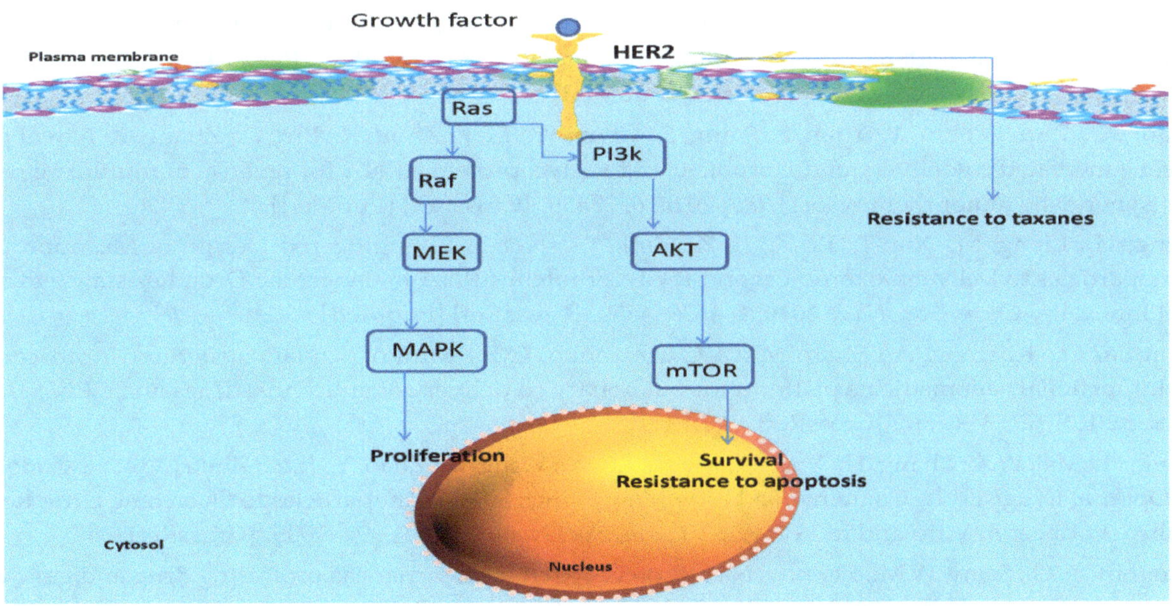

Figure 8. Summary of the ERBB2 and AKT signaling cascades regulating the cell's proliferation, survival, and resistance to apoptosis and treatment.

As revealed through the extensive experiments on breast cancer cells and animal models plus protein expression studies, simultaneous knock down of AKT1 and ERBB2 expression in the presence of paclitaxel or docetaxel leads to a substantial increase in cellular response to the chemotherapeutic agent both in culture and an animal model. Synergistic interactions in target protein knock down have been documented via western blotting in the cells treated with these combinations, which would shed light on the underlying mechanisms of the enhanced sensitivity of the cells to treatment. Taken together, with a favorable in vitro profile and also superior in vivo efficacy, co-administration of genetic materials and classical chemotherapeutics could propose a promising platform for improved strategies against cancer cells in upcoming practice.

Supplementary Materials:

Figure S1. Cell viability assessment in 4T1 cells treated with siRNA loaded carbonate apatite. Figure S2. Carbonate apatite facilitated delivery of ERBB2 (A) and ROS1 (B) siRNA to MCF-7 cells. Figure S3. Effect of single pathway silencing on cytotoxicity of paclitaxel on 4T1 cells. Figure S4. Effect of single pathway silencing on cytotoxicity of docetaxel on 4T1 cells. Figure S5. Effect of single pathway silencing on cytotoxicity of mitomycin C on 4T1 cells. Figure S6. Effect of single pathway silencing on cytotoxicity of topotecan on 4T1 cells. Figure S7. Effects of single pathway silencing on paclitaxel cytotoxicity in MDA-MB-231. Figure S8. Effects of single pathway silencing on docetaxel cytotoxicity. Figure S9. Effects of silencing AKT and ERBB2 oncogenes on drugs cytotoxicity in 4T1. Figure S10. Cell viability assay on MDA-MB-231 cells treated with carbonate apatite complexed with paclitaxel and two siRNAs.

Author Contributions: T.F. carried out experiments and data analysis under the supervision of H.R.M. and E.H.C., H.R.M. provided resources while E.H.C. originally designed the project and provided the resources.

References

1. Holohan, C.; Van Schaeybroeck, S.; Longley, D.B.; Johnston, P.G. Cancer drug resistance: An evolving paradigm. *Nat. Rev. Cancer* **2013**, *13*, 714–726. [CrossRef] [PubMed]
2. Zhang, L.; Lu, Z.; Zhao, Q.; Huang, J.; Shen, H.; Zhang, Z. Enhanced Chemotherapy Efficacy by Sequential Delivery of siRNA and Anticancer Drugs Using PEI-Grafted Graphene Oxide. *Small* **2011**, *7*, 460–464. [CrossRef] [PubMed]
3. Zhu, C.; Jung, S.; Luo, S.; Meng, F.; Zhu, X.; Park, T.G.; Zhong, Z. Co-delivery of siRNA and paclitaxel into cancer cells by biodegradable cationic micelles based on PDMAEMA–PCL–PDMAEMA triblock copolymers. *Biomaterials* **2010**, *31*, 2408–2416. [CrossRef] [PubMed]
4. Zhang, C.; Zhu, W.; Liu, Y.; Yuan, Z.; Yang, S.; Chen, W.; Li, J.; Zhou, X.; Liu, C.; Zhang, X. Novel polymer micelle mediated co-delivery of doxorubicin and P-glycoprotein siRNA for reversal of multidrug resistance and synergistic tumor therapy. *Sci. Rep.* **2016**, *6*, 23859. [CrossRef] [PubMed]
5. Meng, H.; Liong, M.; Xia, T.; Li, Z.; Ji, Z.; Zink, J.I.; Nel, A.E. Engineered Design of Mesoporous Silica Nanoparticles to Deliver Doxorubicin and P-Glycoprotein siRNA to Overcome Drug Resistance in a Cancer Cell Line. *Am. Chem. Soc. Nano* **2010**, *4*, 4539–4550. [CrossRef] [PubMed]
6. Taratula, O.; Kuzmov, A.; Shah, M.A.; Garbuzenko, O.B.; Minko, T. Nanostructured lipid carriers as multifunctional nanomedicine platform for pulmonary co-delivery of anticancer drugs and siRNA. *J. Control. Release* **2013**, *171*, 349–357. [CrossRef]
7. Meng, H.; Mai, W.X.; Zhang, H.; Xue, M.; Xia, T.; Lin, S.; Wang, X.; Zhao, Y.; Ji, Z.; Zink, J.I.; et al. Codelivery of an Optimal Drug/siRNA Combination Using Mesoporous Silica Nanoparticles to Overcome Drug Resistance in Breast Cancer in Vitro and in Vivo. *Am. Chem. Soc. Nano* **2013**, *7*, 994–1005. [CrossRef]
8. Elzoghby, A.O.; Samy, W.M.; Elgindy, N.A. Protein-based nanocarriers as promising drug and gene delivery systems. *J. Control. Release* **2012**, *161*, 38–49. [CrossRef]
9. Liu, C.F.; Chen, R.; Frezzo, J.A.; Katyal, P.; Hill, L.K.; Yin, L.; Srivastava, N.; More, H.T.; Renfrew, P.D.; Bonneau, R.; et al. Efficient Dual siRNA and Drug Delivery Using Engineered Lipoproteoplexes. *Biomacromolecules* **2017**, *18*, 2688–2698. [CrossRef]
10. Fatemian, T.; Chowdhury, E.H. Cytotoxicity Enhancement in Breast Cancer Cells with Carbonate Apatite-Facilitated Intracellular Delivery of Anti-Cancer Drugs. *Toxics* **2018**, *6*, E12. [CrossRef]
11. Tiash, S.; Chua, M.J.; Chowdhury, E.H. Knockdown of ROS1 gene sensitizes breast tumor growth to doxorubicin in a syngeneic mouse model. *Int. J. Oncol.* **2016** *48*, 2359–2366. [CrossRef] [PubMed]

12. Tiash, S.; Chowdhury, E.H. siRNAs targeting multidrug transporter genes sensitize breast tumor to doxorubicin in a syngeneic mouse model. *J. Drug Target.* **2018**, *27*, 325–337. [CrossRef] [PubMed]
13. Knuefermann, C.; Lu, Y.; Liu, B.; Jin, W.; Liang, K.; Wu, L.; Schmidt, M.; Mills, G.B.; Mendelsohn, J.; Fan, Z. HER2/PI-3K/Akt activation leads to a multidrug resistance in human breast adenocarcinoma cells. *Oncogene* **2003**, *22*, 3205–3212. [CrossRef] [PubMed]
14. Tiash, S.; Kamaruzman, N.I.B.; Chowdhury, E.H. Carbonate apatite nanoparticles carry siRNA(s) targeting growth factor receptor genes, EGFR1 and ERBB2 to regress mouse breast tumor. *Drug Deliv.* **2017**, *24*, 1721–1730. [CrossRef] [PubMed]
15. Knowlden, J.M.; Hutcheson, I.R.; Jones, H.E.; Madden, T.; Gee, J.M.; Harper, M.E.; Barrow, D.; Wakeling, A.E.; Nicholson, R.I. Elevated levels of epidermal growth factor receptor/c-erbB2 heterodimers mediate an autocrine growth regulatory pathway in tamoxifen-resistant MCF-7 cells. *Endocrinology* **2003**, *144*, 1032–1044. [CrossRef]
16. Kumar, R.; Mandal, M.; Lipton, A.; Harvey, H.; Thompson, C.B. Overexpression of HER2 modulates bcl-2, bcl-XL, and tamoxifen-induced apoptosis in human MCF-7 breast cancer cells. *Clin. Cancer Res.* **1996**, *2*, 1215–1219.
17. De Iuliis, F.; Salerno, G.; Giuffrida, A.; Milana, B.; Taglieri, L.; Rubinacci, G.; Giantulli, S.; Terella, F.; Silvestri, I.; Scarpa, S. Breast cancer cells respond differently to docetaxel depending on their phenotype and on survivin upregulation. *Tumor Biol.* **2016**, *37*, 2603–2611. [CrossRef]
18. Manandhar, S.; Choi, B.H.; Jung, K.A.; Ryoo, I.G.; Song, M.; Kang, S.J.; Choi, H.G.; Kim, J.A.; Park, P.H.; Kwak, M.K. NRF2 inhibition represses ErbB2 signaling in ovarian carcinoma cells: Implications for tumor growth retardation and docetaxel sensitivity. *Free Radic. Biol. Med.* **2012**, *52*, 1773–1785. [CrossRef]
19. Kim, S.H.; Juhnn, Y.S.; Song, Y.S. Akt Involvement in Paclitaxel Chemoresistance of Human Ovarian Cancer Cells. *Ann. N. Y. Acad. Sci.* **2007**, *1095*, 82–89. [CrossRef]
20. Guo, D.D.; Hong, S.H.; Jiang, H.L.; Kim, J.H.; Minai-Tehrani, A.; Kim, J.E.; Shin, J.Y.; Jiang, T.; Kim, Y.K.; Choi, Y.J.; et al. Synergistic effects of Akt1 shRNA and paclitaxel-incorporated conjugated linoleic acid-coupled poloxamer thermosensitive hydrogel on breast cancer. *Biomaterials* **2012**, *33*, 2272–2281. [CrossRef]
21. Hung, D.Y.; Chie, M. Overexpression of ErbB2 in cancer and ErbB2-targeting strategies. *Oncogene* **2000**, *19*, 6115–6121.
22. Echeverria, C.G.; Sellers, W.R. Drug discovery approaches targeting the PI3K/Akt pathway in cancer. *Oncogene* **2008**, *27*, 5511–5526. [CrossRef] [PubMed]
23. Kunz, C.; Borghouts, C.; Buerger, C.; Groner, B. Peptide Aptamers with Binding Specificity for the Intracellular Domain of the ErbB2 Receptor Interfere with AKT Signaling and Sensitize Breast Cancer Cells to Taxol. *Mol. Cancer Res.* **2006**, *4*, 983–998. [CrossRef] [PubMed]
24. Mori, N.; Kyo, S.; Nakamura, M.; Hashimoto, M.; Maida, Y.; Mizumoto, Y.; Takakura, M.; Ohno, S.; Kiyono, T.; Inoue, M. Expression of HER-2 affects patient survival and paclitaxel sensitivity in endometrial cancer. *Br. J. Cancer* **2010**, *103*, 889–898. [CrossRef] [PubMed]
25. Orr, G.A.; Verdier-Pinard, P.; McDaid, H.; Horwitz, S.B. Mechanisms of Taxol resistance related to microtubules. *Oncogene* **2003**, *22*, 7280–7295. [CrossRef] [PubMed]
26. Zhao, Y.H.; Liu, H.; Liu, Z.; Ding, Y.; Ledoux, S.P.; Wilson, G.L.; Voellmy, R.; Lin, Y.; Lin, W.; Nahta, R.; et al. Overcoming trastuzumab resistance in breast cancer by targeting dysregulated glucose metabolism. *Cancer Res.* **2011**, *71*, 4585–4597. [CrossRef]
27. Shattuck, D.L.; Miller, J.K.; Carraway, K.L.; Sweeney, C. Met receptor contributes to trastuzumab resistance of Her2-overexpressing breast cancer cells. *Cancer Res.* **2008**, *68*, 1471–1477. [CrossRef]

2

Development and Evaluation of a Reconstitutable Dry Suspension Containing Isoniazid for Flexible Pediatric Dosing

Oluwatoyin A. Adeleke [1,2,*], Rose K. Hayeshi [2,3] and Hajierah Davids [4]

1 Division of Pharmaceutical Sciences, School of Pharmacy, Sefako Makgatho Health Sciences University, Pretoria 0208, South Africa
2 Council for Scientific and Industrial Research, Pretoria 0001, South Africa
3 DST/NWU Preclinical Drug Development Platform, Faculty of Health Sciences, North-West University, Potchefstroom 2531, South Africa; rose.hayeshi@nwu.ac.za
4 Department of Physiology, Nelson Mandela University, Port Elizabeth 6031, South Africa; Hajierah.Davids@mandela.ac.za
* Correspondence: Oluwatoyin.adeleke@fulbrightmail.org or oluwatoyin.adeleke@smu.ac.za;

Abstract: Tuberculosis (TB) is a major cause of childhood death. Despite the startling statistics, it is neglected globally as evidenced by treatment and clinical care schemes, mostly extrapolated from studies in adults. The objective of this study was to formulate and evaluate a reconstitutable dry suspension (RDS) containing isoniazid, a first-line anti-tubercular agent used in the treatment and prevention of TB infection in both children and adults. The RDS formulation was prepared by direct dispersion emulsification of an aqueous-lipid particulate interphase coupled with lyophilization and dry milling. The RDS appeared as a cream-white free-flowing powder with a semi-crystalline and microparticulate nature. Isoniazid release was characterized with an initial burst up to 5 min followed by a cumulative release of 67.88% ± 1.88% (pH 1.2), 60.18% ± 3.33% (pH 6.8), and 49.36% ± 2.83% (pH 7.4) over 2 h. An extended release at pH 7.4 and 100% drug liberation was achieved within 300 min. The generated release profile best fitted the zero order kinetics (R^2 = 0.976). RDS was re-dispersible and remained stable in the dried and reconstituted states over 4 months and 11 days respectively, under common storage conditions.

Keywords: pediatric drug delivery; tuberculosis; reconstitutable dry suspension; isoniazid; polymer-lipid; microparticulate; direct emulsification

---

1. Introduction

Tuberculosis (TB) remains a major global health problem present in every country in the world, regardless of the availability of standard treatment guidelines [1,2]. It is the leading cause of death from a single infectious agent, ranking above the Human Immunodeficiency Virus (HIV) with about 10 million new active infections and 1.5–2 million fatalities annually [1,3–5]. TB is an airborne, highly contagious disease often spread by coughing and sneezing. It is caused by strains of bacteria known as *Mycobacterium tuberculosis* (Mtb), which primarily infects the lungs (pulmonary TB) and, occasionally, other body parts (extra-pulmonary TB) [1,5–7]. TB has been identified as a key cause of economic devastation, revolving poverty and illness that has entrapped families, societies, and even entire countries, with women, children, and HIV patients being the most vulnerable [2].

Tuberculosis is a major cause of childhood death. The World Health Organization (WHO) recently estimated that 10%–11% of the global population infected with TB are children, with about 233,000 childhood deaths each year [1,3,6]. The TB mortality rate is 70% higher in children under the age of five than it is in adults in high burden areas [1,8]. Research indicates that children serve as reservoirs for active TB infection later in life, evidenced by the fact that globally, about 67 million children under the age of 15 have latent TB [1,9]. Latent TB infection is known as a state of persistent immune responses to stimulation by Mtb antigens with no evidence of clinical manifestations associated with active infection or symptoms of illness. Nevertheless, latent TB can develop into full-blown, active infection later [1].

Thus far, the greatest challenge to the successful treatment of TB in children is the significant shortage of efficient pediatric pharmaceutical formulations [1,10–12]. Despite the alarming statistics reported on the number of active TB cases in children, it is indeed shocking to note that to date, childhood TB has been generally neglected worldwide, evidenced by treatment and clinical care schemes mostly extrapolated from studies in adults [1,13–15]. Over the years, children have been largely excluded from clinical trials resulting in weak evidence-based treatment of pediatric TB infection. With the shortage of suitable child-friendly anti-TB pharmaceutical formulations, it is common global practice to split adult fixed-dose combination (FDC) preparations: (i) into fractions; (ii) crushed to be taken with food, milk, and other liquids; or (iii) extemporaneous compounding to allow for easy use as needed per child. These practices can lead to dose inaccuracies, reduced active drug potencies, impaired dosage stability, irregular bioavailability, and poor compliance [14–16]. Consequently, there is an urgent need for innovative treatment strategies that can contribute towards combating the TB epidemic in pediatric patients.

Isoniazid is the most widely used first-line anti-tubercular agent for the treatment and prevention of TB infection in both children and adults. It is a drug of choice as it is bactericidal, easily administered, inexpensive, and relatively non-toxic in children. Isoniazid is almost completely absorbed from the gastrointestinal tract and penetrates all body fluid cavities, in which drug levels are similar to serum levels [12,15]. Although subject to considerable hepatic metabolism (or first-pass effect) after oral dosing, it reaches concentrations well above the minimum inhibitory levels of Mtb in most tissues and TB lesions when given in standard doses [17]. Isoniazid is considered a class III drug according to the Biopharmaceutics Classification System (BCS) [18], meaning that it is highly hydrophilic (aqueous solubility = 125 mg/mL at 25 °C) [18,19] but not very permeable (log P = −0.64 at 25 °C) [19]. It is weakly basic, crystalline in nature, and does not display polymorphism [20]. The aim of this study was, therefore, to develop and characterize a microparticulate reconstitutable dry suspension containing isoniazid as a model drug. To date, there is not much detailed in literature on the use of anti-tubercular micro-suspensions for pediatric TB treatment or prophylaxis. Conventional dry suspensions are powder mixtures that require the addition of water at the time of dispensing. They are often widely acceptable, intended for oral administration, and usually choice alternatives when drug stability is a major concern. Dry suspensions are easy to use by any age group (particularly children) and, therefore, enhance patient compliance [13,21]. In this study, microparticulate dry suspensions as micro-structuring remains an ideal way of manufacturing highly efficient, rate-modulated pharmaceutical formulations that are beneficial to patients. Generally, microparticulate drug carriers are known to have high stability with excellent drug loading capacities for hydrophobic and hydrophilic drug moieties, enhanced bioavailability, and decreased toxicity [22]. The reconstitutable dry suspension (RDS) was prepared by blending liquid and solid interphases of drug and excipient into a homogenous mix that was lyophilized and pulverized to produce an isoniazid-loaded free-flowing powdery formulation. Formulation evaluation involved zeta potential and polydispersity index analyses, particle sizing, drug loading, dissolution testing, thermal behavior, structural transitions, surface morphology, crystallinity determinations, cytotoxicity, hydro- and environmental- stability testing.

2. Materials and Methods

2.1. Materials

Polyethylene glycol, poly (vinyl alcohol) 87%–89% hydrolyzed, coconut oil, ethylcellulose, hydrochloric acid, anhydrous sodium phosphate dibasic, 3-(4,5-dimethylthiazol-2-yl)-2,5-diphenyltetrazolium bromide (MTT), Trypsin—EDTA, trypan blue, dimethylsulfoxide (DMSO), camptothecin, potassium dihydrogen phosphate monobasic buffer salt, isoniazid, and phosphate buffered saline powder were purchased from Sigma Chemical Company (St. Louis, MO, USA). D-fructose was obtained from Merck Chemicals (Darmstadt, Germany). The human breast cancer (MCF-7) cell line was purchased from American Type Culture Collection (ATCC, Manassas, VA, USA). Dulbecco's Modified Eagle's Medium (DMEM) and fetal bovine serum (FBS) were procured from BD Biosciences (San Jose, CA, USA). All other reagents utilized were of analytical grade and used as received from the supplier.

2.2. Formulation of the Reconstitutable Dry Suspension Employing a Direct Dispersion Emulsification Method

The RDS was prepared using a direct dispersion emulsification technique coupled with lyophilization and dry milling. This involved emulsification of the aqueous phase, which contained 2%$^{w}/_{w}$ polyethylene glycol, 9%$^{w}/_{w}$ poly (vinyl alcohol), 4%$^{w}/_{w}$ D-fructose, 10%$^{w}/_{w}$ isoniazid dispersed in water with the non-aqueous phase made up of 3%$^{w}/_{w}$ ethylcellulose in coconut oil under constant mechanical blending (Silverson Machines, Inc., East Longmeadow, MA, USA) at 6000 rpm over 5–10 min until a monophasic emulsion was produced. With D-fructose as a lyoprotectant and sweetener, the mono-phased emulsion was exposed to liquid nitrogen for 15 min until completely frozen. Thereafter, the frozen sample was lyophilized (Benchtop Pro Freeze Dryer, VirTis, SP Scientific, Stone Ridge, NY, USA) at a temperature of −60 ± 2 °C and pressure of 124 ± 2 mTorr over 96 h to produce a solid lyophilisate that was then dry milled using a laboratory scale grinder (Kinematica GMBH, Eschbach, Germany). The RDS was stored away in airtight, opaque containers until further testing.

2.3. Formulation Yield

The formulation yield was calculated by relating the total formulation weight (actual yield) to the mass of the component excipients used in the preparation of the formulation (theoretical yield). The constituting excipient plus the model drug and produced RDS formulation were weighed as separate entities using a laboratory scale balance (Kern EG 620-3NM, Kern and Sohn, GmbH, Balingen, Germany). The percentage yield was calculated using Equation (1) below:

$$\%\text{Yield} = \frac{\text{Actual yield (g)}}{\text{Theoretical yield (g)}} \times 100 \tag{1}$$

2.4. Physicochemical Characterization of the Reconstitutable Dry Suspension

2.4.1. Particle Size, Polydispersity Index, and Zeta Potential

Measurement of particle size (PS) and polydispersity index (PDI) was based on the principle of dynamic light scattering using the Nano series Zetasizer (Malvern Instruments Ltd, Malvern, UK). For each quantification, RDS samples were re-dispersed in deionized water, appropriately diluted, and sonicated (Table-type Supersonic Cleaner KQ118, Nanjing T-Bota Scietech Instruments and Equipment, Co, Ltd., Nanjing, China) for 15 min at 37 ± 0.5 °C. All measurements were performed as three independent replicates with 10 readings per sample at a measurement angle of 173° and temperature of 25 °C. Zeta potential (ZP) is an indicator of particle surface charge, which determines particle stability in dispersions [23,24]. It was computed based on the Smoluchowski equation [25] using the Nano series Zetasizer with RDS samples dispersed in deionized water and placed in disposable folded capillary zeta cells maintained at 25 °C. For statistical relevance, samples were measured in triplicate with 20 runs per measurement cycle.

2.4.2. Visualization of Surface Morphology

The surface microstructure of the RDS was observed under a JEOL Transmission Electron Microscope (TEM) (JEM-2100 LaB6 200 kV Transmission Electron Microscope, JEOL, MA, USA). About 1 mg of the test sample was dispersed in ethanol and spotted on a carbon coated copper grid. Ethanol was allowed to evaporate under atmospheric conditions prior to sample loading into the TEM viewing stage (JEOL JEM-2100 LaB6 200 kV Massachusetts, USA). The Gatan Digital Micrograph Software was used to facilitate sample viewing.

2.4.3. Thermal Analysis

The thermal behavior of the drug loaded RDS and pure isoniazid (reference) was characterized using a differential scanning calorimetry (DSC) machine equipped with a 50-position automatic sampler (Q2000 Differential Scanning Calorimeter TA Instruments, New Castle, DE, USA). Separate aluminum crucibles containing about 9 mg of each sample were analyzed under an inert nitrogen flow of 25 mL/minute and heating rate of 10 °C.min^{-1} while an empty crucible subjected to the same testing condition served as the reference. All measurements were performed in triplicate per sample under three heating cycles at a temperature range of 0–220 °C.

2.4.4. Determination of Crystallinity

The crystalline nature of the RDS formulation and pure isoniazid were evaluated under ambient conditions (25 ± 2 °C) using an X-ray diffractometer equipped with the X'Pert PRO data collector software (PANalytical Inc. MA, USA). Each sample (about 3 mg) analysis was performed at a voltage and current of 45 kV and 40 mA, respectively, and a 2θ range of 5 to 90° using a continuous scan mode with a scan step size of 0.03.

2.4.5. Structural Elucidation

The RDS formulation and pure isoniazid chemical backbone structural transitions were determined using the Fourier transform infrared (FTIR) spectrophotometric approach. The FTIR spectra of each test sample was generated on a Perkin Elmer Spectrum 100 Series FTIR Spectrophotometer coupled with Spectrum V 6.2.0 software (Beaconsfield, UK). Initially, blank background measurements were taken, and then, about 5 mg of each test sample was placed on a clean holder situated on the test stage of the machine for structural analysis that was recorded at a frequency range of 650–4000 cm^{-1}, scan time = 32 scans and resolution of 4 cm^{-1}.

2.5. Drug Loading Efficiency

To determine the amount of isoniazid loaded in the RDS formulation, 10 mg sample was placed in 100 mL phosphate buffered saline (pH 7.4) with continuous stirring over 4 h (Five-Position Hot Plate/Stirrer, Model 51450 series, Cole-Parmer, IL, USA), to ensure complete dissolution and release of all entrapped drug molecules. The resulting solution was then appropriately diluted with distilled water and passed through a 0.45 µm nylon membrane Corning® syringe filter (Corning Incorporated, NY, USA). The actual drug content was analyzed using Ultraviolet (UV) Spectrophotometry (PerkinElmer Lambda 35, UV/Vis Spectrometer, Perkin Elmer, Singapore) at a maximum wavelength of absorption for isoniazid, λ_{max} = 262 nm. The percentage of isoniazid load in the RDS formulation was mathematically computed with reference to the originally added amount (Equation (2)). Tests were conducted as three replicate samples.

$$\%\text{Drug loading efficiency} = \frac{\text{Actual drug amount (g)}}{\text{Theoretical drug amount (g)}} \times 100 \quad (2)$$

2.6. In Vitro Dissolution Studies

In vitro dissolution studies were performed on an RDS formulation sample size containing an equivalent of 100 mg isoniazid. The study was carried out using the dissolution tester (Ewreka GmbH, DT 820 series, Heusenstamm, Germany). The RDS formulation was contained in a gelatin capsule (CapsCanada, Ontario, Canada), which was placed in a basket holder attached to the dissolution tester stirring shaft (United States Pharmacopeia Apparatus 1). The basket was then immersed into separate dissolution jars containing 500 mL of either pH 7.4 or pH 6.8 or pH 1.2 pre-heated buffered solution maintained at 37 ± 0.5 °C with continuous rotation at 100 rpm. Samples (5 mL) were removed at the end of the 2-h time-point for quantification. Furthermore, at pH 7.4, drug loaded RDS formulation underwent an extended release testing up to a point when 100% isoniazid liberation was observed. Briefly, samples (5 mL) were removed at pre-determined time intervals and replaced with 5 mL freshly prepared preheated, buffered solution (pH 7.4, 37 ± 0.5 °C). All experiments were performed in triplicate under sink conditions and isolated samples were appropriately diluted, filtered using a 0.45 μm nylon membrane Corning® syringe filter (Corning Incorporated, NY, USA) and analyzed spectrophotometrically (PerkinElmer Lambda 35, UV/Vis Spectrometer, Perkin Elmer, Singapore) at λ_{max} of 262, 263, and 267 nm for pH 7.4, 6.8, and 1.2 buffered solutions, respectively, to determine the amount of isoniazid contained in each sample per time against buffer blanks. The actual quantity of isoniazid released per unit time was calculated using the linear polynomial calibration equations as follows: (a) pH 7.4: $y = 39.38x$; $R^2 = 0.98$; (b) pH 6.8: $y = 32.96x$; $R^2 = 0.99$, and (c) pH 1.2: $y = 45.77x$; $R^2 = 0.98$ where x and y, respectively, represent concentration (mg/mL) and absorbance. Percentage cumulative drug release [26] was computed relative to the total amount of isoniazid present in each medium at the end of the 2-h period. To get an indication of the release kinetics of the RDS formulation, the pH 7.4 release profile was selected for further mathematical model fitting over an extended period when 100% drug release was achieved. Resulting data were further analyzed using the KientDS version 3.0 open source software, which aided the selection of the model of best fit, which was based on mathematical computations, such as the zero, first, and second order kinetics, Higuchi, Korsmeyer-Peppas, Michaelis-Menten and Weibull approaches [19,24,27].

2.7. *Stability Evaluations*

2.7.1. Short-Term Stability Testing under Different Environmental Conditions

The physicochemical stability of the RDS formulation (500.0 mg ± 2 mg per test) was monitored under different storage conditions over four months. A set of samples were placed in an enclosed glass holder that was transferred into the stability tester (Labcon PSIE RH 40 Chamber Standard Incubator, Laboratory Marketing Services, Maraisburg, South Africa) fixed at 30 °C ± 2 °C and a relative humidity of 65% ± 3% adapted from the WHO stability testing scheme for pharmaceutical products containing well established drug substances [28]. Another sample group was stored in airtight, opaque glass vials under standard room conditions (temperature: 25 °C ± 5 °C and humidity: 55% ± 5%). The last sample set was stored in airtight, opaque glass vials and placed in the refrigerator (Sanya Labcool Pharmaceutical Refrigerator, MPR-720R, Sanyo Electrical Biomedical Co. Ltd, CA, USA) at 4 °C ± 1 °C. Formulation stability was monitored at 0, 1, and 4 month intervals for changes in particle size, polydispersity index, zeta potential, and drug content. Samples were also physically examined for any changes in physical appearance or color changes. All tests were conducted in triplicate.

2.7.2. In Vitro Aqueous Stability Assessment

The stability of the RDS formulation in aqueous solution (mimicking the re-constitution process) was evaluated. RDS samples (500 ± 2 mg) were placed in airtight, opaque containers and dispersed in 50 mL sterile deionized water. Hydrated samples were prepared in triplicate per test conditions. Test conditions included placement under ambient conditions (25 ± 5 °C), as well as in the refrigerator (4 ± 2 °C) for 11 days. Hydrated samples (2 mL) were collected from each test vessel for isoniazid content quantification at 0, 1, 5, and 11 days using UVspectrophotometry, as described earlier. Samples were manually agitated daily and before collection to ensure uniform re-dispersion. All tests were carried out in triplicate.

2.8. Preliminary Formulation Toxicity Assessment

The human breast adenocarcinoma (MCF-7) cell line was used for preliminary evaluation of the RDS formulation biocompatibility. The sample was dissolved in double-distilled water to a final stock concentration of 2 mg/mL, filter-sterilized through a 0.22 μm Cameo acetate membrane filter (Millipore Co., Bedford, Massachusetts), and stored at 4 °C until used. The negative control was 1% DMSO while 100 μM camptothecin, a known chemotherapeutic agent, was used as the positive control. The MCF-7 cell line was routinely maintained in Dulbecco's Modified Eagle's Medium (DMEM) supplemented with 10% heat-inactivated fetal bovine serum (FBS), at 5% carbon dioxide and 37 °C ± 0.1 °C. Cells were seeded into 96-well plates at a final concentration of 15,000 cells/well. Test samples were added at final well concentrations of 100, 50, 25 μg/ml, and incubated for 24 h. Thereafter, the spent medium was replaced with 200 μL of 0.05 mg/mL 3-(4,5-dimethylthiazol-2-yl)-2,5-diphenyltetrazolium bromide) (MTT) solution and incubated at 37 °C ± 0.1 °C for 3 h. The MTT was then aspirated from the cells and replaced with 200 μL DMSO to dissolve the formazan crystals. The absorbance was read at a maximum wavelength of 540 nm against DMSO as a blank using a microtiter plate reader (BioTek Powerwave XS, Winooski, VT, USA). The absorbance readings obtained were used to compute the number of viable cells present in the media. All results are presented as the mean reading ± standard deviation, and the statistical significance of all experimental data was evaluated using the GraphPad Prism 7 software (GraphPad, San Diego, CA, USA) using a two-way Analysis of Variance (ANOVA). The number of viable cells in both test and control samples were determined using Equation (3), and all tests were conducted in triplicate.

$$\%\text{Cell viability} = \frac{\text{Number of viable test cells}}{\text{Number of viable control cells}} \times 100 \quad (3)$$

3. Results and Discussions

3.1. Formulation Synthesis and Yield

The isoniazid-loaded RDS formulation was developed using a combination of the direct dispersion emulsification technique, lyophilization, and dry milling. A cream-white, free flowing isoniazid loaded RDS powder with an average yield of 87.43% ± 0.13% was obtained.

3.2. Size, Polydispersity Index, and Zeta Potential Determination and Morphology

The RDS powder formulation showed an average particle size of 1.63 ± 0.20 μm, indicating its intrinsic micro-structure. The PDI can be described as a ratio that provides information about homogeneity of particle size distribution as it relates to a particular system serving as a useful reflection of the quality of the particulate system/dispersion ranging from 0.0–1.0 with values ≤0.1 relating to the highest quality of particulate dispersion, ≤0.3 as optimum, ≤0.5 as generally acceptable [24]. A generally acceptable PDI value of 0.37 ± 0.04 was recorded for the RDS powder, indicating that the particles were mostly homogenous and well dispersed within the formulation. The measured ZP was −41.10 ± 5.57 mV, showing a stable system, where a ZP value of ±30 mV is considered a stable and satisfactory formulation [24,29]. Representative graphs based on an independent measurement of the zeta potential and particle size distribution are shown in Figure 1a,b. Researchers have shown that TEM imaging is an effective and powerful tool for characterizing the morphology of nano- and micro-structured biomaterials and drug carriers as it uses more powerful beams to produce higher resolution images with more details and information [30,31]. The TEM micrographs showed minimally aggregated, dispersed RDS particles that appeared as darker areas relative to the background, with rounded outer morphologies (Figure 1c,d).

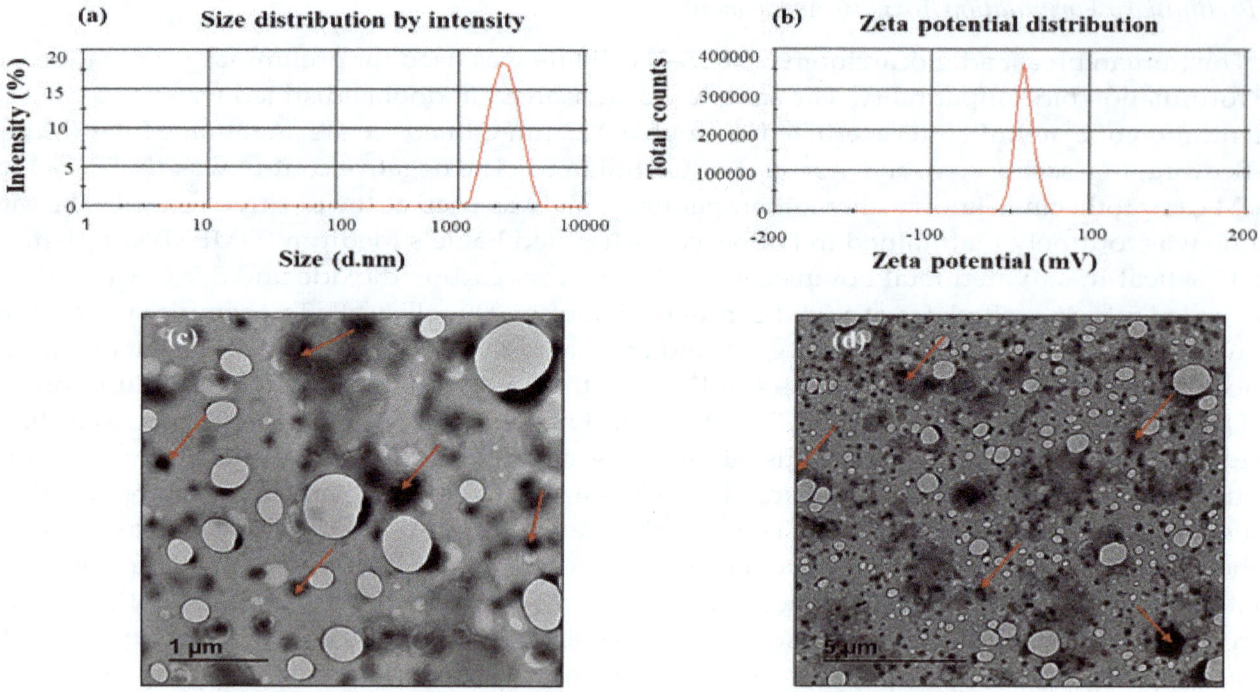

Figure 1. Representative graphs displaying: (**a**) particle size distribution, (**b**) zeta potential distribution, as well as TEM micrographs showing different surface topographies and characteristics of the reconstitutable dry suspension (RDS) particles at different scales: (**c**) 1µm and (**d**) 5 µm, respectively.

3.3. Thermal Behavior

Salient changes in the thermal behavior of isoniazid relative to that of the RDS formulation were studied using conventional DSC methods. The recorded melting peak of pure, unformulated isoniazid was 171.7 °C, which compared well to literature [32]. The melting peak of isoniazid (Figure 2a) was characterized by its sharp and defined geometry confirming its purity and crystalline nature. The RDS thermogram was typified by the presence of multiple distinct sharp or broad peaks showing its physicochemically stable and multi-component state. The RDS formulation showed an intermittent appearance of sharp and blunt peaks representing its semi-crystalline nature (Figure 2b,c). The isoniazid melting peak identified on the RDS formulation thermogram (171.1 °C) was similar to that of the pure drug (171.7 °C), showing its stability within the excipient matrix. However, the formulated isoniazid peak presented as a broad band, which can be related to physical transitioning from crystalline into amorphous structures attributable to solvation and encapsulation of drug molecules into the processed polymeric carrier. A significant change in heat flow from −36.4 mW (unformulated isoniazid) to −3.7 mW (isoniazid in RDS) (Figure 2b,c) was seen, further supporting the likely drug encapsulation in the amorphous state, coupled with stable molecular dispersions within the polymeric chains [24]. Overall, the thermograms (Figure 2a–c) demonstrate the absence of any destructive/irreversible physicochemical interactions between isoniazid and the excipients during the RDS preparation process.

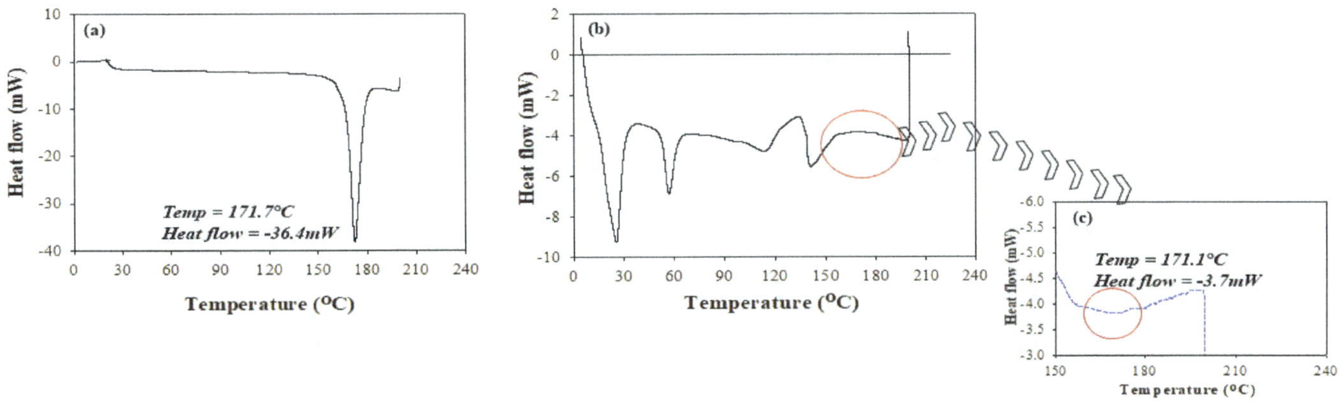

Figure 2. Differential scanning calorimetry (DSC) thermograms of (**a**) unformulated isoniazid, (**b**) RDS formulation, and (**c**) an expanded segment of the RDS thermograms showing the transitions that occurred with formulated isoniazid.

3.4. X-ray Diffractometry

The changes in matrix crystallinity between pure isoniazid and the RDS formulation was further confirmed using X-ray diffraction analysis (XRD) with recorded diffractograms presented in Figure 3a,b. Diffractograms recorded for pure isoniazid showed high intensity, well-defined sharp peaks between 9.3θ and 32.3θ, with intensities as high as 39,885.7 validating the crystalline nature of isoniazid (Figure 3a). This trend differs from that observed for the RDS formulation, which presents broader, not so well-defined peaks between 13.9θ and 28.1θ at a maximum intensity of 11,142.9, which is much lower relative to the isoniazid diffractogram. Furthermore, low intensity (less than 4288.1) plateau-like, broad-banded sections were also identified between 5.3θ—14.6θ and 28.5θ—90.1θ, further confirming that the RDS formulation consists of more than one component, characterized with intermittent, mostly amorphous and minimal crystalline domains, i.e., a semi-crystalline nature (Figure 3b). These findings agree with the outcomes of the DSC analysis.

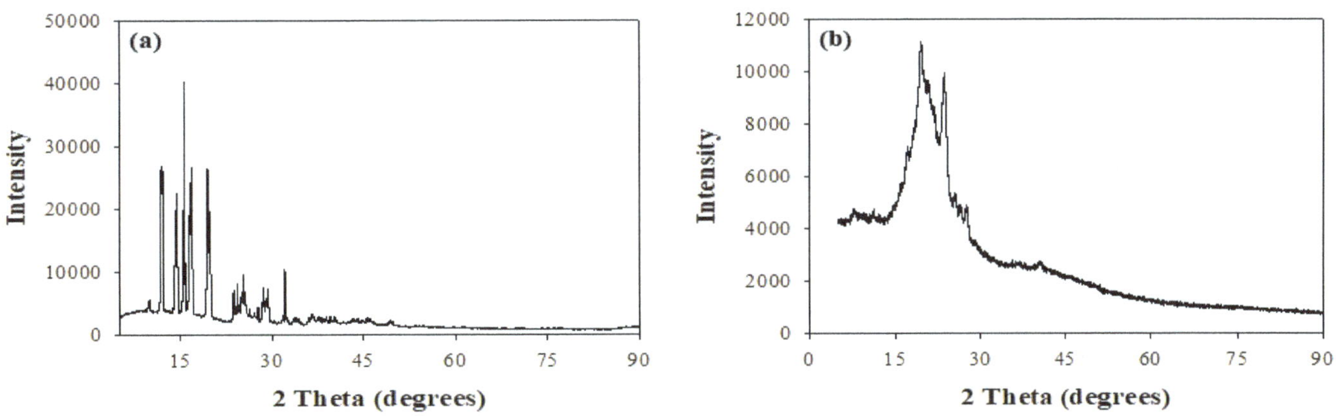

Figure 3. X-ray diffractograms of (**a**) unformulated isoniazid and (**b**) isoniazid loaded RDS formulation.

3.5. Structural Analysis

FTIR spectrum depicting characteristic vibrational frequencies of isoniazid in its unformulated state and encapsulated within the RDS formulation were compared (Figure 4). The vibrational band assignments for formulated and unformulated isoniazid were executed based on their positions, nature, magnitudes, and intensities relative to each characteristic functional group. The key bands plus wavenumbers identified and compared for both the RDS formulation and isoniazid in its pure state are presented in Table 1. The vibrational frequencies of key functional groups as it relates to the chemical backbone structure of isoniazid compares well for both pure drug and RDS formulation, with characteristic peaks presenting with varying intensities. The isoniazid loaded RDS formulation appeared overly dominant in most regions with some of its peaks suppressing those of pure isoniazid. This suggests physical solid–liquid/solid–solid dispersion and significant drug encapsulation. The O–H stretch recorded at 3676 cm^{-1} for the RDS formulation further supports the physically dispersed state in the water/oil medium, followed by snap-freezing and lyophilization.

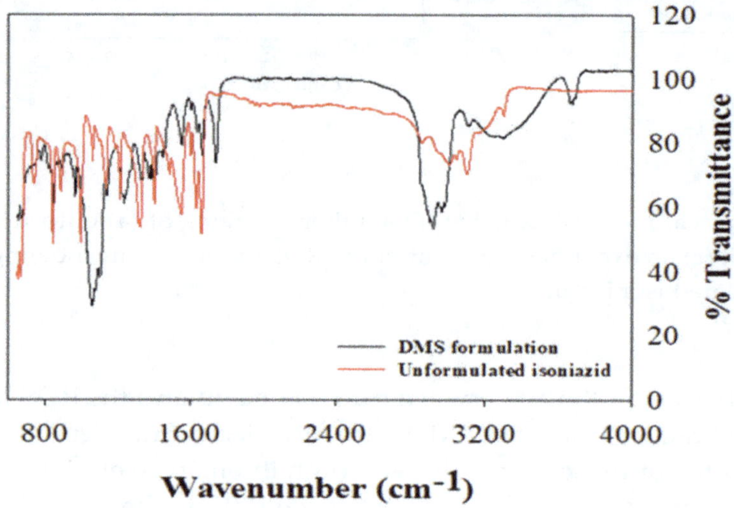

Figure 4. The Fourier transform infrared (FTIR) spectrum of the unformulated isoniazid and RDS formulation, showing different characteristic vibrational bands.

Table 1. FTIR vibrational frequencies representing formulated and unformulated isoniazid key functional groups.

Functional Groups and Remarks	Vibrational Frequencies (cm^{-1})	
	Unformulated Isoniazid	**Isoniazid Loaded RDS Formulation**
C–C–C–C and C–N–C–C torsion	653	665
NH_2 rock	677	677
C–C–C out of plane bending	746	757
C–C–H out of plane bending	850 and 1022	850 and 1023
C–N–C and C–C–C in plane bending	1063	1062
Aromatic C–N stretching	1344	1330
C–C–H in plane bending	1210	1212
O=C-N in plane bending	1330	1333
C–N–H in plane bending	1411	1408
C–C stretching	1477	1471
C=O stretching	1558	1552
NH_2 scissoring	1632	1635
Aromatic C–H stretching	3052	3054
N–H stretching	3307	3308
O–H stretching	-	3676

3.6. Drug Content

The percentage content of isoniazid encapsulated within the RDS formulation matrix was computed relative to the theoretical drug content, totaling 94.12% ± 2.10%. This indicates that there was minimal drug loss during the RDS manufacturing and processing phases.

3.7. Drug Release Behavior

To understand the in vitro drug release behavior and kinetics, dissolution studies were carried out on the RDS formulation containing an equivalence of 100 mg isoniazid in pH 7.4, 6.8, and 1.2 buffered solution over two hours under biorelevant conditions. Percentage cumulative drug release (%CDR) was calculated as the total amount of isoniazid liberated from the RDS formulation matrix, with an increase or decrease in %CDR representing a respective rise or decline in the release rates. %CDR varied for each dissolution media (pH 1.2 = 67.88% ± 1.88%, pH 6.8 = 60.18% ± 3.33%, and pH 7.4 = 49.36% ± 2.83%). Isoniazid release decreased as media pH increased. In other words, a reduction in the pH of the aqueous micro-environment seemed to impact the processes of formulation wetting, pore formation and closure, water penetration, phase transitioning, drug-excipient dissolution and degradation, changes in drug-excipient physical interaction and solubility process, and eventual diffusion of drug molecules coupled with gradual matrix geometry transitions (erosion or swelling) [33]. The RDS formulation demonstrated the potential to stabilize and release the isoniazid molecules in different dissolution media with significant differences in the percentage of drug released under these different conditions.

In addition, isoniazid release at pH 7.4 was selected for further mathematical model fitting to understand the RDS formulation release kinetics over a period when 100% drug liberation was achieved (Figure 5). In vitro isoniazid release from the RDS formulation at pH 7.4 was characterized with an initial burst at 5 min (7.51 ± 0.72 %), followed by a relatively consistent increase in drug release over time, until complete release (100%) was recorded at approximately 300 min.

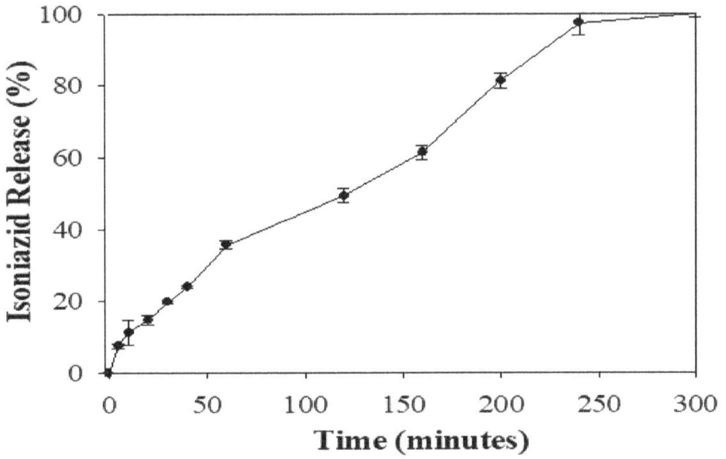

Figure 5. Graphical profile showing 100% isoniazid release from the RDS formulation over time.

The generated profile (Figure 5) was further analyzed using mathematical kinetic models employing the KinetDS, version 3.0 open source freeware. Release profile analysis and model of best fit selection was based on a combination of robust validation quantities, namely the correlation coefficient (R^2) closest to one and lowest Akaike Information Criterion (AIC) numerical value (Table 2) [31]. On this basis, the zero order kinetic model provided the best fit parameters (R^2 = 0.976 and AIC = 74.080) for the isoniazid release data depicted in Figure 5. This indicates that isoniazid release from the RDS formulation is consistent over time, irrespective of the initial drug concentration. In principle, zero order drug release mechanism is beneficial for achieving continuous drug plasma and biological fluid levels, reducing dosing frequency, and improving patient compliance, aiding desired pharmacotherapeutic efficacy [34].

Table 2. Representative mathematical models and their respective fit parameters.

Mathematical Models	R^2	AIC
Zero order	0.976	74.080
First order	0.159	176.881
Second order	0.091	129.633
Korsmeyer-Peppas	0.997	110.291
Weibull	0.990	92.616
Michaelis-Menten	1.000	120.737
Higuchi	-0.341	127.138

3.8. Short-Term Formulation Stability Assessment

3.8.1. Stability Evaluation under Varying Storage Conditions

Evaluation of formulation stability was performed in triplicate per sample under multiple storage conditions: Stability tester—30 °C ± 2 °C and 65% ± 3%; Room—25 °C ± 5 °C and 55% ± 5%; and Refrigerator—4 °C ± 1 °C; over four months employing particle size, polydispersity index, zeta potential, and drug content as indicators of stability. Results showed minimal numerical differences in indicators measured, indicating that the isoniazid loaded RDS formulation can be described as stable under the prescribed environmental storage conditions (Table 3). A slight alteration in physical appearance relating to a color change from white to cream-white was observed at four months, under accelerated storage in the stability chamber (30 °C ± 2 °C; 65% ± 3%) and room conditions (25 °C ± 5 °C; 55% ± 5%). Despite the fact that stability indicators remain closely related, the slight color change is undesirable, considering patient acceptance, making these environments unsuitable for the storage of the RDS formulation. Therefore, the most ideal storage setting for the RDS formulation is, thus, at 4 ± 1 °C as stability indicators are comparable with no color change observed (Table 3).

Table 3. Stability indicators measured under the different storage conditions.

RDS Formulation Test Conditions	Time (Months)	Stability Indicators				
		PDI [a]	ZP [b] (mV)	PS [c] (μm)	DC [d] (%)	Color
Stability tester	0	0.37	−41.10	1.63	94.12	No change
	1	0.40	−42.59	1.58	94.07	No change
	4	0.39	−43.60	1.82	93.76	Slight change
Room	0	0.37	−41.10	1.63	94.12	No change
	1	0.44	−42.71	1.69	93.95	No change
	4	0.46	−40.51	1.97	91.05	Slight change
Refrigerator	0	0.37	−41.10	1.63	94.12	No change
	1	0.39	−41.65	1.61	93.95	No change
	4	0.38	−40.91	1.70	94.02	No change

[a] Particle Size (standard deviation ≤ 0.13 μm in all cases), [b] Polydispersity Index (standard deviation ≤ 0.03 in all cases), [c] Zeta Potential (standard deviation ≤ 1.03 mV in all cases), [d] Drug Content (standard deviation ≤ 0.99% in all cases).

3.8.2. Formulation Stability in an Aqueous Environment

The stability of the drug loaded RDS formulation in an aqueous medium was investigated under select storage conditions (room and refrigeration) over 11 days, mimicking storage duration for commonly reconstituted antibiotic solutions/suspensions. Percentage drug content was chosen as the hydrostability indicator, and overall, there were insignificant changes in its numerical values under room or refrigerated storage conditions, with no visible color changes (Table 4). Summarily, the RDS formulation is stable in the aqueous medium over 11 days, either refrigerated or stored under ambient conditions, suggesting that the RDS formulation is a potentially useful preparation for re-constitution purposes, especially in pediatrics.

Table 4. Hydrostability indicators at different time-points, under ambient and refrigerated conditions.

Test Conditions	Time-Points (Days)	Drug Content (%)	Discoloration
Room/Ambient	0	94.12	None
	1	93.18	None
	5	93.61	None
	11	92.89	None
Refrigerator	0	94.12	None
	1	93.33	None
	5	93.79	None
	11	92.56	None

3.9. Cell Viability Assessment

Preliminary assessment of the effects of the RDS formulation on viability was performed on MCF-7 cell lines. Tests were conducted over 24 h using different concentrations of the RDS ranging from 0 μg/mL (negative control) to 100 μg/mL. This cell line is routinely used as a prototype for assessing the biocompatibility of drugs, delivery systems, and biologicals that are non-specific for treating carcinomas [35–37]. Graphical representations of the impact of different test formulation concentrations on cell viability relative to camptothecin (positive control) and the negative control are presented in Figure 6. The RDS lowest concentration (25 μg/mL) caused significant MCF-7 cell proliferation ($p < 0.0500$: $p = 0.0001$). The increased viability may signify that the RDS formulation supported cell growth at a low concentration (25 μg/mL) and can be considered an indication of biocompatibility. This may be attributed to the drug or excipient concentration or a combination of both. In contrast, the 50 and 100 μg/mL reduced cell viability, although not significantly ($p > 0.0500$: 50 μg/mL—$p = 0.0056$; 100 μg/mL—$p = 0.0001$). Nevertheless, higher concentrations of the RDS (50 and 100 μg/mL) did not reduce cell viability as much as the camptothecin that decreased it to 48.93% ± 3.99%. In general, the RDS was well-tolerated by the MCF-7 cells at all test concentrations. Cellular responses following exposure to the formulation can be described as biphasic and dose-dependent, a phenomenon associated with hormesis (a two-phased adaptive response of cells and organisms to increasing or decreasing amounts of external stress, e.g., drug, chemical substances, and disease state) [38,39]. It is not unusual for cells to exhibit hormetic effects as they are biological systems known to be dynamic and constantly evolving. These initial findings form a baseline for future work on understanding the biocompatibility of the RDS formulation and its components (active drug and excipients) in vitro and in vivo.

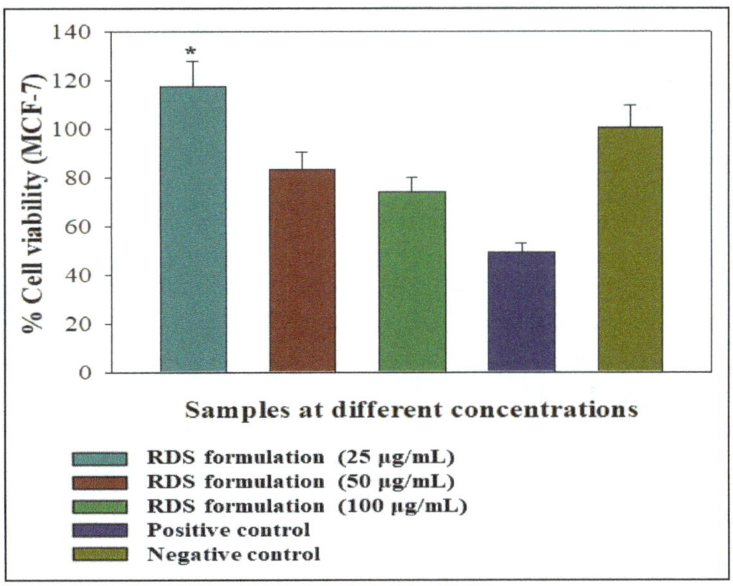

Figure 6. Graphical illustration of the percentage cell viability 24-h post-exposure to the RDS formulation in the human breast cancer (MCF-7) cell lines as a prototype. Statistical difference between two data sets was considered significant when $p < 0.05$.

4. Conclusions and Future Work

In this study, isoniazid loaded reconstitutable dry suspension was prepared using the direct dispersion emulsification technique, coupled with lyophilization and dry milling. The direct dispersion technique produced a relatively high yield (87.43% ± 0.13%) of RDS particles with good drug loading capabilities (94.12% ± 2.10%). The RDS formulation showed no significant evidence of toxicity supported by outcomes from viability studies in the MCF-7 cells. The formulation was physicochemically stable, mostly amorphous, with marginal intermittent crystalline domains, and had no irreversible alterations in its backbone chemical structure. It demonstrated the ability to regulate isoniazid release in a controlled, zero order manner, and was environmentally stable under common storage conditions, either as a dry powder or in the hydrated form. The findings from this work may contribute towards improving flexible pediatric dosing for tuberculosis drug treatment, considering the current global shortage of such preparations, especially for the first-line anti-tubercular drugs.

To establish a course for further investigations, we identified the need to extend biocompatibility testing for the RDS formulation and its components to normal cells and tissue isolates from animal models (e.g., mice, rabbit, or pigs) employing cytotoxicity assays and histopathological techniques, respectively. Further preclinical evaluation of pharmacokinetics, efficacy, and eventual optimization of isoniazid dosing and absorption from the RDS formulation, in animal models similar to humans, such as pigs, are important next steps. Considering the hydrophilic/hydrophobic and particulate nature of the RDS, we anticipate that it can find extensive use as an effective carrier for other anti-tubercular drugs (e.g., pyrazinamide, rifampicin) suitable for pediatrics irrespective of their solubilities and molecular weights. For implementation purposes, a range of these bioactives would need to be tested in vitro/in vivo and optimized to ensure desirable drug loading, controlled release, and absorption for the intended pharmacotherapeutic application. Overall, the RDS formulation reported herein has the potential for improving tuberculosis treatment within the pediatric population.

Author Contributions: Conceptualization, O.A.A.; methodology, O.A.A., R.K.H., H.D.; formal analysis, O.A.A., R.K.H.; investigation, O.A.A., R.K.H., H.D.; writing-original draft preparation, O.A.A.; writing, review and editing, O.A.A., R.K.H., H.D.; project administration, O.A.A., R.K.H.; resources, O.A., R.K.H., H.D.; funding acquisition, O.A.A., R.K.H. All authors have read and agreed to the published version of the manuscript.

Acknowledgments: We thank the National Centre for Nano-structured Materials, Council for Scientific and Industrial Research, South Africa, for sample characterization. We thank the CSIR National Centre for Nano-structured Materials for sample characterization. Opinions, findings and conclusions or recommendations expressed in this publication are that of the authors. The funders accept no liabilities whatsoever in this regard.

References

1. World Health Organization. WHO Global TB Report. 2018. Available online: http://www.who.int/tb/publications/global_report/en/ (accessed on 10 December 2019).
2. TB Alliance. The Pandemic. 2019. Available online: https://www.tballiance.org/why-new-tb-drugs/global-pandemic (accessed on 2 December 2019).
3. Suárez-González, J.; Santoveña-Estévez, A.; Soriano, M.; Fariña, J.B. Design and optimization of a child-friendly dispersible tablet containing Isoniazid, Pyrazinamide and Rifampicin for treating Tuberculosis in pediatrics. *Drug Dev. Ind. Pharm.* **2020**, *46*, 309–317. [CrossRef] [PubMed]
4. Venturini, E.; Turkova, A.; Chiappini, E.; Gali, L.; de Martino, M.; Thorne, C. Tuberculosis and HIV co-infection in children. *BMC Infect. Dis.* **2014**, *14*, 1–10. [CrossRef] [PubMed]
5. Sinha, P.; Shenoi, S.V.; Friedland, G.H. Opportunities for community health workers to contribute to global efforts to end tuberculosis. *Glob. Public Health* **2020**, *15*, 474–484. [CrossRef] [PubMed]
6. Chan, J.G.Y.; Chan, H.K.; Prestidge, C.A.; Denman, J.A.; Young, P.M.; Traini, D. A novel dry powder inhalable formulation incorporating three first-line anti-tubercular antibiotics. *Eur. J. Pharm. Biopharm.* **2013**, *83*, 285–292. [CrossRef]
7. Hussain, A.; Shakeel, F.; Singh, S.K.; Alsarra, I.A.; Faruk, A.; Alanazi, F.K.; Christoper, G.P. Solidified SNEDDS for the oral delivery of rifampicin: Evaluation, proof of concept, in vivo kinetics, and in silico GastroPlusTM simulation. *Int. J. Pharm.* **2019**, *566*, 203–217. [CrossRef]
8. Hamzaoui, A.; Yalaoui, A.; Cherif, F.A.; Slim, L.; Barraies, A. Childhood tuberculosis: A concern for the modern world. *Eur. Respir. Update Tuberc.* **2014**, *23*, 278–291. [CrossRef]
9. Jenkins, H.E. Global burden of childhood tuberculosis. *Pneumonia* **2016**, *8*, 24. [CrossRef]

10. Peña, M.J.M.; García, B.S.; Baquero-Artigao, F.; Pérez, D.M.; Pérez, R.P.; Echevarría, A.M.; Amador, J.T.R.; Durán, D.G.P.; Julian, A.N.; Tuberculosis, W.G.; et al. Tuberculosis treatment for children: An update. *An. Pediatr.* **2018**, *88*, 52.e1–52.e12.
11. Pérez, R.P.; García, B.S.; Fernández-Llamazares, C.M.; Artigao, F.B.; Julia, A.N.; Péna, M.J.M. The challenge of administering anti-tuberculosis treatment in infants and pre-school children. *An. Pediatr.* **2016**, *8*, 4–12.
12. Samad, A.; Sultana, Y.; Khar, R.K.; Aqil, M.; Chuttani, K.; Mishra, A.K. Reconstituted powder for formulation of antitubercular drugs formulated as microspheres for paediatric use. *Drug Discov. Ther.* **2008**, *2*, 108–114.
13. Shanbhag, P.P.; Bhalerao, S.S. Development and evaluation of oral reconstitutable systems of cephalexin. *Int. J. Pharm. Tech. Res.* **2010**, *2*, 502–506.
14. Pouplin, T.; Phuong, P.N.; Van Toi, P.; Pouplin, J.N.; Farrar, J. Isoniazid, pyrazinamide and rifampicin content variation in split fixed-dose combination tablets. *PLoS ONE* **2014**, *9*, e102047. [CrossRef] [PubMed]
15. Lopez, F.L.; Ernest, T.B.; Tuleu, C.; Gul, M.O. Formulation approaches to paediatric oral drug delivery: Benefits and limitations of current platforms. *Expert Opin. Drug Deliv.* **2015**, *12*, 1727–1740. [CrossRef] [PubMed]
16. Long, S.S.; Prober, C.G.; Fischer, M. *Principles and Practice of Pediatric Infectious Diseases E-Book*, 5th ed.; Elsevier Health Sciences: Amsterdam, The Netherlands, 2017.
17. Grange, J.M.; Schaaf, H.S.; Zumla, A. *Tuberculosis: A Comprehensive Clinical Reference*; Saunders/Elsevier: Philadelphia, PA, USA, 2009.
18. Moretton, M.A.; Cagel, M.; Bernabeu, E.; Gonzalez, L.; Chiappetta, D.A. Nanopolymersomes as potential carriers for rifampicin pulmonary delivery. *Colloids Surf. B Biointerfaces* **2015**, *136*, 1017–1025. [CrossRef]
19. Adeleke, O.A.; Tsai, P.C.; Karry, K.M.; Monama, N.O.; Michniak-Kohn, B.B. Isoniazid-loaded orodispersible strips: Methodical design, optimization and in vitro-in silico characterization. *Int. J. Pharm.* **2018**, *547*, 347–359. [CrossRef]
20. Brennan, P.J.; Young, D.B. Handbook of Anti-Tuberculosis Agents. *Tuberculosis* **2008**, *88*, 112–116.
21. Fülöp, V.; Jakab, G.; Bozó, T.; Tóth, B.; Endrésik, D.; Balogh, E.; Kellermayer, M.; Antal, I. Study on the dissolution improvement of albendazole using reconstitutable dry nanosuspension formulation. *Eur. J. Pharm. Sci.* **2018**, *123*, 70–78. [CrossRef]
22. Anselmo, A.C.; Mitragotri, S. An overview of clinical and commercial impact of drug delivery systems. *J. Control. Release* **2014**, *190*, 15–28. [CrossRef]
23. Yin Win, K.; Feng, S. Effects of particle size and surface coating on cellular uptake of polymeric nanoparticles for oral delivery of anticancer drugs. *Biomaterials* **2005**, *26*, 2713–2722. [CrossRef]
24. Öztürk, A.A.; Yenilmez, E.; Özarda, M.G. Clarithromycin-Loaded Poly (Lactic-co-glycolic acid) (PLGA) Nanoparticles for Oral Administration: Effect of Polymer Molecular Weight and Surface Modification with Chitosan on Formulation, Nanoparticle Characterization and Antibacterial Effects. *Polymers* **2019**, *11*, 1632. [CrossRef]
25. Kodama, T.; Tomita, N.; Horie, S.; Sax, N.; Iwasaki, H.; Suzuki, R.; Maruyama, K.; Mori, S.; Manabu, F. Morphological study of acoustic liposomes using transmission electron microscopy. *J. Electron Microsc.* **2009**, *59*, 187–196. [CrossRef] [PubMed]
26. Jermy, B.R.; Alomari, M.; Ravinayagam, V.; Almofty, S.A.; Akhtar, S.; Borgio, J.F.; AbdulAzeez, S. SPIONs/3D SiSBA-16 based Multifunctional Nanoformulation for target specific cisplatin release in colon and cervical cancer cell lines. *Sci. Rep.* **2019**, *9*, 1–12. [CrossRef] [PubMed]
27. Yang, X.; Trinh, H.M.; Agrahari, V.; Sheng, Y.; Pal, D.; Mitra, A.K. Nanoparticle-based topical ophthalmic gel formulation for sustained release of hydrocortisone butyrate. *AAPS Pharm. Sci. Tech.* **2016**, *17*, 294–306. [CrossRef]
28. World Health Organization (WHO). Guidelines for Stability Testing of Pharmaceutical Products Containing Well-Established Drug Substances in Conventional Dosage Forms. WHO Technical Report Series 863, Annex 5. 1996. Available online: https://apps.who.int/medicinedocs/pdf/s5516e/s5516e.pdf (accessed on 24 February 2020).
29. Dodiya, S.; Chavhan, S.; Korde, A.; Sawant, K.K. Solid lipid nanoparticles and nanosuspension of adefovir dipivoxil for bioavailability improvement: Formulation, characterization, pharmacokinetic and biodistribution studies. *Drug Dev. Ind. Pharm.* **2013**, *39*, 733–743. [CrossRef] [PubMed]
30. Manaia, E.B.; Abuçafy, M.P.; Chiari-Andréo, B.G.; Silva, B.L.; Junior, J.A.O.; Chiavacci, L.A. Physicochemical characterization of drug nanocarriers. *Int. J. Nanomed.* **2017**, *12*, 4991. [CrossRef]

31. Maciel, V.B.; Yoshida, C.M.; Pereira, S.M.; Goycoolea, F.M.; Franco, T.T. Electrostatic self-assembled chitosan-pectin nano-and microparticles for insulin delivery. *Molecules* **2017**, *22*, E1707. [CrossRef]
32. Afinjuomo, F.; Barclay, T.G.; Parikh, A.; Chung, R.; Song, Y.; Nagalingam, G.; Triccas, J.; Wang, L.; Liu, L.; Hayball, J.D.; et al. Synthesis and Characterization of pH-Sensitive Inulin Conjugate of Isoniazid for Monocyte-Targeted Delivery. *Pharmaceutics* **2019**, *11*, 555. [CrossRef]
33. Siepmann, J.; Siepmann, F. Mathematical modeling of drug delivery. *Int. J. Pharm.* **2008**, *364*, 328–343. [CrossRef]
34. Paolino, D.; Tudose, A.; Celia, C.; Di Marzio, L.; Cilurzo, F.; Mircioiu, C. Mathematical Models as Tools to Predict the Release Kinetic of Fluorescein from Lyotropic Colloidal Liquid Crystals. *Materials* **2019**, *12*, 693. [CrossRef]
35. Bácskay, I.; Nemes, D.; Fenyvesi, F.; Váradi, J.; Vasvári, G.; Fehér, P.; Vecsernyés, M.; Ujhelyi, Z. Role of Cytotoxicity Experiments in Pharmaceutical Development. In *Cytotoxicity*; Çelik, T.A., Ed.; InTech: London, UK, 2018; ISBN 978-1-78923-430-5.
36. Senthilraja, P.; Kathiresan, K. In vitro cytotoxicity MTT assay in Vero, HepG2 and MCF-7 cell lines study of Marine Yeast. *J. Appl. Pharm. Sci.* **2015**, *5*, 80–84. [CrossRef]
37. Garcia-Fernandez, J.; Turiel, D.; Bettmer, J.; Jakubowski, N.; Panne, U.; Rivas García, L.; Llopis, J.; Sánchez González, C.; Montes-Bayón, M. In vitro and in situ experiments to evaluate the biodistribution and cellular toxicity of ultrasmall iron oxide nanoparticles potentially used as oral iron supplements. *Nanotoxicology* **2020**, *20*, 1–16. [CrossRef] [PubMed]
38. Calabrese, E.J. Hormesis: Path and progression to significance. *Int. J. Mol. Sci.* **2018**, *19*, 2871. [CrossRef] [PubMed]
39. Kloner, R.A. Remote Ischemic Conditioning as a Form of Hormesis. In *The Science of Hormesis in Health and Longevity*; Academic Press: Amsterdam, The Netherlands, 2019.

3

Therapeutic Applications of Solid Dispersions for Drugs and New Molecules: In Vitro and In Vivo Activities

Verônica da Silva Oliveira [1], Amanda Silva de Almeida [2], Ingrid da Silva Albuquerque [2], Fernanda Ílary Costa Duarte [1], Bárbara Cristina Silva Holanda Queiroz [1], Attilio Converti [3] and Ádley Antonini Neves de Lima [1,2,*]

1 Postgraduate Program in Pharmaceutical Sciences, Health Sciences Center, Federal University of Rio Grande do Norte, Natal-RN 59012-570, Brazil; veronicasoliver47@gmail.com (V.d.S.O.); fernandailary@gmail.com (F.Í.C.D.); barbaracqueiroz@gmail.com (B.C.S.H.Q.)
2 Department of Pharmacy, Universidade Federal do Rio Grande do Norte, Natal-RN 59012-570, Brazil; amandasdealmeida@gmail.com (A.S.d.A.); ingridmariaalbuquerque@gmail.com (I.d.S.A.)
3 Department of Civil, Chemical and Environmental Engineering, Pole of Chemical Engineering, Genoa University, I-16145 Genoa, Italy; converti@unige.it
* Correspondence: adleylima13@gmail.com

Abstract: This review aims to provide an overview of studies that address the use, in therapeutic applications, of solid dispersions (SDs) with biological activities in vitro and/or in vivo mainly made up of polymeric matrices, as well as to evaluate the bioactive activity of their constituents. This bibliographic survey shows that the development of solid dispersions provides benefits in the physicochemical properties of bioactive compounds, which lead to an increase in their biological potential. However, despite the reports found on solid dispersions, there is still a need for biological assay-based studies, mainly in vivo, to assist in the investigation and to devise new applications. Therefore, studies based on such an approach are of great importance to enhance and extend the use of solid dispersions in the most diverse therapeutic applications.

Keywords: solid dispersions; drug delivery; biological applications

---

1. Introduction

Many drug candidates have low aqueous solubility, which can make their oral absorption inadequate. According to the literature, approximately 40% of marketed drugs are poorly soluble in water, as are, according to the Biopharmaceutical Classification System, about 40–90% of new drug candidates [1–4].

The slow dissolution rate and low solubility of some drugs lead to unpredictable bioavailability, non-reproducible clinical response or treatment inefficiency due to low therapeutic plasma levels; therefore, their use must be optimized using formulation strategies capable of improving their administration [5].

Several technological strategies have been developed and employed to circumvent this situation such as complexation with cyclodextrins, particle size reduction by micronization, crystal development, nanotechnology [5], salt formation and solid dispersions (SDs) [6,7]. However, some of these strategies have shown disadvantages including the development of active forms in vivo, high execution cost and considerable levels of toxicity. Some of these limits can be overcome by employing solid dispersions, a viable, well-established and widely-used strategy to increase the dissolution rate and solubility of poorly water-soluble drugs [4,6,7].

SDs can be defined as molecular mixtures of drugs that are not soluble in hydrophilic carriers, which exhibit a drug release profile driven by the polymer properties [8]. The so-called first-generation crystalline SDs, which use crystalline carriers such as urea and sugars including sucrose, dextrose and galactose, have the disadvantage of high thermodynamic stability that prevents a quick release of drugs [9]. In second-generation SDs drugs are dispersed in usually polymeric amorphous carriers [8], while the carriers used in third-generation SDs are surfactant or a mixture of amorphous polymers and surfactants [10].

The use of hydrophilic polymeric matrices to develop SDs for the release of commercial drugs or new drugs candidates has been shown to be a promising alternative able to improve their pharmacokinetic properties [7].

This review deals with SDs, mainly those belonging to the second-generation class that use polymers as carriers. It describes the main in vitro and in vivo activities (Figure 1) of SDs having different compositions and various preparation methods, intending to innovate and enhance the release of poorly water-soluble drugs, as well as improving the biological activities of the loaded bioactive compounds.

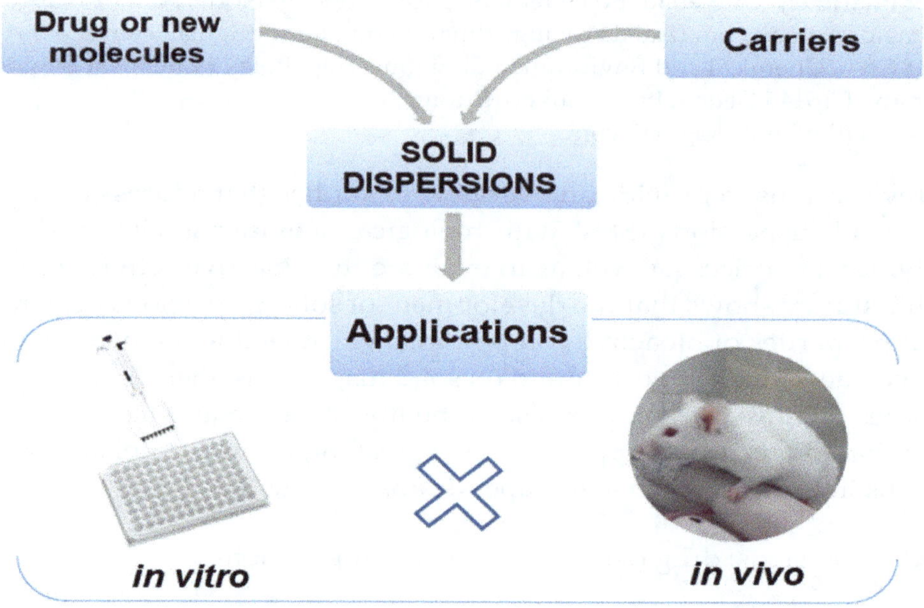

Figure 1. Representation of the application of solid dispersions in biological assays.

2. Methods

This literature search was conducted through the ScienceDirect and PubMed specialized databases, using different combinations of the following keywords: "amorphous solid dispersions" or "in vitro solid dispersions" or "in vivo solid dispersions". Studies performed in the last 10 years in vitro and in vivo were included, in which the biological action and use of solid dispersions to improve the biological performance of substances were investigated.

3. In Vitro Study of Solid Dispersions in Polymeric Matrices

This section deals with solid dispersions (SDs) prepared to improve the properties and release of poorly soluble drugs and drug candidates of natural or synthetic origin. The preparation and use of SDs have been reported in several in vitro studies, which have been numerically quantified and classified in Figure 2 based on the biological activities of their active compounds, while the main information on these studies is summarized in Table 1.

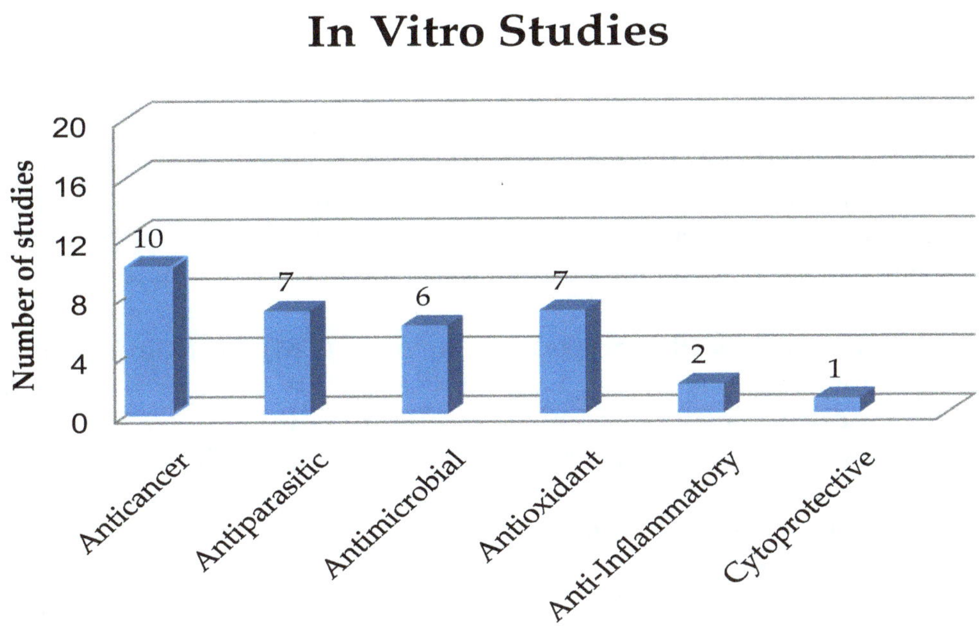

Figure 2. Quantification and classification of in vitro studies on solid dispersions published in the period from 2009 to 2020.

3.1. Anticancer Activities of Solid Dispersions

To improve the solubility and bioavailability of niclosamide, an anthelmintic with promising anticancer activity, a SD of its mixture with the octenylsuccinate hydroxypropyl phytoglycogen (OHPP) biopolymer was prepared by spray drying. In vitro tests by the 3-(4,5-dimethylthiazol-2-yl)-2,5-diphenyltetrazolium bromide (MTT) assay provided half inhibitory concentration (IC50 values) of SD against HeLa (cervical carcinoma), PC-3 (prostate cancer) and A549 (lung cancer) cells of 0.92, 0.68 and 1.18 μg/mL, while those of niclosamide alone were 1.82, 5.93 and 1.46 μg/mL, respectively. These results demonstrated that niclosamide-OHPP SD showed higher cytotoxicity than DMSO-assisted niclosamide solutions, mostly on PC-3 cell line, although OHPP, as the solubilizer, did not contribute to cytotoxicity. In addition, the analysis on OHPP alone is missed [11].

Although paclitaxel (PTX) is a natural compound with powerful antitumor activity against lung, breast and ovarian cancers, its low water solubility poses a challenge for the manufacture and administration of its formulations [12]. There are currently two commercial forms, Taxol® and Abraxane®, which; however, have a high rate of hypersensitivity and side effects.

Considering these drawbacks, Xie and Yao [13] incorporated PTX with OHPP in the form of solid dispersion (PTX-OHPP SD) by spray drying, whose in vitro antitumor activity was tested by the MTT method against HeLa, PC-3 and A549 cells and compared to that of PTX alone. Cytotoxicity was dose dependent and OHPP alone was not cytotoxic to cells, with an inhibition rate lower than 15% at the highest concentration (93.75 μg/mL). The IC50 values of DMSO-assisted PTX solutions against the above tumor cells were 0.02, 0.08 and 0.03 μg/mL, respectively, while PTX-OHPP SD demonstrated the greatest efficacy against cancer cells, with values of 0.008, 0.017 and 0.002 μg/mL, respectively.

In another study conducted by Choi et al. [14], the goal was to develop PTX-containing SDs. Several polymers were tested to increase the drug solubility and, subsequently, to select the best polymer to prepare SDs by the solvent evaporation method. Solubility and dissolution tests allowed to select a SD composed of D-α-tocopheryl polyethylene glycol 1000 succinate (TPGS), polyvinylpyrrolidone/vinyl acetate (PVP/VA), Aerosil®200 and PTX (SD4) and another containing PTX, TPGS and Aerosil®200 (SD9), whose antitumor activities were assessed, at drug concentrations of 0.1, 1, 5, 10 and 20 μg/mL, against breast cancer cells (BT-474, MCF-7 and SK-BR-3) and non-tumor cells by the MTT assay. Whereas both SDs were nontoxic to normal cells, at a dose of 20 μg/mL the cytotoxicity of SD4 and SD9 was 3.0- and 2.8-fold higher than that of PTX alone against BT-474 cells, 4.0- and 4.1-fold against

MCF-7 cells and 5.6- and 5.0-fold against SK-BR-3 cells. These results show greater cytotoxicity of SD4 and SD9 compared to PTX alone at the same concentration of 20 μg/mL.

In order to improve the solubility and absorption of chrysin, a potent inhibitor of breast cancer resistance protein, Lee et al. [15] have developed SD formulations with hydrophilic carriers, including polyoxyethylene (4) lauryl ether (Brij®L4), using the solvent evaporation method. To evaluate the cytotoxicity of chrysin alone and SD in the concentration range of 5–160 μM, the MTT assay against HT29 (human colorectal carcinoma) cells was used. SD displayed a 50% cytotoxic concentration (CC50) of 26.3 μM, while pure chrysin showed low activity even at the highest concentration tested.

Despite its wide variety of bioactive properties, Curcumin (CM), the main bioactive polyphenolic compound in the rhizomes of *Curcuma longa* L., has low solubility in water and; therefore, a limited bioavailability, which reduces its applicability. Based on these limitations, SDs of curcumin were prepared and tested for cytotoxic activity against tumor cells, namely MCF-7, NCIH460 (non-small cell lung carcinoma), HeLa and HepG2 (carcinoma hepatocellular) cells and non-tumor (PLP2) cells [16]. SDs showed cytotoxicity to all tumor cell lines tested, with concentrations causing 50% cell growth inhibition (GI50) of 207 ± 4, 208 ± 3, 259 ± 8 and 240 ± 7 μg/mL against NCIH460, HeLa, HepG2 and MCF-7, respectively, whereas no cytotoxicity was detected to non-tumor cells, with GI50 > 400 μg/mL. The improved CM activity was attributed to its association with copolymer surfactants such as Poloxamer 407 used to prepare SDs, which increased the dissolution rate and bioavailability of this hydrophobic drug.

In another study on CM, SD of zinc(II)-curcumin complex was developed using polyvinylpyrrolidone (PVP K30) [17]. Metal-curcumin complexes are known to exert anticancer activity, but they have low bioavailability and poor solubility in water, which hinder oral formulations. To evaluate the in vitro activity, the MTT assay was used in hepatocellular carcinoma cell lines (HepG2 and SK-HEP1), using different concentrations of SDs containing pure CM (CM-SD) or Zn(II)-curcumin complex (ZnCM-SD). Treatment with CM-SD significantly reduced the viability of HepG2 and SK-HEP1 cells within 48 h, with IC50 of 17.73 and 57.31 nM, respectively, while cells treated with ZnCM-SD exhibited after the same time IC50 of 38.52 and 10.41 nM, respectively, in a dose-dependent manner.

Xiong et al. [18] prepared telaprevir-containing SDs by the co-grinding technique using hydroxypropyl methylcellulose (HPMC), PVP K30 and polyethylene glycol (PEG) 6000 as polymers. SDs were characterized and their cytotoxicity was evaluated in vitro by the MTT method against HepG2 and normal liver cells (LO2) at drug concentrations between 0.1 and 30 μM. Although the viability of HepG2 cells gradually decreased as the drug concentration increased, it was almost the same in the presence of SDs and pure drug; furthermore, the efficacy of telaprevir was maintained even after the addition of polymers and no systems developed were toxic to normal liver cells.

Considering that uterine carcinoma still affects several women worldwide and is responsible for the highest rate of female malignancy [19], a study developed by Jiang et al. [20] sought to evaluate the anticancer activity of *Angelica gigas* Nakai, a medicinal herb containing coumarins, essential oils and polyacetylene that has several biological activities. However, its main components have a hydrophobic character that affects its application in formulations. To overcome this difficulty, these authors developed a SD of the above herb using the Soluplus® polymer and subjected it to shear by hot-melt extrusion. The MTT method was used for the in vitro antiproliferative activity and the developed systems were tested at concentrations of 50, 100 and 200 μg/mL against HeLa cells and normal cells (HEK 293 lineage). All formulations reduced cell viability, but the hot-melt extruded powder led to the lowest HeLa cells viability after 24 h. When these cells were treated for 48 h with the SD, there were a considerable reduction in viability and a higher cytotoxicity compared to the others, with only 17.37% of viability being observed at the concentration of 200 μg/mL. On the other hand, none of the systems tested showed cytotoxicity in 24 or 48 h to HEK 293 cells.

The research developed by Guo et al. [21] aimed at obtaining a SD using a methacrylic acid polymer Eudragit S-100 in association with berberine hydrochloride (HB), which is an isoquinoline-derived alkaloid found widely in the root and stem bark of numerous medicinal plants. Previous in vitro studies did in fact show that berberine decreases the viability of breast cancer cells, lung and hepatocellular carcinoma [22,23]. However, the development of formulations using HB is hampered by the low bioavailability of this compound that causes irritation to the gastrointestinal tract after oral administration. In this context, a SD made up of HB and Eudragit S-100 was prepared by the solvent evaporation method and its antitumor activity evaluated by the MTT method against SW480, HCT116 and Caco-2 colon cancer cells, over time periods of 12, 24 and 48 h, at HB equivalent concentrations from 0 to 100 μM [21]. The IC50 values obtained after 24 h treatment with HB alone against the above cells were 88.64, 67.83 and 89.78 μM, respectively, while those of SD were 52.96, 42.81 and 37.68 μM, respectively. After 48 h treatment, both showed better results, with pure HB IC50 values of 43.10, 34.13 and 32.82 μM and SD IC50 values of 28.15, 22.06 and 15.39 μM against the same cells in the above order. These results showed that cell viability of these strains suffered a dose and time dependent reduction in the presence either of HB or SD.

Kumar et al. [24] developed binary and ternary SDs incorporating IIIM-290, a synthetic chromone alkaloid acting as a potent inhibitor of CDK2/A and CDK9/T1 kinases, whose poor water solubility causes it to be used in high doses. SDs were prepared by solvent casting and evaporation method using PVP K30, PEG-Polypropylene glycol(PPG)-PEG or xanthan gum as polymers. In in vitro cytotoxicity tests against Ehrlich ascites carcinoma cells, IIIM-290 alone and the best drug-containing SD prepared with PVP K30 showed IC50 values of 1.10 ± 0.05 and 1.35 ± 0.02 μg/mL, respectively.

The results summarized in this section demonstrated that the use of SDs not only allowed to increase the solubility and dissolution of the bioactive substances, but also to improve their in vitro antitumor activity, as evidenced mainly by a IC50 reduction; therefore, it can be deduced that this improvement derives from the increase in the solubility of active compounds when present in the dispersed systems. Furthermore, it is important to note that SDs were obtained for a large number of active compounds and that toxicity tests were performed on different cell types, which demonstrates their potential as systems for the release of lipophilic compounds to fight a variety of cancers.

3.2. Antiparasitic Activity of Solid Dispersions

3.2.1. Antichagasic Activity of Solid Dispersions

Chagas disease is an infection that affects around eight million people around the world, mainly in Latin America, which is treated with nifurtimox and benznidazole (BNZ). Although the latter is preferable because of fewer adverse effects than the former, it has low solubility, which limits its effectiveness in treating the disease [25].

One of the first studies developed to obtain BNZ-containing SDs was conducted by Lima et al. [26] with the aim of improving the solubility of this drug. In this work, the use of PEG 6000 and PVP K30 as hydrophilic polymer carriers led to an increase in the solubility of BNZ in aqueous medium. The interaction of BNZ with polymers was evaluated by physicochemical characterization and in vitro dissolution tests. The dissolution profile of all SDs was significantly better than that of BNZ alone, thus demonstrating the solubilizing effect of PEG and PVP. Another work published by the same group [27] aimed to develop SDs with HPMC and β-cyclodextrin inclusion complexes to increase the drug solubility and dissolution.

In a study by Fonseca-Berzal et al. [28], BNZ-containing SDs were prepared by the freeze-drying technique using sodium deoxycholate (NaDC) as surfactant and low-substituted hydroxypropyl cellulose (HPC) as polymer, whose trypanocidal activity was tested in vitro against axenic cultures of *Trypanosoma cruzi*. The results showed greater activity of the 1:3 BNZ:NaDC solid dispersion, with IC50 values of 33.92 ± 6.41 μM for epimastigote and 0.40 ± 0.05 μM for amastigote, compared to pure BNZ (IC50 of 52.95 ± 2.22 and 1.8 ± 0.66 μM, respectively).

To potentiate the effect of the same drug, Simonazzi et al. [25] prepared a BNZ-containing SD using Poloxamer 407 (P407) as polymer, whose in vitro activity was tested by the MTT method against

T. cruzi (Tulahuén lineage) in the epimastigote phase at a concentration of 4 × 107 cells/mL. SD showed higher antiparasitic activity (IC50 of 21.68 ± 1.6 μM) than BNZ alone (32.47 ± 4.9 μM), likely because P407 significantly improved BNZ solubility and consequently increased the rate of its release compared to the other preparations. According to the authors, this SD could be of great help in the treatment of Chagas disease, as it would allow for more effective treatment with fewer adverse effects.

In a study carried out by Eloy et al. [29], a SD has been developed with ursolic acid, a compound that helps to prevent mass loss and muscle atrophy, inhibits fat accumulation and possesses trypanocidal activity, acting as an important ally in treatment of Chagas disease. SD was prepared by the solvent method using ursolic acid, polyoxylglyceride (Gelucire 50/13) as carrier and silica dioxide as drying agent. In in vitro tests against the trypomastigote form obtained through infection of Swiss albino mice by *T. cruzi* (strain Y), SD showed an IC50 value (219.2 μM) 44.7% lower than that of the physical mixture. These data suggest that the surfactant interacted intermolecularly with ursolic acid in the SD, enhancing its trypanocidal activity.

3.2.2. Antischistosomal Activity of Solid Dispersions

Praziquantel (PZQ) is a drug widely used in the treatment of parasitic diseases, especially schistosomiasis, popularly known as "water belly" in Brazil, which is caused by contact of the parasite *Schistosoma mansoni* with the skin of the individual. Despite being the only drug in the treatment of flattened worms, PZQ has several limitations due to its low water solubility, which implies the need to administer it in high doses to patients [30,31].

Solid dispersions were developed by Perissutti et al. [30] to increase the solubility and bioavailability of this drug and then reduce its doses. SDs with PZQ were prepared using different carriers; however, the best results were obtained using PVP (Kollidon K30), PVP/VA, Kollidon-CL-M and sodium starch glycolate as polymers. Adult schistosomes were removed from female mice infected by the infectious form of *S. mansoni* (cercaria) and incubated. A ratio of 1:1 (*w/w*) Kollidon-CL-M:PZQ showed better performance in terms of solubility (642.54 mg/mL) and IC50 value (0.102 μg/mL) than pure PZQ (solubility of 140.30 mg/mL and IC50 of 0.165 μg/mL). According to the authors, PZQ-loaded SDs with Kollidon-CL-M could be a valid candidate for the treatment of schistosomiasis.

In another study performed by Albertini et al. [31] with the aim to improve the antiparasitic activity of PZQ, a SD with PVP K30 was prepared by the mechanochemical activation process and spray congealing technique. For in vitro testing of SDs, newly transformed schistosomula, obtained by mechanical transformation from *S. mansoni* and adult forms of the parasite were used. Adult *S. mansoni* individuals were removed from the hepatic portal and mesenteric veins of infected mice. The IC50 values of the physical mixture, pure PZQ and SD against schistosomula were 3.16, 2.58 and 2.4 μg/mL, respectively, while those of physical mixture and SD against adult parasites were 0.48 and <0.23 μg/mL. These results suggest that the SD contributed to the increase in PZQ solubility thanks to a 70% reduction of its crystallinity, thus reducing its dosage to a level suitable even for pediatric use.

3.2.3. Antimalarial Activity of Solid Dispersions

Malaria is an ancient disease dating back to the fifth century BC, but today it is one of the main public health problems in the world. It is estimated to affect around 200 million people worldwide, particularly individuals living in subtropical and tropical areas, causing 500,000 deaths each year [32]. It is caused by parasites belonging to the genus *Plasmodium*, of which the most aggressive species is *P. falciparum* that multiplies in the bloodstream, whereas *P. vivax* is milder affecting less than 1% of red blood cells and hardly leads individuals to death [33].

Artemether is a drug used in combination with lumefantrine to treat malaria. In the study proposed by Fule et al. [34], SDs were developed to improve the dissolution rate of this drug, as well as to increase its solubility in water. Solid dispersions were prepared by hot-melt extrusion using a combination of several polymers, such as Soluplus, PEG 400, Lutrol F127 and Lutrol F68 and sodium lauryl sulphate as surfactant. In in vitro studies, 15 artemether dispersions formulations were tested for antimalarial activity against the protozoan *P. falciparum* 3D7 (chloroquine-sensitive cell line) in schizont form and against ITG cells (chloroquine-resistant cell line). On average, the IC50 values of SDs, ranging from 0.054 to 0.081 ng/mL, were 39 times less than that of pure artemether and about 70 times less than that of chloroquine, the standard antimalarial drug. Among the formulations, the one formed by 1.0:3.8:0.2 drug, Soluplus and PEG 400, was the most promising with an IC50 value of 0.054 ng/mL.

Lumefantrine is a medicine used in association with artemether in a 6:1 ratio to treat malaria caused by *P. vivax* strains, either sensitive or resistant to chloroquine, as well as cerebral malaria caused by *P. falciparum*. However, it has low oral bioavailability due to its low aqueous solubility, which also affects its dissolution rate. To circumvent this problem and enhance its therapeutic potential, Fule et al. [35] prepared solid dispersions of lumefantrine by hot-melt extrusion using Soluplus, Kollidon VA64 and Plasdone S630 as polymers, which were tested in vitro for their antiparasitic activity against *P. falciparum* 3D7 and ITG cells. SDs showed IC50 values of 0.084–0.213 ng/mL, while pure lumefantrine and chloroquine showed values of 18.2 and 3.8 ng/mL, respectively, which demonstrates the remarkable increase in the antiparasitic activity of this drug induced by the SDs environment.

From the studies cited in this section aimed at antiparasitic activity, it can be concluded that SDs are a valid alternative in the treatment of some parasitic diseases such as Chagas disease, schistosomiasis and malaria. Solid dispersions containing drugs already used for these diseases have in fact shown an increase in their solubility and dissolution rate, as well as a consequent improvement in the activity against parasites, showing IC50 values lower than those of pure drugs. It should also be remembered that a dose reduction can reduce the incidence of toxicity during pharmacotherapy.

3.3. Antimicrobial Activity of Solid Dispersions

In a study conducted by Crucitti et al. [36], the antimicrobial activity of SDs of abietic acid and chitosan prepared in different drug:polymer proportions was checked against *Staphylococcus epidermidis*. Minimum inhibitory concentrations (MICs) of abietic acid, chitosan, 1:1 drug:chitosan mixture and SD containing this mixture were 0.8, 0.5, 1.0 and 0.25 mg/mL, respectively. According to the authors, not only the amorphous state of the drug in SD but also the synergistic effect between the two components may have improved the antimicrobial activity of the bioactive compound.

The low solubility of griseofulvin, which is one of the antimicrobials generally used in the treatment of dermatophytosis caused by the fungus *Trichophyton rubrum*, makes oral administration of its formulation particularly difficult, requiring high doses to reach therapeutic levels. To get around this problem, Al-Obaidi et al. [37] have successfully increased the solubility of this drug developing forms of solvates, also known as pseudopolymorphs, consisting of drug crystals with solvents, stabilized within polymeric matrices. To obtain solid dispersions, different solvated (chloroform) and unsolvated (methanol and acetone) materials were used, including microcrystalline cellulose, PVP K30 and hydroxypropyl methylcellulose acetate succinate (HPMCAS). Griseofulvin solubility in the HPMCAS-based SD (200 μg/mL) was almost seven-fold that of the pure drug. The antifungal potential of griseofulvin and this SD was tested in vitro against *T. rubrum* NCPF 935. Biofilm production and fungal proteolytic activity were significantly reduced in the presence of SDs incorporating either solvated or unsolvated materials when compared to the control. These results demonstrated the role of polymeric dispersion in increasing the antifungal activity of this drug.

Gatifloxacin is an antibiotic used to treat various eye infections such as conjunctivitis, keratitis and keratoconjunctivitis caused by bacteria [38]. The low solubility of this drug promoted the preparation of polymeric micelles incorporating it into Pluronic F127 as polymer by the solvent diffusion method [39]. Among the dispersions obtained, the one prepared at a 0.25:2.52 (*w/w*) drug:polymer ratio showed the best results in terms of particle size, stability and solubility. In the agar diffusion test conducted using *Staphylococcus aureus* as the target microorganism, this dispersion yielded an inhibition zone diameter (10.33 ± 0.57 mm) 18.3% larger than that produced by commercial gatifloxacin.

Among the numerous attempts to exploit the biological potential of CM, the results of studies aimed at the preparation of CM-containing SDs with antibacterial and pesticidal activity are summarized here. Hernandez-Patlan et al. [40] prepared CM-SDs using boric acid and PVP by the solvent evaporation method. In in vitro tests, 1% boric acid, 1% SD containing 10:90 (*w/w*) CM:PVP and a 50:50 (*w/w*) mixture of them were tested against *Salmonella enteritidis* in media simulating culture, intestine and proventriculus. Boric acid led to $\log_{10}$ CFU/mL values of 7.78 ± 00 in culture, 3.81 ± 0.05 in proventriculus and even 0.00 ± 0.00 in intestine, while 1% CM:PVP of 7.73 ± 00, 3.91 ± 0.08 and 5.00 ± 0.55 and their mixture of 7.65 ± 00, 3.71 ± 0.05 and 3.94 ± 0.23, respectively. In summary, the promising results shown by the SD containing CM and PVP were even improved in the presence of boric acid, thanks to its ability to penetrate the cell membrane of the target microorganism.

Solid dispersions were also prepared to enhance the efficacy of CM in antimicrobial photodynamic therapy. Bearing in mind that CM as a photosensitizer has low solubility and phototoxicity limited to Gram-negative bacteria, Hegge et al. [41] prepared SDs using concentrated solutions of hydroxypropyl-β-cyclodextrin/CM by solvent evaporation and then HPMC by lyophilization. The antibacterial activity was tested against *Escherichia coli* (ATCC 25922) (1 × 106 CFU/mL) at concentrations of 10 and 25 µM of CM in SDs exposed to irradiation. The dispersion that showed the best results in dissolution tests was then used in in vitro tests. Since it displayed phototoxicity at both concentrations (10 and 25 µM) at a radiation dose of 5 J/cm^2, one can infer that the dispersion increased the bactericidal power of CM against *E. coli*, so it could play an important role in photodynamic therapy.

Another study was conducted by Alves et al. [42] with the aim of developing a formulation with antimicrobial activity using CM and silver nanoparticles, as both have activity against bacteria, fungi and viruses. For this purpose, CM-containing SDs were prepared by co-precipitation using CM and P407 at 1:1, 1:2 and 2:1 (*w/w*) ratios and then silver nanoparticles were added. Nanoparticles were synthesized and stabilized using polyvinyl alcohol and PVP as polymers and sodium citrate. The antibacterial activity was determined in in vitro tests and expressed as MIC against *E. coli* ATCC 25922, *Pseudomonas aeruginosa* ATCC 9721 and *S. aureus* ATCC 10390. The SD composed of P407/CM/nanoparticles/PVP showed better MIC values against *P. aeruginosa* (50 µg/mL) and *E. coli* (25 µg/mL) compared to those reported in the literature (175 and 163 µg/mL, respectively) [43]. All formulations were less effective against *S. aureus* (Gram-positive) and the best performance was observed for the P407/CM/nanoparticles/citrate system. The different SD activity against Gram-positive and Gram-negative bacteria was probably due to the thinner cell wall of the latter, which may have facilitated SD internalization and cell wall disruption.

In this context, DSs with drugs and antimicrobials showed good results including increased solubility, low MIC values and reduction of bacterial colonies. Although there are currently many antimicrobial drug options on the market, they are still being used indiscriminately leading to the emergence of resistant bacteria as well as other adverse effects. Therefore, SDs not only can be an option to improve their solubility, but also require lower dosages, making antimicrobial treatment safer and more effective.

3.4. *Antioxidant Activity of Solid Dispersions*

Quercetin is a flavonoid that has, among other activities, the ability to capture free radicals. In the study by Costa et al. [44], a solid dispersion of quercetin with PVP K25 was developed with the aim of increasing its solubility and antioxidant activity determined by the 2,2-diphenyl-1-picryl-hydrazyl-hydrate (DPPH) radical assay and expressed as IC50. IC50 values of 0.61 ± 0.03 and 1.00 ± 0.02 µg/mL were obtained for SD dissolved in water and for quercetin dissolved in methanol, respectively, which demonstrates that SD enhanced quercetin antioxidant activity.

The SDs prepared by Crucitti et al. [36] using 1:1 abietic acid:chitosan already discussed in the previous section were also tested for their antioxidant activity with the same method. As expected, the antioxidant activity of chitosan (IC50 of approximately 11 mg/mL) was much lower than that of abietic acid (IC50 of 1.65 mg/mL), but the one of the 1:1 AB/chitosan SD was even stronger (IC50 of

0.61 mg/mL). There are at least two factors that can explain the particularly high antioxidant activity of SDs. First, the amorphous state may have influenced the solubility and availability of the drug compared to its crystalline nature. Secondly, the natural tendency of abietic acid to react with oxygen forming peroxides may have been reduced by its stabilization due to interaction with chitosan.

The previously mentioned CM-SD prepared by Sá et al. [16] using P407 was investigated for possible effect on the activities of acetylcholinesterase (AChE), butyrylcholinesterase (BChE), glutathione S-transferase (GST) and two isoforms (A and B) of monoamine oxidase (MAO). The SD was able to inhibit the activities of AChE, BChE and GST in aqueous medium, which suggests that the hydrophobic nature of CM was overcome by the SD amorphous state. In addition, it inhibited both MAO isoforms at a concentration of 100 μM, while pure CM had no effect at the same concentration, suggesting that CM interaction with P407 in SD was responsible for enzyme inhibition. It is known that the reaction catalyzed by MAO produces hydrogen peroxide, a source of hydroxyl radicals, so MAO inhibitors, as well as this SD, may be usefully exploited to treat pathologies associated with oxidative stress.

Coenzyme Q10 has two main functions, namely the transport of mitochondrial electrons to form phosphate for muscle contraction and the antioxidant activity of its reduced form (ubiquinol). However, its bioavailability is low and variable because of its poor solubility and high molecular weight. A study performed by Ge et al. [45] aimed to investigate the therapeutic potential of water-soluble nanoscale Coenzyme Q10-SDs with mannitol prepared by high-pressure homogenization. To assess the antioxidant activity, intracellular reactive oxygen species (ROS) were detected using myocardial cells divided into three groups treated with SDs with different particle sizes, namely 408, 300 and 146 nm and a control. Myocardial cells were subjected to hypoxia/reoxygenation to detect the free-radical scavenging ability of substances. In vitro tests showed that the ROS level in the control group increased by 96%, while those in the three other groups were reduced by 48.3–87.3%, which proved the strong antioxidant activity of SDs.

To increase water solubility of usnic acid, a secondary metabolite of lichen with antioxidant activity, Fitriani et al. [46] developed SDs with PVP K30 by spray-drying and freeze-drying and determined their antioxidant activity by the DPPH assay. Since the drug and the developed systems showed IC50 values in the range 50–100 ppm, they can be classified as moderate antioxidants, with the lowest value (63.87 μg/mL) detected for the SD prepared by freeze-drying in the proportion 1:2 (usnic acid:polymer).

Luteolin is a compound belonging to the class of biflavonoids, which is found in several plants and has a rich arsenal of therapeutic activities; however, its low solubility and instability in water pose a challenge for its use in pharmaceutical formulations. Therefore, a study promoted the production of luteolin-containing SDs by solvent evaporation, microwave irradiation or fusion using PEG 4000 as polymer [47]. After dissolving the drug (control) and the three different SDs in dimethyl sulfoxide up to a concentration of 5 mg/mL, their antioxidant activity was assessed by the DPPH assay. The antioxidant activity of the drug was 61.12 ± 4.11% and those of the above SDs 61.12 ± 4.11, 94.14 ± 6.11, 88.55 ± 3.98 and 76.23 ± 5.12%, respectively, suggesting that this property increased due to improved solubilization of luteolin in the presence of PEG 4000 as carrier.

In summary, the antioxidant activity of SDs was quantified by different methods including the activities of some enzymes, but with a certain prevalence of the DPPH assay. In the above studies aimed at therapeutic purposes, the best results have always been obtained with SDs, probably thanks to the increase in the solubility of drugs in the administration systems.

3.5. Anti-Inflammatory Activity of Solid Dispersions

α,β-Amyrin (ABAM) is a natural blend of pentacyclic triterpenes that has shown numerous pharmacological properties, including the anti-inflammatory activity [7]. To increase this activity, ABAM-SDs, prepared using PVP K30, PEG 6000 and HPMC by physical mixture, kneading and rotary evaporation, were submitted to the in vitro anti-inflammatory test based on nitric oxide (NO) production by lipopolysaccharide (LPS)-stimulated macrophages J774. The results showed that ABAM inhibited NO production at concentration of 20 μg/mL, although the effect of SDs was stronger than those of the control and the drug alone. Specifically, the ABAM-PVP SD prepared by the kneading method had the greatest effect with 62.49% inhibition, while ABAM showed a value of 44.55%. According to the authors, SDs prepared with hydrophilic polymers were effective in increasing the solubility of ABAM and allowed to enhance its anti-inflammatory activity.

In the cited study of Sá et al. [16], CM-SD was tested for anti-inflammatory activity via inhibition of NO production by LPS-stimulated murine macrophages (RAW 264.7). The SD was able to improve the affinity of water for CM which, in turn, exerted cytotoxic effects in the aqueous medium, with an IC50 value > 400 μg/mL. This result suggests possible SD administration in vivo, avoiding the use of toxic solvents to increase its clinical efficacy.

These studies as a whole demonstrated that the use of SDs containing low water-soluble active ingredients, both natural and synthetic, prepared with different methods, is an effective means to increase their anti-inflammatory activity, which can be evaluated in vitro by quantifying the inhibition of NO production by LPS-stimulated macrophages.

3.6. Cytoprotective Activity on Liver Cells

SDs of CM prepared using HPMC as the polymer have been reported by Shin et al. [48], who studied their possible hepatoprotective action in HepG2 cells treated with tert-butyl hydroperoxide (t-BHP) as a hepatotoxic agent. The survival rate of cells, which in the presence of t-BHP was about 40%, significantly increased after treatment with DSs-CM at concentrations of 10, 20 and 40 μg/mL compared to the treatment with CM alone at equivalent concentrations (2, 4 and 8 μg/mL, respectively). Additionally, the extracellular activity of lactate dehydrogenase, an enzyme released by HepG2 cells under the stress conditions induced by t-BHP, was reduced by treatment with CM-containing SDs more than by that with CM alone, indicating a stronger cytoprotective activity. Treatment with SDs containing 10 and 20 μg/mL CM was also able to inhibit, more effectively than CM alone, the activation of caspase-7, -8 and poly (ADP-ribose) polymerase, responsible for t-BHP-induced apoptosis in HepG2 cells.

In summary, given the hepatoprotective activity of CM-containing SDs, their use can be considered a valid alternative to other therapies, considering that the administration of drugs for long periods and in large doses can cause liver damage, especially in elderly patients. In this sense, further in vitro and in vivo studies on DSs of CM and other bioactive compounds are needed, given the hepatoprotective potential associated with this drug delivery system.

Table 1. In vitro studies on solid dispersions.

Carrier Type	Substance	Cell Type	Activity	Improved Characteristics	Reference
OHPP	Niclosamide	PC-3, HeLa, A549	Anticancer	SDs showed higher cytotoxicity to target cells (lower IC50) than the niclosamide solution.	[11]
OHPP	Paclitaxel	PC-3, HeLa, A549	Anticancer	SDs showed significantly higher cytotoxicity to target cells (lower IC50) than the paclitaxel solution.	[13]
PVP/VA TPGS	Paclitaxel	BT-474, MCF-7, SK-BR-3	Anticancer	SDs showed higher cytotoxicity against cancer cells compared to the pure drug.	[14]
Brij®L4	Chrysin	HT29	Anticancer	The higher solubility of chrysin in SDs compared to water solution increased cytotoxicity.	[15]
Poloxamer 407	Curcumin (CM)	NCIH460, HeLa, HepG2, MCF-7 and PLP2	Anticancer	SDs showed cytotoxicity against all tumor cell lines tested, but no toxic effects on non-tumor cells.	[16]
		AChE, BChE, GST, MAO A-B	Enzyme inhibitory /Antioxidant	SD was able to inhibit the activities of AChE, BChE and GST in aqueous medium.	
		LPS-stimulated murine macrophages (RAW 264.7)	Anti-inflammatory	IC50 (inhibitory concentration of 50% NO production by macrophages) > 400 μg/mL.	
PVP K30	Zn(II)-curcumin complex	HepG2, SK-HEP1	Anticancer	SD of Zn(II)-curcumin complex had a potent anticancer effect.	[17]
HPMC, PVP K30, PEG 6000	Telaprevir	HepG2	Anticancer	The antitumor activity was dose dependent and even with the addition of the polymer the drug maintained its efficacy.	[18]
Soluplus®	Angelica gigas Nakai	HeLa, HEK 293	Anticancer	SD at the concentration of 200 μg/mL showed a significant decrease (to only 17.37%) in cell viability. There was no toxicity to normal cells.	[20]
Eudragit S-100	Berberine hydrochloride (HB)	SW480, HCT116, Caco-2	Anticancer	The release of HB from SDs was effective and cell viability was reduced in a dose and time dependent manner.	[21]
PVP K30	IIIM-290	Ehrlich ascites carcinoma cells	Cytotoxic	Despite the reduced amount of IIIM-290 in SD, the IC50 value of SD was lower than that of IIIM-290 alone.	[24]
Poloxamer 407	Benznidazole	Epimastigotes of *Trypanosoma cruzi*	Antichagasic	SDs enhanced drug solubility, release kinetics and parasitic activity	[25]
Low-substituted HPC	Benznidazole	Epimastigotes and intracellular amastigotes of *T. cruzi* (CL-B5)	Antichagasic	SDs had higher antiparasitic activity against amastigotes than epimastigotes.	[28]
Gelucire 50/13	Ursolic acid	Trypomastigotes of *T. cruzi* Y	Antichagasic	Increased antiparasitic activity.	[29]

Table 1. *Cont.*

Carrier Type	Substance	Cell Type	Activity	Improved Characteristics	Reference
PVP K30,PVP/VA, Kollidon-CL-M, sodium starch glycolate	Praziquantel	Adult Schistosomes of *Schistosoma mansoni*	Antischistosomal	Increased solubility, better bioavailability and stronger antiparasitic activity.	[30]
PVP K30	Praziquantel	Newly transformed schistosomula of *S. mansoni* and adults	Antischistosomal	Increased solubility, reduced dosage especially for children and increased antiparasitic activity.	[31]
Soluplus, PEG 400, Lutrol F127 and Lutrol F68	Artemether	Schizonts of *Plasmodium falciparum* 3D7	Antimalarial	Increased dissolution rate, amorphous form, increased solubility and, mainly, increased antimalarial activity.	[34]
Soluplus, Kollidon VA64, Plasdone S630	Lumefantrine	ITG cells	Antimalarial	Increased antiparasitic activity.	[35]
Chitosan	Abietic acid	*Staphylococcus epidermidis*	Antimicrobial	SD exhibited better MIC values against *S. epidermidis* than chitosan and abietic acid alone.	[36]
		DPPH radical scavenging	Antioxidant	SD had higher antioxidant power (IC50 of 0.61 mg/mL) than abietic acid alone (IC50 of 11 mg/mL).	
PVP K30 and HPMCAS	Griseofulvin	Dermatophytes of *Trichophyton rubrum* NCPF 935	Antimicrobial	SDs significantly reduced biofilm formation when compared to the control.	[37]
Pluronic F127	Gatifloxacin	*Staphylococcus aureus*	Antimicrobial	The gatifloxacin/Pluronic F127 system exhibited antimicrobial efficacy when compared to commercialized eye drops.	[39]
PVP K30	Curcumin	*Salmonella enteritidis*	Antimicrobial	SD had a strong antimicrobial effect on *S. enteritidis*, while CM alone did not show antimicrobial activity in vitro.	[40]
HPMC	Curcumin	*Escherichia coli*	Antimicrobial	SD used to prepare phototoxic supersaturated solutions showed significant bactericidal activity against *E. coli*.	[41]
Polaxamer 407	Curcumin	*E. coli*, *Pseudomonas aeruginosa* and *S. aureus*	Antimicrobial	The association between SD and silver nanoparticles increased CM antimicrobial and antioxidant activities.	[42]
		DPPH radical scavenging	Antioxidant		
PVP K25	Quercetin	DPPH radical scavenging	Antioxidant	Increased quercetin antioxidant activity in SD ($0.61 \pm 0.03 \leq IC50 \leq 1.00 \pm 0.02$ μg/mL).	[44]
Mannitol	Coenzyme Q10	Intracellular ROS level	Antioxidant	The SD with the smallest particle size showed the greatest absorption of UVB radiation as well as the highest antioxidant activity in vitro.	[45]

Table 1. *Cont.*

Carrier Type	Substance	Cell Type	Activity	Improved Characteristics	Reference
PVP K30	Usnic acid	DPPH radical scavenging	Antioxidant	Increased usnic acid solubility and antioxidant activity.	[46]
PEG 4000	Luteolin	DPPH	Antioxidant	Polymers increased luteolin solubility and antioxidant activity.	[47]
PVP K30, PEG 6000 and HPMC	α,β-Amyrin	LPS-stimulated macrophages J774	Anti-inflammatory	SDs enhanced the anti-inflammatory activity of α,β-amyrin.	[7]
HPMC	Curcumin	HepG2	Cytoprotective	SDs showed better cytoprotective activity than pure CM and inhibited cell death induced by *t*-BHP.	[48]

OHPP, Octenylsuccinate hydroxypropyl phytoglycogen; IC50, Half inhibitory concentration; PVP/VA, Polyvinylpyrrolidone/vinyl acetate; TPGS, D-α-toco-pheryl polyethylene glycol-1000-succinate; PVP, Polyvinylpyrrolidone; SD, Solid dispersion; AChE: Acetylcholinesterase; BChE, Butyrylcholinesterase; CM, Curcumin; GST, Glutathione S-transferase; MAO, Monoamine oxidase; LPS, Lipopolysaccharide; NO, Nitric oxide; PEG, Polyethylene glycol; HPMC, Hydroxypropyl methylcellulose; ITG (chloroquine-resistant cell line); DPPH, 2,2-diphenyl-1-picryl-hydrazyl-hydrate; HPMCAS, Hydroxypropyl methylcellulose acetate succinate; MIC, Minimum inhibitory concentration; ROS, Reactive oxygen species; t-BHP, *tert*-Butylhydroperoxide.

4. In Vivo Studies on Solid Dispersions in Polymeric Matrices

As already mentioned, solid dispersions (SDs) have been used as a strategy in pharmaceutical technology to circumvent some limitations presented by drugs and new bioactive compounds such as low solubility and bioavailability. In this sense, this section addresses in vivo studies on SDs with different biological activities, as shown in Figure 3 and quantitatively expressed in Figure 4. The main information about these studies is summarized in Table 2.

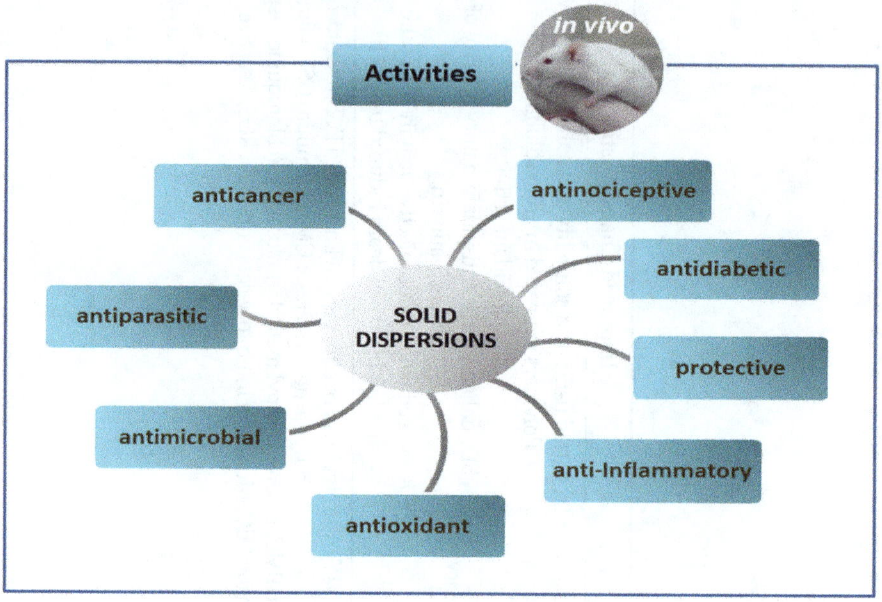

Figure 3. In vivo activities of solid dispersions.

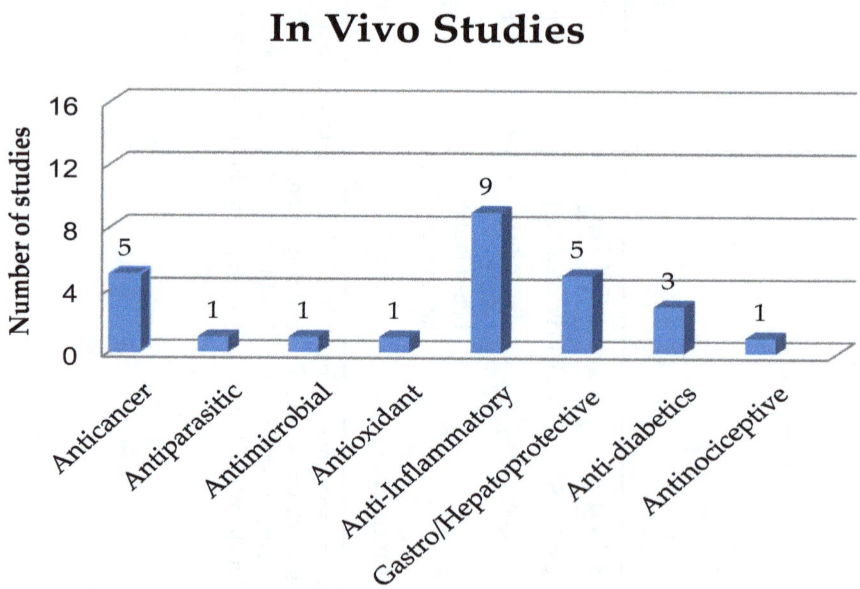

Figure 4. Quantification and classification of in vivo studies on solid dispersions published in the period from 2009 to 2020.

4.1. Anticancer Activity of Solid Dispersions

As previously mentioned, the low solubility of many active compounds complicates oral formulations requiring high doses. Therefore, SDs have been prepared to increase their solubility and, consequently, their therapeutic effects. Most SDs that were successful in in vitro experiments described previously in Section 3 were also assessed in vivo assays, whose results are summarized and critically discussed here together with those of other studies.

The IIIM-290-containing SDs prepared by Kumar et al. [24] with the highest solubility were assessed for in vivo anticancer activity on mice with Ehrlich ascites carcinoma. The animals were divided into four groups to receive treatment and two controls. Group I received only IIIM-290 (50 mg/kg), while groups II, III and IV received SD consisting of PVP K30 and drug at doses of 25, 50 and 75 mg/kg, respectively. While the group that received the drug alone showed a tumor inhibition rate of only 24.75%, the SD reduced tumor growth by 31–43% and ensured better performance even at a half dosage of drug.

To improve the solubility and permeability of 9-nitrocamptothecin, a topoisomerase I inhibitor and potent chemotherapy drug to treat pancreatic cancer, a SD was developed using Soluplus by lyophilization and its antitumor activity was in vivo assessed in mice with sarcoma 180 [49]. SD showed higher tumor growth inhibitory rate (approximately 80%) than the drug alone due to improved oral bioavailability.

(−)-Oleocanthal, a phenolic compound derived from olive oil with anti-inflammatory, antitumor and anti-Alzheimer activities, exerts an irritating action in the oropharyngeal region that limits its use in oral formulations. To improve its taste and dissolution, Qusa et al. [50] developed by the hot-melting method a SD containing 1:7 oleocanthal:xylitol, whose antitumor activity was tested in vivo against human triple-negative breast cancer cells (MDA-MB-231) xenografted in mice. SD administration resulted in a two-day delay and 49% tumor growth rate when compared with the group treated only with placebo. Additionally, in the recurrence test the SD-treated group showed recurrence-free survival in two days, with only two of the five animals suffering from recurrent but smaller tumors, while in the control group a 100% tumor reappearance rate was observed.

Stimulated by the promising results obtained in vitro, Wu et al. [17] also tested in vivo the antitumor effect of Zn(II)-curcumin (CM) SDs with PVP K30. Hepatic xenografts of H22 and HepG2 cells were performed in male BALB/c mice and female B-NDG mice, respectively. BALB/c mice were divided into three groups, in which each received a dose of PVP K30 (700 mg/kg), or CM-SD or Zn-CM-SD (equivalent doses of 100 mg/kg CM and ZnCM), while B-NDG mice were treated with the same formulations except CM-SD at the same doses. Using H22 cells, while the untreated group had tumors weighing over 3 g and volume of 2000 mm^3, tumors in animals treated with Zn-CM-SD weighed less than 2 g and had a volume of less than 1000 mm^3. In addition, greater extension of necrotic tissue but no reduction in animal body weight was reported.

Selaginella doederleinii Hieron is a widely distributed medicinal herb in southern China that has traditionally been used as a folk medicine for cancer, especially lung cancer. However, its total biflavonoid extract (TBESD) has low water solubility, gastrointestinal permeability and oral absorption that limit its use in therapeutic formulations [51,52].

To overcome these difficulties, Chen et al. [53] prepared a solid dispersion of TBESD with the polymer PVP K30 (TBESD-SD) by the solvent evaporation method. To assess the in vivo antitumor effect, mice with xenograft of A549 cells derived from human alveolar basal epithelial cell adenocarcinoma were treated with doses of 200 mg/kg TBSED and TBESD-SD and 2 mg/kg doxorubicin. Tumor growth inhibition rates in the TBESD, TBESD-SD and pure drug groups were 29.48, 46 and 58.44%, respectively and the respective reduction rates of tumor angiogenesis 24.30, 52.20 and 59.91%. However, the drug group, unlike the other two, showed significant body weight loss. Therefore, the dispersion developed in this study proved to be a promising formulation for the treatment of tumors.

In summary, it can be concluded, despite the limited number of studies concerning the in vivo antitumor activity, that the use of SDs allowed a higher rate of tumor inhibition than the isolated compounds, also corroborating the results obtained in vitro in other studies.

4.2. Antiparasitic Activity of Solid Dispersions

The Benznidazole (BNZ)-containing SDs developed by Fonseca-Berzal et al. [28] using sodium deoxycholate (NaDC) as surfactant and low-substituted hydroxypropyl cellulose (HPC) as polymer were also tested in vivo for trypanocidal activity. For this purpose, parasites of *Trypanosoma cruzi* (strain Y) isolated from human individuals in the acute phase of the disease were used in their trypomastigote form to infect mice, which were administered at a 25 mg/kg/day oral dosage. The percentage reductions in the area under the parasitic curve were 91.93, 96.65 and 95.27% administering SD with 1:3 BNZ:NaDC, SD with 1:3 BNZ-HPC and BNZ alone, with the best anti-interference performance obtained for the second formulation, while the survival rate of in the control group was only 44.44%. None of the mice treated with SDs or BNZ alone died, which indicates no toxic effects at the established dosage. Although these SDs have shown great potential in in vivo tests, further studies are needed because BNZ has a reduced pharmacological activity in the chronic phase of Chagas disease and has several side effects.

4.3. Antimicrobial Activity of Solid Dispersions

In the study developed by Hernandez-Patlan et al. [40], the antibacterial activity of CM-loaded SDs prepared using PVP K30 and boric acid was evaluated against *Salmonella enteritidis*. In vivo tests were performed to determine the effects of (a) SD with 10/90 (*w/w*) CM/PVP, (b) boric acid and (c) 50/50 (*w/w*) CM/PVP plus boric acid administered orally to broiler chickens treated with 10^7 CFU/mL *S. enteritidis* each. While boric acid had no significant effect, the CM/PVP plus boric acid triad significantly reduced the number of colonies in the intestine of animals compared to CM/PVP, revealing a synergistic effect. Since such a reduction occurred only in the above CM/PVP proportion in SD, it can be concluded that this effect was the result of the increase in CM solubility. Although this in vivo antimicrobial activity of CM-SDs would allow for equivalent or even greater therapeutic effects than the drug alone in lower doses, further studies involving other species of target microorganisms and animals are needed.

4.4. Antioxidant Activity of Solid Dispersions

Some studies have revealed that zinc plays an important role in maintaining redox balance as well as protecting against oxidative stress and damage induced by ethanol, a compound capable of reducing the defenses of the gastric mucosa and inducing gastric ulcers [54,55]. Taurine is an amino acid that participates in numerous physiological reactions and can exert a cytoprotective effect against lesions of the stomach mucosa [56] thanks to its antioxidant activity [57].

In this sense, SDs of the taurine-zinc complex with the PVP K30 were prepared by Yu et al. [58] in the 1:6 (*w/w*) proportion by spray drying. In the in vivo study, the gastric mucosa of rats with ethanol-induced lesions was examined. The treatment with SD taurine-zinc (200 mg/kg) led to a 46% increase in the superoxide dismutase (SOD) activity and a 3.9-fold increase in the level of glutathione in the gastric mucosa compared to the model group (28.40 U/mg protein and 0.81 ± 0.56 mg/g protein, respectively), which suggests a direct relationship between endogenous level of this antioxidant and SOD activity to be exploited for better therapeutic response. Unlike in vitro activity, we found in the databases only this study published on in vivo antioxidant activity of SDs, which highlights the need for further research in this field.

4.5. Anti-Inflammatory Activity of Solid Dispersions

In an anti-inflammatory study conducted by Gou et al. [59], a solid dispersion of triacetylated andrographolide (TA) with Kollidon (VA64) had its in vivo anti-inflammatory activity assessed in mice ulcerative colitis model through parameters such as length, weight and levels of inflammatory cytokines (IL-2, IL-6) and SOD activity in the colon. Reduced length and increased weight of the colon indicated severe edema in the model group and in the group administered with TA suspension. Significant differences were also observed in these parameters between the model/crude TA group and the groups treated with TA-SD at different doses. While high a dose (200 mg/kg/day) of TA-SD remarkably reduced colon weight, low (50 mg/kg/day), or medium (100 mg/kg/day) doses showed a therapeutic effect against ulcerative colitis comparable to that of andrographolide pills (commercial anti-inflammatory drug). In addition, a reduction in the levels of IL-2 and IL-6 cytokines was observed in both the TA-SD and pill groups compared to the model group and the crude TA group. Finally, SOD activity significantly decreased in the model group compared to the normal one, while administration of TA-SD at medium and high doses caused an increase in SOD activity comparable to that induced by andrographolide pills. These results taken together demonstrated the anti-inflammatory effect of TA-SD.

Different solid dispersions of curcumin with PVP K30, Poloxamer 188 or 2-hydroxypropyl-β-cyclodextrin (HP-β-CD) were prepared by the solvent evaporation method and their anti-inflammatory activity was tested in mouse ear edema model [60]. The histological cuts of the ears revealed a decrease in the number of inflammatory cells infiltrated when mice were submitted to treatment with curcumin and CM-PVP. The results of ELISA assay showed a stronger anti-inflammatory activity of SDs compared to pure CM, revealed by a reduction in the expression of matrix metallopeptidase 9 as well as the levels of IL-1β and IL-6 cytokines.

Still regarding curcumin, Teixeira et al. [61], with the aim of improving its solubility, prepared atomized ternary SDs using Gelucire®50/13-Aerosil®, which provided important results in terms of anti-inflammatory activity in vivo. Administration of SDs containing 40% CM in a dose of 100 mg/kg showed a greater capacity to reduce rat paw edema than indomethacin (5 mg/kg). This anti-inflammatory activity, which appeared to be dose-dependent in the 10–100 mg/kg range, was ascribed to the increase in gastrointestinal absorption of SDs observed in the study.

In another research, Chuah et al. [62] investigated the bioavailability and bio-efficacy of CM in a solid dispersion prepared using HPMC, lecithin and isomalt by hot-melt extrusion for possible application in food products. To test the bio-efficacy of CM-SD on male Sprague-Dawley rats, they used the in vivo LPS-induced lung inflammation model and a dose of 5 mg/kg in 0.25% carboxymethylcellulose as vehicle administered for 21 days by oral gavage. Administration of LPS resulted in acute inflammatory lung injury and septic shock. Because the bioavailability of CM was increased by more than 10 times in solid dispersion, its efficacy was tested at a concentration 10 times lower than that of unformulated CM. While the treatment with CM alone at 50 mg/kg for 21 days reduced the leukocyte count marginally, that with CM-SD at only 5 mg of CM/kg significantly reduced the counts of both bronchoalveolar lavage fluid leukocytes and neutrophils. Damages in the lung tissues were less pronounced in CM-SD treated rats compared to those treated with LPS or CM alone. CM-SD, but not unformulated CM, was also able to downregulate the levels of IL-1, IL-6 and IL-8 inflammatory cytokines significantly. In summary, despite a 10 times lower dose, CM-SD was responsible for greater anti-inflammatory activity than CM alone. This study, which is the first report on CM-SDs suitable for food, demonstrated that the use of CM in solid dispersion in significantly low doses does not affect its efficacy and may improve color, taste and smell of foods.

Aceclofenac, chemically [2-(2′,6′-dichlorophenyl)amino] phenylacetoxyacetic acid, is used as a non-steroidal anti-inflammatory drug in the symptomatic treatment of pain and inflammation. However, like other drugs of this class, its oral administration is associated with gastrointestinal side effects like gastric ulceration, gastrointestinal bleeding and liver and kidney trouble. For these reasons, aceclofenac is increasingly administered by topical route. In this context, Carbopol gels offer a good alternative to oil-based topical formulations [63] and crospovidone has been used as a carrier of SDs of various drugs to improve their aqueous solubility [64]. In the study performed by Jana et al. [65], an attempt was made to develop Carbopol 940 gel for topical application containing SDs of aceclofenac using crospovidone as carrier to improve the skin permeation profile of this drug. The aceclofenac-crospovidone (1:4) SD was prepared by the solvent evaporation technique and tested in vivo for anti-inflammatory activity on male Sprague-Dawley rats using carrageenan-induced rat-paw edema model. The results obtained applying 1 g of optimized gel on the skin (1 cm^2) back of rats showed that SDs increased the rate of permeation of the drug, increased the intensity of response and gave results comparable with those of a marketed gel without leading to any skin irritation.

Another non-steroidal anti-inflammatory drug widely used in the treatment of mild-to-moderate pain and fever is ibuprofen ([2RS]-1[4-(2-methyl propyl) phenyl] propionic acid). Ofokansi et al. [66] tested in vivo the anti-inflammatory activity of ibuprofen-loaded PEG 8000 SDs prepared by the fusion method. The paw edema test was applied on Wister rats by orally administering ibuprofen-SD doses equivalent to 20 mg/kg body weight, while the reference group received 20 mg/kg of pure drug and the control one 1% (*w*/*v*) PEG 8000 suspension used as vehicle. Thirty minutes after treatment, paw edema was induced by injection of egg albumin. All SDs showed good anti-inflammatory properties being able to inhibit up to 90% of edema after 6 h versus only 77% of inhibition observed with the drug alone. This study clearly demonstrated that the use of hydrophilic carriers such as PEG 8000 can improve the drug pharmacological activity.

To understand and improve the dissolution behavior of poorly water-soluble drugs from SDs, flurbiprofen, a phenylalkanoic acid derivative belonging to the non-steroidal anti-inflammatory drugs, was used as a model [67]. SDs were prepared by the fusion method using urea and mannitol as hydrophilic carriers. Microspheres were also prepared by the solvent evaporation method using Eudragit L-100 (EL100) and Eudragit RS PO (ERS) as rate-controlling polymers. Flurbiprofen:urea-SDs and microspheres were used to develop controlled-release formulations by mixing them in different proportions. In in vivo anti-inflammatory tests, the pure drug and formulations were administered orally at a dose of 11.69 mg/kg body weight. The formulation that showed the best inhibition of rat paw edema up to 16 h was identified as a suitable product for controlled drug delivery.

Still within this context, meloxicam is a potent nonsteroidal anti-inflammatory drug belonging to the selective cyclo-oxygenase II inhibitors with the advantage of being safer in the gastrointestinal tract; however, it is poorly water-soluble and highly permeable (class II). A study by Al-Remawi et al. [68] aimed to improve meloxicam solubility and maximizing its pharmacological activity by preparing, by rotary evaporation and freeze drying, binary SDs with paracetamol, a highly water-soluble and poorly permeable drug. The anti-inflammatory effect was also investigated by measuring the changes in tail volume of edema induced by carrageenan injection. The formulation prepared by lyophilization using ethanol as a solvent and a meloxicam:paracetamol ratio of 1:10 (*w*/*w*) showed a decrease of more than 50% in the volume of carrageenan-induced tail edema compared to the physical mixture.

Chelerythrine (CHE), a quaternary benzo[c]phenanthridine alkaloid widely distributed in the Papaveraceae and Rutaceae families of plants, is a medicine officially listed in the Chinese Pharmacopoeia. Although this drug has shown a wide range of biological activities, its use in formulations is hampered by its poor water solubility. With the aim of improving CHE solubility and bioavailability, Li et al. [69] prepared solid dispersions with PVP K30 by the solvent evaporation method. Their anti-inflammatory activity was assessed in LPS-induced endotoxic shock experiments after single dose administration of dispersions (CHE-SDs) to mice in comparison with the CHE solution. CHE-SDs (10 mg/kg) significantly improved the bioavailability and anti-inflammatory activity of CHE by reducing the levels of TNF-α, IL-6 and NO in mice serum.

In summary, most in vivo studies on the anti-inflammatory activity used the paw edema test in rats, which revealed a significant increase in the biological activity of drugs in SDs compared to pure drugs, reducing lesion size and inflammatory cytokines production. These results corroborate those of tests often carried out by the same authors on solubility, bioavailability and physicochemical properties of drugs, which are directly related to the pharmacokinetic characteristics of SDs.

4.6. Gastro and Hepatoprotective Activity of Solid Dispersions

Among the activities and effects reported in the literature for SDs, the gastroprotective and hepatoprotective ones were also found.

Regarding the gastroprotective effect, a dispersion of the zinc taurine complex with PVP K30, already mentioned in the section on antioxidant activity, was also tested in vivo for its gastroprotective effect in experiments conducted on rats with ethanol-induced lesions in the gastric mucosa [58]. The gastric mucosa pretreated with taurine-zinc SD had an almost normal appearance, while that of the untreated group exhibited severe hemorrhagic ulcers. In addition, administration of SD reduced the ulcer index from 124.63 ± 26.72 in the untreated group to no more than 13.25 ± 4.77 in that treated with 200 mg/kg of SD. The gastroprotective effect of SDs was confirmed by a reduction in serum NO levels and a significant increase in gastric prostaglandin E2 compared to the untreated group.

Instead, Shin et al. [48] tested in vivo the hepatoprotective activity of CM-containing SDs with HPMC against tert-butyl hydroperoxide (t-BHP)-treated mice by administering 80 mg/kg of CM (positive control) or an equivalent dose of SD (400 mg/kg). Levels of alanine aminotransferase (ALT) and aspartate aminotransferase (AST), which indicate liver damage in response to t-BHP, were reduced by SD, while CM alone had no statistically significant effect. In the same study, the hepatoprotective effects of dispersion in liver tissues of mice were also evaluated. The liver section of the CM-administered group showed a slightly reduced necrotic region and decreased cellular infiltration, whereas these effects were much more marked in the SD-administered groups (200 and 400 mg/kg), with consequent improvement of the histological damage caused to the liver.

Solid dispersions of nobiletin and hydroxypropyl cellulose were also developed with the aim of improving drug solubility and bioavailability, as well as detecting possible hepatoprotective properties. Nobiletin is a polymethoxylated flavone with pharmacological activities such as anti-inflammatory, anti-apoptotic, anti-dementia, anti-oxidative and anti-tumor activities. The method used by Onoue et al. [70] to prepare nobiletin-SD was wet-milling followed by freeze drying. The evaluation of hepatoprotective activity was conducted in a rat model with acute liver damage induced by carbon tetrachloride (CCl_4). Administration of 2 mg/kg of SD led to a significant decrease in liver damage, evidenced by 60 and 43% reductions in ALT and AST levels and to greater hepatoprotective efficacy compared to the crystalline drug.

Silymarin is an extract of *Silybum marianum* seeds, used in the treatment of liver diseases, which however has low solubility in water. SDs and spherical agglomerates of silymarin were developed by Balata and Shamrool [71] to investigate their therapeutic effects on liver and kidney diseases. SDs with PVP K30 were prepared by the solvent evaporation method in 1:2, 1:4 and 1:8 (*w/w*) extract:polymer proportions. In vivo liver tests were conducted on albino rats with CCl_4-induced hepatotoxicity. The group treated with the SD with the lowest extract content significantly reduced the serum activities of ALT, AST and ALP as well as the level of total bilirubin, but increased the activity of alkaline phosphatase compared to the untreated group. In summary, this SD improved biomarker rates and had a significantly better therapeutic effect than the commercial extract. Furthermore, the results of histopathological studies confirmed the SD potential to reverse the chemically induced liver toxicity.

Another study with silymarin developed by Hwang et al. [72] aimed to evaluate a new system of SDs prepared using PVP K30 and Tween 80 by spray drying. Adhesion of the former ingredient to the outer surface of the drug led to a 650-fold increase in silymarin solubility. The hepatoprotective activity was determined on male rats and the tested substances were administered before and after exposure to CCl_4. The level of AST, which had been increased by exposition to CCl_4, was significantly reduced by the administration of silymarin-containing SD, while both the raw powder and commercial product did not show any appreciable hepatoprotective effect. These results agree with those of the histopathological study.

In summary, with regard to gastro and hepatoprotection, an evident increase in the biological activity of drugs was observed when they were incorporated into polymers, which reduced the level of damage more than the isolated drugs, thus demonstrating that SD have advantages that go beyond the increase in aqueous solubility and improvement of physicochemical properties of pharmacologically active molecules.

4.7. *Antidiabetic Activity of Solid Dispersions*

Diabetes mellitus is an endocrine-metabolic disorder characterized by chronic hyperglycemia, which can cause microvascular damage (retinopathy, nephropathy and neuropathy) and macrovascular damage (ischemic heart disease, stroke and peripheral vascular disease) [5,73].

Repaglinide, a hypoglycemic drug indicated for the treatment of patients with type 2 diabetes mellitus, was used by Zawar and Bari [74] to develop dispersions with Poloxamer 188 in the 1:3 (*w*/*w*) drug:polymer proportion by the conventional fusion or microwave method. In vivo experiments conducted on Wistar rats showed that the SD prepared by the microwave method reduced the serum glucose level determined by the glucose-oxidase method to 88 ± 0.73 mg/dL within 2 h, while the pure drug and the control led to glucose levels of 94 ± 2.63 and 120 ± 2.1 mg/dL, respectively. This study has shown that SDs can be an effective way to increase the solubility and bioavailability of repaglinide, leading to an enhancement of its antihyperglycemic activity and that the microwave method can be a green and effective alternative to obtain them.

Among the substances used in the treatment of non-insulin dependent diabetes mellitus is glimepiride, one of the sulfonylurea antidiabetics responsible for stimulating insulin secretion. These drugs have low solubility and high permeability and their use in the treatment of diabetes has been impaired by side effects [75]. In this sense, glimepiride-SDs were prepared by the solvent evaporation method using mixtures of Soluplus1 and PEG 4000 as polymers in different proportions and their antidiabetic activity in vivo was determined by changes in blood glucose concentrations in albino rats [5]. Glycemia was reduced by as much as 90.2–91.0% after 3 h in rats treated with the most effective SDs compared to the pure drug (38%) and commercial formulation (Amaryl1) (85%) and glucose in blood remained within the normoglycemic level for 9–12 h.

Pioglitazone is an antidiabetic drug that acts reducing glucose production in the liver and increasing insulin-dependent glucose availability. However, limitations related to its low water solubility and dissolution have led Pokharkar et al. [76] to prepare solid dispersions using different polymers such as HPMC E3, PVP K17, PVP K30, Soluplus and surfactants including Tween 80, Poloxamer 407 and Labrasol. The PVP K17-SD showed a better dissolution profile in vitro compared to pure pioglitazone, therefore it was chosen to assess hypoglycemic activity in vivo. This dispersion exerted an anti-hyperglycemic effect that resulted within 10 h in a serum glucose level (270.50 ± 4.47 mg/dL) approximately 20% lower than that observed using pure pioglitazone or a commercial drug, corresponding to a 33.85% reduction in concentration versus about 17%. The results of this study showed that SD was effective in improving the physicochemical properties of pioglitazone and may contribute to medical treatments as a hypoglycemic drug.

4.8. *Antinociceptive Activity of Solid Dispersions*

Neuropathic pain is a state of chronic pain caused by lesions or diseases of the somatosensory nervous system [77], for the treatment of which different drugs are used, which; however, have shown inconsistent results. To develop alternative therapies, among the pharmacological activities attributed to hecogenin acetate, the analgesic one has proven interesting in the treatment of chronic pain [78]. In this context Moreira et al. [77] developed solid dispersions with hydrophilic polymers, namely PVP K30, PEG 6000, HPMC, Soluplus® and PVP/VA 64, to increase the solubility of this drug and improve its dissolution profile. In this study, the anti-hyperalgesic activity of SDs was evaluated in vivo in mice selected as a neuropathic pain model. To assess the hyperalgesia of formulations, after induction of damage in mice by crushing the sciatic nerve, hecogenin acetate or its SD prepared with HPMC were administered and the parameters of mechanical and thermal hyperalgesia as well as grip strength were evaluated. The thermal hyperalgesia test on groups treated with SD showed that the incorporation of the drug in the HPMC matrix significantly improved its antinociceptive activity, while mice treated with hecogenin acetate and SD-HPMC only showed a significant effect on nociceptive behavior after mechanical and thermal stimulus testing.

Table 2. In vivo studies on solid dispersions.

Carrier Type	Substance	Animal	Dose	Activity	Improved Characteristics	References
PVP K30	IIIM-290	Swiss male mice (18–23 g)	25, 50 and 75 mg/kg	Anticancer	SD was able to reduce the IIIM-290 dose by at least 1.5-fold thanks to its efficiency in Ehrlich solid tumor model.	[24]
Soluplus®	9-Nitrocamptothecin	Male Sprague-Dawley rats (20 ± 2 g)	4 mg/kg	Anticancer	SD showed higher tumor growth inhibitory rate than the pure compound due to improved oral bioavailability	[49]
(+)-Xylitol	(−)-Oleocanthal	Athymic nude mice	10 mg/kg	Anticancer	Treatment with SD showed prevention, lower growth rate and less recurrence of tumor.	[50]
PVP K30	Zinc(II)-curcumin complex	B-NDG, BALB/c mice	100 mg/kg	Anticancer	SD reduced tumor size and weight in animals.	[17]
PVP K30	*Selaginella doederleinii* Hieron	BALB/c mice	200 mg/kg	Anticancer	SD reduced tumor size as well as the level of tumor angiogenesis.	[53]
Low substituted HPC	Benznidazole	Female NMRI mice (25 ± 2 g)	25 mg/kg/day	Antichagasic	The best SD showed a 96.65% trypanocidal activity, expressed as percentage reduction in the area under the parasitic curve.	[28]
PVP K30	Curcumin (CM)	Male Cobb-Vantress broiler chickens	1 g/kg of feed	Antimicrobial	The synergistic effect of 0.05% CM/PVP SD with 0.05% boric acid reduced colonization of *Salmonella enteritidis* in crop and ceca-cecal tonsils.	[40]
PVP K30	Taurine-zinc complex	Female Sprague-Dawley rats (240–260 g)	100 and 200 mg/kg/day	Antioxidant Gastroprotective	SDs protected rat gastric mucosa from ethanol-induced injury and increased SOD activity and glutathione level.	[58]
Kollidon (VA64)	Triacetylated andrographolide (TA)	Male Kunming mice	50, 100 and 200 mg/kg/day	Anti-inflammatory	TA-SD prepared with VA64 significantly improved the drug activity against ulcerative colitis.	[59]
PVP K30, Poloxamer 188	Curcumin	Female CD-1 mice	100 mg/kg oral doses	Anti-inflammatory	CM-SD prepared with PVP decreased matrix metallo-peptidase 9 expression and levels of IL-1β and IL-6 cytokines.	[60]
Gelucire®50/13-Aerosil®	Curcumin	Rat	10 to 100 mg/kg	Anti-inflammatory	A CM-SD dose of 100 mg/kg was more effective than 5 mg/kg indomethacin in reducing edema.	[61]
HPMC, lecithin and isomalt	Curcumin	Male Sprague-Dawley rats	5 mg/kg	Anti-inflammatory	A CM-SD dose of 5 mg/kg had greater anti-inflammatory activity than 50 mg/kg curcumin alone.	[62]
Crospovidone	Aceclofenac	Male Sprague-Dawley rats	1 g/cm^2 (topical)	Anti-inflammatory	The enhanced drug permeation increased the intensity of the anti-inflammatory response.	[65]
PEG 8000	Ibuprofen	Wistar rats	20 mg/kg	Anti-inflammatory	All SDs showed better anti-inflammatory activity than the pure drug, allowing up to 90% edema inhibition after 6 h.	[66]
Urea and mannitol	Flurbiprofen	Rat	11.69 mg/kg	Anti-inflammatory	SD showed better inhibition of rat paw edema up to 16 h.	[67]

Table 2. *Cont.*

Carrier Type	Substance	Animal	Dose	Activity	Improved Characteristics	References
Paracetamol	Meloxicam	Rat	-	Anti-inflammatory	SDs reduced by more than 50% the volume of carrageenan-induced tail edema compared to the physical mixture.	[68]
PVP K30	Chelerythrine (CHE)	Mice	10 mg/kg	Anti-inflammatory	SD enhanced CHE anti-inflammatory effect by reducing the levels of TNF-α, IL-6 and NO in mice serum.	[69]
HPMC	Curcumin	Male BABL/c mice	200 and 400 mg/kg	Hepatoprotective	The best SD increased the hepatoprotective efficacy of CM.	[48]
HPC	Nobiletin	Male Sprague-Dawley rats(220 g)	2 mg of drug/kg	Hepatoprotective	SD was more effective than the crystalline drug in rats with acute liver injury.	[70]
PVP K30	Silymarin	Adult male albino rats (150–200 g)	25 mg/kg	Hepatoprotective	The best SD improved biomarker rates and had a significantly better hepatoprotective effect than the commercial extract.	[71]
PVP K30	Silymarin	Male Sprague-Dawley rats (190–210 g)	50 mg/kg	Hepatoprotective	SD improved drug solubility and hepatoprotective activity, reducing the AST levels.	[72]
Poloxamer 188	Repaglinide	Wistar rats (150–250 g)	(1 mg of drug)	Antihyperglycemic	SD obtained by the microwave method improved the drug anti-hyperglycemic activity.	[74]
Soluplus1 and PEG 4000	Glimepiride	Albino Wistar rats (200–250 g)	0.0285 mg of drug/kg	Anti-diabetic	SD reduced the glucose level in rats more than the pure drug and a commercial product.	[5]
PVP K17	Pioglitazone	Male Swiss albino mice (25–30 g)	30 mg/kg SD	Antihyperglycemic	SD reduced the mean glucose level in mice more than the pure drug and a commercial product.	[76]
HPMC	Hecogenin acetate	Male Swiss mice (28–35 g)	40 mg/kg	Antinociceptive	Both the drug alone and its SD with HPMC-reduced mechanical and thermal hyperalgesia induced by crushing of the sciatic nerve in mice.	[77]

PVP, Polyvinylpyrrolidone; SD, Solid dispersion; HPC, Hydroxypropyl cellulose; CM, Curcumin; CM/PVP SD, curcumin/polyvinylpyrrolidone solid dispersion; SOD, Superoxide dismutase; PEG, Polyethylene glycol; TNF-α, tumor necrosis factor alpha; IL, interleukin; NO, Nitric oxide; HPMC, Hydroxypropyl methylcellulose; AST, Aspartate aminotransferase.

5. Critical Analysis

In this review, the main studies on the biological activities of solid dispersions (SDs) have been examined to make a comparison of the results of in vitro and in vivo tests carried out in the last 10 years. In vitro studies have demonstrated the ability of SDs incorporating various types of active compounds to enhance their antitumor, antiparasitic, antimicrobial, antioxidant, anti-inflammatory, or cytoprotective activities, while additional activities, such as the gastroprotective, hepatoprotective, antidiabetic, or antinociceptive ones, have been highlighted by in vivo studies.

Most of the articles published and cited in this review, for a total of 33, refer to in vitro studies particularly addressed to the antitumor activity of active compounds (cell viability or cytotoxicity), while the in vivo ones were relatively fewer in number, equal to 26 and mostly devoted to their anti-inflammatory activity.

Although SDs have already been studied and cited in the literature, the number of studies published on them with this focus is still relatively small, considering the great potential of these formulations in pharmaceutical technology and the possibility of preparing both amorphous and crystalline ones for the most diverse applications. In this review, different processes, carriers and drugs to prepare SDs were also discussed, a variety that can be of great value in the field of pharmaceutical technology to develop new SDs for the release of a large number of different drugs.

The results of biological activity studies have shown that SDs, as a tool of drug release, do not constitute a limiting factor for the execution of in vitro and in vivo tests; indeed, they stand out as a promising system in which the active principle and the vector interact allowing, in most cases, an increase in the pharmacological potential of the former as a consequence of changes in the physicochemical properties of the constituents. Similarly, SDs can enhance the biological properties of the incorporated bioactive compounds, making them more effective against a wide variety of pathogens such as bacteria and protozoa.

As a final remark, SDs could play a role in various biological mechanisms, thus representing a safe and effective alternative for the development and improvement of drugs targeting a wide range of pharmacological treatments.

6. Conclusions

Solid dispersions are a technological strategy to improve the pharmacological potential of natural or synthetic bioactive molecules, thanks to an increase in their solubility and bioavailability, thus leading to possible enhancement of their biological activities. In this context, this review sought to summarize and critically examine studies conducted with this approach both in vitro and in vivo, which have provided evidence of a significant therapeutic potential that solid dispersions could offer in the context of the most diverse biological activities.

As poorly water-soluble active ingredients incorporated in solid dispersions exhibited improved physicochemical and pharmacological properties, these systems can be targeted in the pharmaceutical industry as possible therapeutic alternatives for certain diseases, with greater selectivity, safety and efficacy than the existing treatments.

Author Contributions: All authors collaborated in data collection, analysis and writing of the review. All authors have read and agreed to the published version of the manuscript.

Acknowledgments: The authors thank CNPq and CAPES for their support and Federal University of Rio Grande do Norte.

Abbreviations

AChE, Acetylcholinesterase; ALT, Alanine aminotransferase; AST, Aspartate aminotransferase; BChE, Butyrylcholinesterase; BNZ, Benznidazole; CC50, 50% Cytotoxic concentration; CFU, Colony forming units; CHE, Chelerythrine; CM, Curcumin; DPPH, 2,2-diphenyl-1-picryl-hydrazyl-hydrate; GI50, Concentration causing 50% cell growth inhibition; GST, Glutathione S-transferase; HB, Berberine hydrochloride; HPMC, Hydroxypropyl methylcellulose; HPMCAS, Hydroxypropyl methylcellulose acetate succinate; IC50, Half inhibitory concentration; LPS, Lipopolysaccharide; HPC, Hydroxypropyl cellulose; MAO, Monoamine oxidase; MIC, Minimum inhibitory concentration; MTT, 3-(4,5-dimethylthiazol-2-yl)-2,5-diphenyltetrazolium bromide; NaDC, Sodium deoxycholate; NO, Nitric oxide; OHPP, Octenylsuccinate hydroxypropyl phytoglycogen; P407, Poloxamer 407; PEG, Polyethylene glycol; PPG, Polypropylene glycol; PTX, Paclitaxel; PVP, Polyvinylpyrrolidone; PVP/VA, Polyvinylpyrrolidone/vinyl acetate; PZQ, Praziquantel; ROS, Reactive oxygen species; SD, Solid dispersion; SOD, Superoxide dismutase; TA, Triacetylated andrographolide; TBESD, Total biflavonoids extract of *Selaginella doederleinii*; t-BHP, *tert*-Butylhydroperoxide; TPGS, D-α-toco-pheryl polyethylene glycol-1000-succinate.

References

1. Kambayashi, A.; Kiyota, T.; Fujiwara, M.; Dressman, J.B. PBPK modeling coupled with biorelevant dissolution to forecast the oral performance of amorphous solid dispersion formulations. *Eur. J. Pharm. Sci.* **2019**, *135*, 83–90. [CrossRef] [PubMed]
2. Jermain, S.V.; Brough, C.; Williams, R.O. Amorphous solid dispersions and nanocrystal technologies for poorly water-soluble drug delivery—An update. *Int. J. Pharm.* **2018**, *535*, 379–392. [CrossRef] [PubMed]
3. Loftsson, T.; Brewster, M.E. Pharmaceutical applications of cyclodextrins: Basic science and product development. *J. Pharm. Pharmacol.* **2010**, *62*, 1607–1621. [CrossRef] [PubMed]
4. Worku, Z.A.; Aarts, J.; Singh, A.; Mooter, G.V.D. Drug–Polymer Miscibility across a Spray Dryer: A Case Study of Naproxen and Miconazole Solid Dispersions. *Mol. Pharm.* **2014**, *11*, 1094–1101. [CrossRef]
5. Reginald-Opara, J.N.; Attama, A.; Ofokansi, K.; Umeyor, C.; Kenechukwu, F. Molecular interaction between glimepiride and Soluplus®-PEG 4000 hybrid based solid dispersions: Characterisation and anti-diabetic studies. *Int. J. Pharm.* **2015**, *496*, 741–750. [CrossRef]
6. Danda, L.J.D.A.; Batista, L.D.M.; Melo, V.C.S.; Sobrinho, J.L.S.; Soares, M.F.D.L.R. Combining amorphous solid dispersions for improved kinetic solubility of posaconazole simultaneously released from soluble PVP/VA64 and an insoluble ammonio methacrylate copolymer. *Eur. J. Pharm. Sci.* **2019**, *133*, 79–85. [CrossRef]
7. Júnior, W.F.D.S.; Pinheiro, J.G.D.O.; De Menezes, D.L.B.; Silva, N.E.D.S.E.; De Almeida, P.D.O.; Lima, E.S.; Veiga-Junior, V.F.; De Azevedo, E.P.; Lima, E.S. Development, Physicochemical Characterization and In Vitro Anti-Inflammatory Activity of Solid Dispersions of α,β Amyrin Isolated from Protium Oilresin. *Molecules* **2017**, *22*, 1512. [CrossRef]
8. Vasconcelos, T.; Sarmento, B.; Costa, P.C. Solid dispersions as strategy to improve oral bioavailability of poor water soluble drugs. *Drug Discov. Today* **2007**, *12*, 1068–1075. [CrossRef]
9. Leuner, C. Improving drug solubility for oral delivery using solid dispersions. *Eur. J. Pharm. Biopharm.* **2000**, *50*, 47–60. [CrossRef]
10. Zhang, Z.; Chen, Y.; Deng, J.; Jia, X.-B.; Zhou, J.; Lv, H. Solid dispersion of berberine–phospholipid complex/TPGS 1000/SiO2: Preparation, characterization and in vivo studies. *Int. J. Pharm.* **2014**, *465*, 306–316. [CrossRef]
11. Xie, Y.; Yao, Y. Octenylsuccinate hydroxypropyl phytoglycogen enhances the solubility and in-vitro antitumor efficacy of niclosamide. *Int. J. Pharm.* **2018**, *535*, 157–163. [CrossRef] [PubMed]
12. Steed, H.; Sawyer, M.B. Pharmacology, pharmacokinetics and pharmacogenomics of paclitaxel. *Pharmacogenomics* **2007**, *8*, 803–815. [CrossRef] [PubMed]
13. Xie, Y.; Yao, Y. Incorporation with Dendrimer-Like Biopolymer Leads to Improved Soluble Amount and In Vitro Anticancer Efficacy of Paclitaxel. *J. Pharm. Sci.* **2019**, *108*, 1984–1990. [CrossRef] [PubMed]
14. Choi, J.-S.; Cho, N.H.; Kim, D.-H.; Park, J.-S. Comparison of paclitaxel solid dispersion and polymeric micelles for improved oral bioavailability and in vitro anti-cancer effects. *Mater. Sci. Eng. C* **2019**, *100*, 247–259. [CrossRef] [PubMed]

15. Lee, S.H.; Lee, Y.-S.; Song, J.G.; Han, H.-K. Improved In vivo Effect of Chrysin as an Absorption Enhancer Via the Preparation of Ternary Solid Dispersion with Brij®L4 and Aminoclay. *Curr. Drug Deliv.* **2018**, *16*, 86–92. [CrossRef] [PubMed]
16. De Sá, I.S.; Peron, A.P.; Leimann, F.V.; Bressan, G.N.; Krum, B.N.; Fachinetto, R.; Pinela, J.; Calhelha, R.C.; Barreiro, M.F.; Ferreira, I.C.; et al. In vitro and in vivo evaluation of enzymatic and antioxidant activity, cytotoxicity and genotoxicity of curcumin-loaded solid dispersions. *Food Chem. Toxicol.* **2019**, *125*, 29–37. [CrossRef]
17. Wu, R.; Mei, X.; Ye, Y.; Xue, T.; Wang, J.; Sun, W.; Lin, C.; Xue, R.; Zhang, J.; Xu, D. Zn(II)-curcumin solid dispersion impairs hepatocellular carcinoma growth and enhances chemotherapy by modulating gut microbiota-mediated zinc homeostasis. *Pharmacol. Res.* **2019**, *150*, 104454. [CrossRef]
18. Xiong, X.; Zhang, M.; Hou, Q.; Tang, P.; Suo, Z.; Zhu, Y.; Li, H. Solid dispersions of telaprevir with improved solubility prepared by co-milling: Formulation, physicochemical characterization and cytotoxicity evaluation. *Mater. Sci. Eng. C* **2019**, *105*, 110012. [CrossRef]
19. Lewinska, A.; Adamczyk, J.; Pajak, J.; Stoklosa, S.; Kubis, B.; Pastuszek, P.; Slota, E.; Wnuk, M. Curcumin-mediated decrease in the expression of nucleolar organizer regions in cervical cancer (HeLa) cells. *Mutat. Res. Toxicol. Environ. Mutagen.* **2014**, *771*, 43–52. [CrossRef]
20. Jiang, Y.; Piao, J.; Cho, H.-J.; Kang, W.-S.; Kim, H. Improvement in antiproliferative activity of Angelica gigas Nakai by solid dispersion formation via hot-melt extrusion and induction of cell cycle arrest and apoptosis in HeLa cells. *Biosci. Biotechnol. Biochem.* **2015**, *79*, 1635–1643. [CrossRef]
21. Guo, S.; Wang, G.; Wu, T.; Bai, F.; Xu, J.; Zhang, X. Solid dispersion of berberine hydrochloride and Eudragit® S100: Formulation, physicochemical characterization and cytotoxicity evaluation. *J. Drug Deliv. Sci. Technol.* **2017**, *40*, 21–27. [CrossRef]
22. Wang, L.; Li, H.; Wang, S.; Liu, R.; Wu, Z.; Wang, C.; Wang, Y.; Chen, M. Enhancing the Antitumor Activity of Berberine Hydrochloride by Solid Lipid Nanoparticle Encapsulation. *AAPS PharmSciTech* **2014**, *15*, 834–844. [CrossRef] [PubMed]
23. Patil, J.B.; Kim, J.; Jayaprakasha, G.K. Berberine induces apoptosis in breast cancer cells (MCF-7) through mitochondrial-dependent pathway. *Eur. J. Pharmacol.* **2010**, *645*, 70–78. [CrossRef] [PubMed]
24. Kumar, V.; Mintoo, M.J.; Mondhe, D.M.; Bharate, S.B.; Vishwakarma, R.A.; Bharate, S.S. Binary and ternary solid dispersions of an anticancer preclinical lead, IIIM-290: In vitro and in vivo studies. *Int. J. Pharm.* **2019**, *570*, 118683. [CrossRef]
25. Simonazzi, A.; Davies, C.; Cid, A.G.; Gonzo, E.; Parada, L.; Bermúdez, J.M. Preparation and Characterization of Poloxamer 407 Solid Dispersions as an Alternative Strategy to Improve Benznidazole Bioperformance. *J. Pharm. Sci.* **2018**, *107*, 2829–2836. [CrossRef] [PubMed]
26. Lima, Á.A.; Soares-Sobrinho, J.L.; Silva, J.L.; Corrêa-Júnior, R.A.; Lyra, M.A.; Santos, F.L.; Oliveira, B.G.; Hernandes, M.Z.; Rolim, L.A.; Rolim-Neto, P.J. The Use of Solid Dispersion Systems in Hydrophilic Carriers to Increase Benznidazole Solubility. *J. Pharm. Sci.* **2011**, *100*, 2443–2451. [CrossRef]
27. Lima, Á.A.N.; Sobrinho, J.L.S.; De Lyra, M.A.M.; Dos Santos, F.L.A.; Figueirêdo, C.B.M.; Neto, P.J.R. Evaluation of in vitro dissolution of benznidazole and binary mixtures: Solid dispersions with hydroxypropylmethylcellulose and β-cyclodextrin inclusion complexes. *Int. J. Pharm. Pharm. Sci.* **2015**, *7*, 371–375.
28. Fonseca-Berzal, C.; Palmeiro-Roldán, R.; Escario, J.A.; Torrado, S.; Arán, V.J.; Torrado-Santiago, S.; Gómez-Barrio, A. Novel solid dispersions of benznidazole: Preparation, dissolution profile and biological evaluation as alternative antichagasic drug delivery system. *Exp. Parasitol.* **2015**, *149*, 84–91. [CrossRef]
29. Eloy, J.O.; Saraiva, J.; De Albuquerque, S.; Marchetti, J.M. Solid Dispersion of Ursolic Acid in Gelucire 50/13: A Strategy to Enhance Drug Release and Trypanocidal Activity. *AAPS PharmSciTech* **2012**, *13*, 1436–1445. [CrossRef]
30. Perissutti, B.; Passerini, N.; Trastullo, R.; Keiser, J.; Zanolla, D.; Zingone, G.; Voinovich, D.; Albertini, B. An explorative analysis of process and formulation variables affecting comilling in a vibrational mill: The case of praziquantel. *Int. J. Pharm.* **2017**, *533*, 402–412. [CrossRef]
31. Albertini, B.; Perissutti, B.; Bertoni, S.; Zanolla, D.; Franceschinis, E.; Voinovich, D.; Lombardo, F.; Keiser, J.; Passerini, N. Combining Mechanochemistry and Spray Congealing for New Praziquantel Pediatric Formulations in Schistosomiasis Treatment. *Int. J. Mol. Sci.* **2019**, *20*, 1233. [CrossRef] [PubMed]
32. White, J.; Rathod, P.K. Indispensable malaria genes. *Science* **2018**, *360*, 490–491. [CrossRef] [PubMed]

33. Abreu, T.P.; Silva, L.D.S.; Takiya, C.M.; Souza, M.C.; Henriques, M.D.G.M.O.; Pinheiro, A.A.S.; Caruso-Neves, C. Mice Rescued from Severe Malaria Are Protected against Renal Injury during a Second Kidney Insult. *PLoS ONE* **2014**, *9*, e93634. [CrossRef] [PubMed]
34. Fule, R.A.; Meer, T.A.; Sav, A.R.; Amin, P. Artemether-Soluplus Hot-Melt Extrudate Solid Dispersion Systems for Solubility and Dissolution Rate Enhancement with Amorphous State Characteristics. *J. Pharm.* **2013**, *2013*, 1–15. [CrossRef]
35. Fule, R.; Meer, T.; Sav, A.; Amin, P. Solubility and dissolution rate enhancement of lumefantrine using hot melt extrusion technology with physicochemical characterisation. *J. Pharm. Investig.* **2013**, *43*, 305–321. [CrossRef]
36. Crucitti, V.C.; Migneco, L.M.; Piozzi, A.; Taresco, V.; Garnett, M.; Argent, R.H.; Francolini, I. Intermolecular interaction and solid state characterization of abietic acid/chitosan solid dispersions possessing antimicrobial and antioxidant properties. *Eur. J. Pharm. Biopharm.* **2018**, *125*, 114–123. [CrossRef]
37. Al-Obaidi, H.; Kowalczyk, R.M.; Kalgudi, R.; Zariwala, M.G. Griseofulvin solvate solid dispersions with synergistic effect against fungal biofilms. *Colloids Surfaces B Biointerfaces* **2019**, *184*, 110540. [CrossRef]
38. Gorle, A.P.; Gattani, S.G. Development and evaluation of ocular drug delivery system. *Pharm. Dev. Technol.* **2010**, *15*, 46–52. [CrossRef]
39. Kanoujia, J.; Kushwaha, P.S.; Saraf, S.A. Evaluation of gatifloxacin pluronic micelles and development of its formulation for ocular delivery. *Drug Deliv. Transl. Res.* **2014**, *4*, 334–343. [CrossRef]
40. Hernandez-Patlan, D.; Solis-Cruz, B.; Pontin, K.P.; Latorre, J.D.; Baxter, M.F.A.; Hernandez-Velasco, X.; Merino-Guzman, R.; Méndez-Albores, A.; Hargis, B.M.; Lopez-Arellano, R.; et al. Evaluation of a Solid Dispersion of Curcumin With Polyvinylpyrrolidone and Boric Acid Against Salmonella Enteritidis Infection and Intestinal Permeability in Broiler Chickens: A Pilot Study. *Front. Microbiol.* **2018**, *9*, 1289. [CrossRef]
41. Hegge, A.B.; Vukićević, M.; Bruzell, E.; Kristensen, S.; Tønnesen, H. Solid dispersions for preparation of phototoxic supersaturated solutions for antimicrobial photodynamic therapy (aPDT). *Eur. J. Pharm. Biopharm.* **2013**, *83*, 95–105. [CrossRef] [PubMed]
42. Alves, T.; Chaud, M.; Grotto, D.; Jozala, A.F.; Pandit, R.; Rai, M.; Dos Santos, C.A. Association of Silver Nanoparticles and Curcumin Solid Dispersion: Antimicrobial and Antioxidant Properties. *AAPS PharmSciTech* **2017**, *19*, 225–231. [CrossRef] [PubMed]
43. Gunes, H.; Gulen, D.; Mutlu, R.; Gumus, A.; Tas, T.; Topkaya, A.E. Antibacterial effects of curcumin. *Toxicol. Ind. Health* **2013**, *32*, 246–250. [CrossRef] [PubMed]
44. Costa, A.R.D.M.; Marquiafável, F.S.; Vaz, M.M.D.O.L.L.; Rocha, B.A.; Bueno, P.C.P.; Amaral, P.L.M.; Barud, H.D.S.; Berreta-Silva, A.A. Quercetin-PVP K25 solid dispersions. *J. Therm. Anal. Calorim.* **2010**, *104*, 273–278. [CrossRef]
45. Ge, Y.; Zhao, X.; Wang, S.; Zu, Y.; Zhao, T.; Sang, M.; Sui, X.; Wang, K. 10 (CoQ10) Prepared by Heat Melt and High-pressure Homogenization Method. *Curr. Nanosci.* **2014**, *10*, 292–296. [CrossRef]
46. Fitriani, L.; Rismawati, E.; Umar, S.; Zaini, E. Solid dispersion of usnic acid-PVP K30 and evaluation of antioxidant activity. *Rasayan J. Chem.* **2018**, *11*, 1643–1648. [CrossRef]
47. Alshehri, S.; Imam, S.S.; Altamimi, M.A.; Hussain, A.; Shakeel, F.; Elzayat, E.M.; Mohsin, K.; Ibrahim, M.; Alanazi, F. Enhanced Dissolution of Luteolin by Solid Dispersion Prepared by Different Methods: Physicochemical Characterization and Antioxidant Activity. *ACS Omega* **2020**, *5*, 6461–6471. [CrossRef]
48. Shin, M.-S.; Yu, J.S.; Lee, J.; Ji, Y.S.; Joung, H.J.; Han, Y.-M.; Yoo, H.H.; Kang, K.; Shin, Y. A Hydroxypropyl Methylcellulose-Based Solid Dispersion of Curcumin with Enhanced Bioavailability and its Hepatoprotective Activity. *Biomolecules* **2019**, *9*, 281. [CrossRef]
49. Lian, X.; Dong, J.; Zhang, J.; Teng, Y.; Lin, Q.; Fu, Y.; Gong, T. Soluplus® based 9-nitrocamptothecin solid dispersion for peroral administration: Preparation, characterization, in vitro and in vivo evaluation. *Int. J. Pharm.* **2014**, *477*, 399–407. [CrossRef]
50. Qusa, M.H.; Siddique, A.B.; Nazzal, S.; El Sayed, K. Novel olive oil phenolic (−)-oleocanthal (+)-xylitol-based solid dispersion formulations with potent oral anti-breast cancer activities. *Int. J. Pharm.* **2019**, *569*, 118596. [CrossRef]
51. Yang, S.; Shi, P.; Huang, X.; Zhao, M.; Li, S.; Wu, Y.; Lin, X.-H.; Yao, H. Pharmacokinetics, Tissue Distribution and Protein Binding Studies of Chrysocauloflavone I in Rats. *Planta Med.* **2015**, *82*, 217–223. [CrossRef] [PubMed]

52. Chen, B.; Wang, X.; Zou, Y.; Chen, W.; Wang, G.; Yao, W.; Shi, P.; Li, S.; Lin, S.; Lin, X.-H.; et al. Simultaneous quantification of five biflavonoids in rat plasma by LC-ESI–MS/MS and its application to a comparatively pharmacokinetic study of Selaginella doederleinii Hieron extract in rats. *J. Pharm. Biomed. Anal.* **2018**, *149*, 80–88. [CrossRef] [PubMed]
53. Chen, B.; Wang, X.; Zhang, Y.; Huang, K.; Liu, H.; Xu, D.; Li, S.; Liu, Q.; Huang, J.; Yao, H.; et al. Improved solubility, dissolution rate and oral bioavailability of main biflavonoids from Selaginella doederleinii extract by amorphous solid dispersion. *Drug Deliv.* **2020**, *27*, 309–322. [CrossRef] [PubMed]
54. Zhang, W.-H.; Wu, X.-J.; Niu, J.-X.; Yan, H.; Wang, X.-Z.; Yin, X.-D.; Pang, Y. Serum zinc status and Helicobacter pylori infection in gastric disease patients. *Asian Pac. J. Cancer Prev.* **2012**, *13*, 5043–5046. [CrossRef] [PubMed]
55. Zhong, W.; Zhao, Y.; Sun, X.; Song, Z.; McClain, C.J.; Zhou, Z. Dietary Zinc Deficiency Exaggerates Ethanol-Induced Liver Injury in Mice: Involvement of Intrahepatic and Extrahepatic Factors. *PLoS ONE* **2013**, *8*, e76522. [CrossRef] [PubMed]
56. Ma, N.; Sasaki, T.; Sakata-Haga, H.; Ohta, K.-I.; Gao, M.; Kawanishi, S.; Fukui, Y. Protective effect of taurine against nitrosative stress in the stomach of rat with water immersion restraint stress. In *Advances in Experimental Medicine and Biology*; Springer Science and Business Media LLC: Berlin/Heidelberg, Germany, 2009; Volume 643, pp. 273–283.
57. Marcinkiewicz, J.; Kontny, E. Taurine and inflammatory diseases. *Amino Acids* **2012**, *46*, 7–20. [CrossRef]
58. Yu, C.; Mei, X.-T.; Zheng, Y.-P.; Xu, D. Gastroprotective effect of taurine zinc solid dispersions against absolute ethanol-induced gastric lesions is mediated by enhancement of antioxidant activity and endogenous PGE2 production and attenuation of NO production. *Eur. J. Pharmacol.* **2014**, *740*, 329–336. [CrossRef]
59. Gou, J.; Fei, S.; Xue, B.; Zhang, J.; Zhang, Y.; Wang, X.; Zhang, Y.; Yin, T.; He, H.; Tang, X. Triacetylated andrographolide solid dispersions: Preparation, stability study and in vivo anti-inflammation in mice ulcerative colitis model. *J. Drug Deliv. Sci. Technol.* **2019**, *51*, 91–100. [CrossRef]
60. He, Y.; Liu, H.; Bian, W.; Liu, Y.; Liu, X.; Ma, S.; Zheng, X.; Du, Z.; Zhang, K.; Ouyang, D. Molecular Interactions for the Curcumin-Polymer Complex with Enhanced Anti-Inflammatory Effects. *Pharmaceutics* **2019**, *11*, 442. [CrossRef]
61. Teixeira, C.C.C.; Mendonça, L.M.; Bergamaschi, M.M.; Queiroz, R.H.C.; Souza, G.E.P.; Antunes, L.M.G.; Freitas, L. Microparticles Containing Curcumin Solid Dispersion: Stability, Bioavailability and Anti-Inflammatory Activity. *AAPS PharmSciTech* **2015**, *17*, 252–261. [CrossRef]
62. Chuah, A.M.; Jacob, B.; Jie, Z.; Ramesh, S.; Mandal, S.; Puthan, J.K.; Deshpande, P.; Vaidyanathan, V.V.; Gelling, R.W.; Patel, G.; et al. Enhanced bioavailability and bioefficacy of an amorphous solid dispersion of curcumin. *Food Chem.* **2014**, *156*, 227–233. [CrossRef] [PubMed]
63. Chakraborty, S.; Khandai, M.; Sharma, A.; Khanam, N.; Patra, C.; Dinda, S.; Sen, K. Preparation, in vitro and in vivo evaluation of algino-pectinate bioadhesive microspheres: An investigation of the effects of polymers using multiple comparison analysis. *Acta Pharm.* **2010**, *60*, 255–266. [CrossRef] [PubMed]
64. Fujii, M.; Okada, H.; Shibata, Y.; Teramachi, H.; Kondoh, M.; Watanabe, Y. Preparation, characterization and tableting of a solid dispersion of indomethacin with crospovidone. *Int. J. Pharm.* **2005**, *293*, 145–153. [CrossRef] [PubMed]
65. Jana, S.; Ali, S.A.; Nayak, A.K.; Sen, K.K.; Basu, S.K. Development of topical gel containing aceclofenac-crospovidone solid dispersion by "Quality by Design (QbD)" approach. *Chem. Eng. Res. Des.* **2014**, *92*, 2095–2105. [CrossRef]
66. Kenechukwu, F.C.; Ofokansi, K.C.; Ezugwu, R.O.; Attama, A.A. Improved dissolution and anti-inflammatory activity of ibuprofen-polyethylene glycol 8000 solid dispersion systems. *Int. J. Pharm. Investig.* **2016**, *6*, 139–147. [CrossRef]
67. Malipeddi, V.R.; Dua, K.; Awasthi, R. Development and characterization of solid dispersion-microsphere controlled release system for poorly water-soluble drug. *Drug Deliv. Transl. Res.* **2016**, *6*, 540–550. [CrossRef]
68. Al-Remawi, M.; Ali, A.M.A.; Khames, A.; Hamaidi, M. Meloxicam-Paracetamol Binary Solid Dispersion Systems with Enhanced Solubility and Dissolution Rate:Preparation, Characterization and In Vivo Evaluation. *J. Pharm. Innov.* **2017**, *12*, 206–215. [CrossRef]
69. Li, W.; Qing, S.; Zhi, W.; Yao, H.; Fu, C.; Niu, X. The pharmacokinetics and anti-inflammatory effects of chelerythrine solid dispersions in vivo. *J. Drug Deliv. Sci. Technol.* **2017**, *40*, 51–58. [CrossRef]

70. Onoue, S.; Nakamura, T.; Uchida, A.; Ogawa, K.; Yuminoki, K.; Hashimoto, N.; Hiza, A.; Tsukaguchi, Y.; Asakawa, T.; Kan, T.; et al. Physicochemical and biopharmaceutical characterization of amorphous solid dispersion of nobiletin, a citrus polymethoxylated flavone, with improved hepatoprotective effects. *Eur. J. Pharm. Sci.* **2013**, *49*, 453–460. [CrossRef]
71. Balata, G.; Shamrool, H. Spherical agglomeration versus solid dispersion as different trials to optimize dissolution and bioactivity of silymarin. *J. Drug Deliv. Sci. Technol.* **2014**, *24*, 478–485. [CrossRef]
72. Hwang, D.H.; Kim, Y.-I.; Cho, K.H.; Poudel, B.K.; Choi, J.Y.; Kim, D.-W.; Shin, Y.-J.; Bae, O.-N.; Yousaf, A.M.; Yong, C.S.; et al. A novel solid dispersion system for natural product-loaded medicine: Silymarin-loaded solid dispersion with enhanced oral bioavailability and hepatoprotective activity. *J. Microencapsul.* **2014**, *31*, 619–626. [CrossRef] [PubMed]
73. Heydari, I.; Radi, V.; Razmjou, S.; Amiri, A. Chronic complications of diabetes mellitus in newly diagnosed patients. *Int. J. Diabetes Mellit.* **2010**, *2*, 61–63. [CrossRef]
74. Zawar, L.R.; Bari, S.B. Preparation, characterization and in vivo evaluation of antihyperglycemic activity of microwave generated repaglinide solid dispersion. *Chem. Pharm. Bull.* **2012**, *60*, 482–487. [CrossRef] [PubMed]
75. Li, H.; Ma, L.; Li, X.; Cui, X.; Yang, W.; Shen, S.; Chen, M. A simple and effective method to improve bioavailability of glimepiride by utilizing hydrotropy technique. *Eur. J. Pharm. Sci.* **2015**, *77*, 154–160. [CrossRef]
76. Pokharkar, V.; Kutwal, M.; Mandpe, L. Pioglitazone Solid Dispersion System Prepared by Spray Drying Method: In Vitro and In Vivo Evaluation. *PDA J. Pharm. Sci. Technol.* **2013**, *67*, 23–34. [CrossRef]
77. Moreira, C.D.L.D.F.A.; Pinheiro, J.G.D.O.; Da Silva-Júnior, W.F.; Barbosa, E.G.; Lavra, Z.M.M.; Pereira, E.W.M.; Resende, M.M.; De Azevedo, E.P.; Quintans-Júnior, L.J.; Araújo, A.A.D.S.; et al. Amorphous solid dispersions of hecogenin acetate using different polymers for enhancement of solubility and improvement of anti-hyperalgesic effect in neuropathic pain model in mice. *Biomed. Pharmacother.* **2018**, *97*, 870–879. [CrossRef]
78. Gama, K.B.; Quintans, J.S.; Antoniolli, A.R.; Quintans-Júnior, L.J.; Santana, W.A.; Branco, A.; Soares, M.B.P.; Villarreal, C.F. Evidence for the Involvement of Descending Pain-Inhibitory Mechanisms in the Antinociceptive Effect of Hecogenin Acetate. *J. Nat. Prod.* **2013**, *76*, 559–563. [CrossRef]

4

Polymeric Nanoparticles Based on Tyrosine-Modified, Low Molecular Weight Polyethylenimines for siRNA Delivery

Alexander Ewe [1], Sandra Noske [1,2], Michael Karimov [1] and Achim Aigner [1,*]

1 Rudolf-Boehm-Institute for Pharmacology and Toxicology, Faculty of Medicine, Clinical Pharmacology, Leipzig University, 04107 Leipzig, Germany; alexander.ewe@medizin.uni-leipzig.de (A.E.); sandra.noske@medizin.uni-leipzig.de (S.N.); michael.karimov@medizin.uni-leipzig.de (M.K.)
2 Faculty of Chemistry, Technical University Kaiserslautern, 67663 Kaiserslautern, Germany
* Correspondence: achim.aigner@medizin.uni-leipzig.de

Abstract: A major hurdle for exploring RNA interference (RNAi) in a therapeutic setting is still the issue of in vivo delivery of small RNA molecules (siRNAs). The chemical modification of polyethylenimines (PEIs) offers a particularly attractive avenue towards the development of more efficient non-viral delivery systems. Here, we explore tyrosine-modified polyethylenimines with low or very low molecular weight (P2Y, P5Y, P10Y) for siRNA delivery. In comparison to their respective parent PEI, they reveal considerably increased knockdown efficacies and very low cytotoxicity upon tyrosine modification, as determined in different reporter and wildtype cell lines. The delivery of siRNAs targeting the anti-apoptotic oncogene survivin or the serine/threonine-protein kinase PLK1 (polo-like kinase 1; PLK-1) oncogene reveals strong inhibitory effects in vitro. In a therapeutic in vivo setting, profound anti-tumor effects in a prostate carcinoma xenograft mouse model are observed upon systemic application of complexes for survivin or PLK1 knockdown, in the absence of in vivo toxicity. We thus demonstrate the tyrosine-modification of (very) low molecular weight PEIs for generating efficient nanocarriers for siRNA delivery in vitro and in vivo, present data on their physicochemical and biological properties, and show their efficacy as siRNA therapeutic in vivo, in the absence of adverse effects.

Keywords: poly(ethylene) imine; PEI; RNA; siRNA delivery; tyrosine-modification; tumor xenograft

---

1. Introduction

The induction of RNA interference (RNAi) by small interfering RNAs (siRNAs) [1] has great potential, allowing for the downregulation of pathophysiologically over-expressed genes on the post-transcriptional level. Since siRNAs can be specifically directed against virtually any target gene, including otherwise "undruggable" genes, they offer novel avenues towards customized therapies against many diseases, for example, the treatment of cancer (see, e.g., [2] for review). Today, siRNAs can be easily designed and chemically synthesized to target a gene of interest in a sequence-specific manner. By harnessing the cellular enzyme machinery, siRNAs are incorporated in the RNA-induced silencing complex (RISC) and, upon activation, the siRNA guide strand binds to its complementary target mRNA, leading to mRNA cleavage, degradation, and thus long-lasting gene knockdown. This is a unique characteristic of RNAi which cannot be achieved with small molecules or anti-sense oligonucleotides [3,4].

While it is thus necessary and sufficient to deliver siRNAs to the cell for inducing RNAi-mediated gene knockdown, the physicochemical properties of siRNAs, i.e., relatively high molecular weight, high polyanionic charge density, hydrophilic properties, and their instability/susceptibility to nuclease degradation, largely prevent their use in an unmodified form for therapeutic approaches [5]. Beyond chemical modifications of the siRNA, delivery systems are required [6,7]. Apart from siRNA conjugates specifically suited for liver uptake, a variety of different cationic lipids, polymeric materials, and other nanoscale systems have been developed to adsorb, electrostatically interact with or incorporate siRNA and mediate cellular uptake [8–12]. For in vitro application several compounds have been commercialized as transfection reagents and are able to induce a potent gene knockdown at low siRNA concentrations in cell culture [13]. However, they are generally not suited for in vivo applications and clinical translation is still challenging, and thus require the development of novel delivery systems. On the other hand, the feasibility of siRNA therapeutics has been shown when the first siRNA drug, ONPATTRO® (Patisiran), was approved by the US Food and Drug Administration (FDA) and European Medicines Agency (EMA) in 2018. ONPATTRO® is a lipid-based siRNA nanoparticle designed to downregulate transthyretin in the liver for treatment of the polyneuropathy of hereditary transthyretin-mediated amyloidosis (hATTR) [14,15]. Despite this success, it might be assumed that one delivery platform cannot address all diseases, especially when it comes to target tissues other than the liver [16].

Polymeric reagents are another well studied class of materials for the delivery of nucleic acids (for review, see [17,18]). A highly investigated cationic polymer is polyethylenimine (PEI), which is able to efficiently deliver nucleic acids in vitro and in vivo. PEIs are available in branched and linear topologies over a wide range of molecular weights (0.8–100 kDa) (for review, see [19,20]). While higher molecular weight PEIs show biological activity but are associated with toxicity, low molecular weight PEIs are more biocompatible but essentially lack transfection efficacy, especially in the case of smaller oligonucleotides like siRNA. Branched PEIs are more efficient for the delivery of siRNA than their linear counterparts [21–23]. Since the commercially available 25 kDa branched PEI shows some efficacy but is also attributed to toxic effects, the lower molecular weight PEI F25-LMW (branched; 4–10 kDa) has been introduced for siRNA delivery in vitro and in vivo [24]. Still, further improvements are warranted and various approaches have been explored to optimize transfection efficacies of low molecular weight PEIs and/or to decrease the toxicity of high molecular weight PEIs. These include the covalent modification of PEI with polyethylene glycol (PEG) [25–27], the cross-linking of small PEIs with hydrolysable linkers, e.g., esters, ketals, or reductive cleavable disulfide groups leading to the reversible formation of higher molecular weights ([28–31]; see [32] for review), the copolymerization/grafting with other polymers like polycaprolactone (PCL), starch or polyvinylalcohol (PVA) [33–35], the modification with lipophilic molecules, e.g., fatty acids, alkanes or cholesterol ([36,37], see [38] for review), or the combination of PEI-based complexes with liposomes [39–42].

The chemical modification of PEI with amino acids offers another very promising approach for nucleic acid delivery in vivo. In previous studies, the grafting of arginine, lysine, or leucine onto PEI showed increased β-galactosidase activity in tumor-bearing mice upon i.v. injection of modified PEI/pDNA complexes [43]. In another report, a library of twenty amino acids conjugated to a poly(amidoamine) (PAMAM G5) dendrimer was characterized for pDNA delivery in vitro and identified cationic and hydrophobic amino acids as most effective [44]. The triple modification of PAMAM G5 with arginine, histidine, and phenylalanine revealed synergistically enhanced pDNA reporter gene expression in vitro and in vivo as compared to their mono-functionalized derivatives [45]. Amino acid modifications have also been shown to improve the delivery of siRNA. Derivatives of a branched 25 kDa PEI with leucine, tryptophan, phenylalanine, or tyrosine were evaluated in vitro and identified the tyrosine-modified PEI as efficient for siRNA transfection [46]. The same high molecular weight 25 kDa branched PEI modified with *N*-acetyl-leucine was used for the delivery of miR34a, significantly improving bone regeneration in an orthodontic in vivo model [47]. The incorporation of histidine and tyrosine also improved in vitro siRNA transfection efficacy in the case of oligoamino amides, a new class of polymers prepared by solid phase synthesis, and decreased the EG5 mRNA expression upon i.v. injection of siEG5 nanoparticles in tumor bearing mice [48,49].

It becomes apparent from these studies that for the successful modification of cationic polymers with amino acids a balanced hydrophobicity and hydrophilicity is of great importance. This may then also allow for exploring lower molecular weight PEIs which are insufficiently active in the unmodified form, especially for the delivery of small nucleic acid molecules like siRNAs, but show significantly improved bioactivities upon introducing modifications. In a recent study, we selected a low molecular 10 kDa branched PEI for tyrosine modification. This new PEI derivative (P10Y) showed excellent in vitro siRNA transfection efficacies and increased complex stability upon serum contact. Moreover, P10Y/siRNA complexes decreased tumor growth in an aggressively growing melanoma xenograft mouse model [50,51]. Based on these results, we extended this approach towards even smaller 2 kDa and 5 kDa branched PEIs. Initial data indicated high knockdown efficacies of these small tyrosine-modified derivatives compared to their otherwise inactive parent PEIs [51]. In this study, we comprehensively explore these small tyrosine-PEIs in various cell lines, for targeting different reporter genes as well as endogenous genes. We identify P5Y as particularly active, and thus also studied this most efficient derivative in a tumor xenograft mouse model.

2. Materials and Methods

2.1. Cells and Cell Culture

Cell culture plastics and consumables were from Sarstedt (Nümbrecht, Germany). Cell culture media were from Sigma-Aldrich (Taufkirchen, Germany) and fetal calf serum was purchased from Biochrom (Berlin, Germany). The cell lines HCT116 (colorectal carcinoma), H441 (lung adenocarcinoma), PC3 (prostate carcinoma), Saos-2 (osteosarcoma), and MV3 (melanoma) were obtained from ATCC/LGC Promochem (Wesel, Germany), and G55T2 (glioblastoma) was a kind gift from Katrin Lamszus (University Clinic Hamburg-Eppendorf, Hamburg, Germany). All cell lines were cultivated in a humid atmosphere at 37 °C and 5% CO_2. HCT116, PC3, G55T2 cells were grown in IMDM medium, H441 and MV3 cells were grown in RPMI 1640 medium, and Saos-2 cells were grown in McCoy's 5a medium. All media were supplemented with 10% FCS and 2 mM alanyl-glutamine.

Reporter cell lines were stably transduced by lentiviral transduction. The EGFP/luciferase plasmid pCCLc-MNDU3-Luciferase-PGK-EGFP-WPRE was a gift from Fernando Fierro (University of California, Davis, CA, USA; Addgene plasmid # 89608) [52]) and the luciferase plasmid pLenti PGK V5-LUC Puro (w543-1) was a gift from Eric Campeau and Paul Kaufman (University of Massachusetts, Worchester, MA, USA; Addgene plasmid # 19360) [53]. Cell lines were cultivated in the above mentioned media and stable reporter cells were selected by either using puromycin (luciferase plasmid) or sorted by FACS (EGFP/luciferase plasmid).

2.2. Synthesis of Tyrosine-Modified PEIs

Branched polyethylenimines were obtained from the following suppliers: 2 kDa PEI (Sigma-Aldrich, Taufkirchen, Germany), 5 kDa PEI (a kind gift from BASF, Ludwigshafen, Germany), and 10 kDa PEI (Polysciences, Eppelheim, Germany). *N*-Boc-tyrosine-OH, *N*-hydroxysuccinimide, EDC·HCl were from Carbolution Chemicals (Saarbrücken, Germany). Dry *N*,*N*-Dimethylformamide (DMF) was from VWR (Darmstadt, Germany), Trifluoroacetic acid (TFA), ethanol, and methanol were from Carl Roth (Karlsruhe, Germany).

For the tyrosine modification, *N*-Boc (*tert*-butyloxycarbonyl) protected tyrosine (0.65 g, 2.3 mmol) and *N*-hydroxysuccinimide (0.27 g, 2.3 mmol) were dissolved in 3 mL dry DMF in a glass vial, followed by addition of EDC·HCl (0.45 g, 2.3 mmol), and stirred for 4 h under a nitrogen atmosphere at RT. In a second vial, PEI (0.2 g, 4.65 mmol in ethylenimine) was dissolved in 3 mL dry DMF, and the pre-activated tyrosine mixture was added and further stirred under nitrogen for 3 d. The reaction mixture was purified by dialysis (1 kDa MWCO regenerated cellulose, Serva, Heidelberg, Germany) against methanol for 10 h with intermediate solvent replacement to remove by-products. Next, the methanol was removed in vacuo and the viscous polymer was dissolved in 3 mL TFA, prior to stirring overnight for Boc-deprotection. Excess TFA was removed by co-evaporation with ethanol. Finally, the crude polymer was dissolved in 0.1 M HCl and excessively purified by dialysis against 0.05 M HCl for 24 h, then against water for 48 h. Lyophilization yielded the tyrosine-modified PEIs as yellowish fluffy powders. The degree of functionalization (~25–30% based on ethylenimine monomer) was confirmed by ^{1}H-NMR (Mercury plus, 300 MHz, Varian Agilent Technologies, Santa Clara, CA, USA) as described previously [50,51].

2.3. Polyplex Preparation

The polyplexes were prepared based on polymer/siRNA mass ratios. Typically, the P5Y- and P10Y-based complexes were prepared at a mass ratio of 2.5 unless indicated otherwise. For P2Y, a mass ratio of 10 was used. For standard transfection experiments in a 24 well plate, 30 pmol (0.4 µg) siRNA per well was diluted in 12.5 µL HN buffer (150 mM NaCl, 10 mM HEPES (4-(2-hydroxyethyl)-1-piperazineethanesulfonic acid), pH 7.4). In a separate tube, the calculated amount of the polymer was diluted in 12.5 µL HN buffer and the siRNA solution was added to the polymer solution, thoroughly mixed by pipetting up and down and incubated for 30 min at RT. For serum stability studies, the prepared polyplexes were additionally incubated with different volumes of FCS.

For in vivo experiments, the polyplexes were prepared as above, with slight modifications. Per dose for injection, 10 µg siRNA was diluted in 75 µL HN buffer and 25 µg (mass ratio 2.5) of the polymer (P5Y) was diluted in 75 µL 5% (*w/v*) glucose, 10 mM HEPES pH 7.4. The complexation was performed as described above.

2.4. Polyplex Characterization

The hydrodynamic diameters and zeta potentials were measured by dynamic light scattering (DLS) and phase analysis light scattering (PALS) with a Brookhaven ZetaPALS system (Brookhaven Instruments, Holtsville, NY, USA). Polyplexes containing 5 µg siRNA in 250 µL were prepared as described above and diluted to 1.7 mL with millipore water. The data were analyzed using the manufacturer's software, with applying the viscosity and refractive index of pure water at 25 °C. For the size determination, polyplexes were measured in five runs with a run duration of 1 min per experiment. Zeta potentials were analyzed in ten runs, with each run containing ten cycles using the Smoluchowski model. Additionally, polyplex sizes were analyzed by nanoparticle tracking (NTA) using a NanoSight LM10 (Malvern, Wiltshire, UK) equipped with a 640 nm sCMOS camera, software NTA 3.0, and a siRNA concentration of 1 µg/mL.

Complex stabilities were determined by a heparin displacement assay. The complexes based on the different tyrosine-modified PEIs were prepared at their optimal mass ratios as described above, prior to further incubation in FCS (50%, *v/v*) for 1 h. The complexes were then subjected to the polyanion heparin at different concentrations (units), as indicated in Figure S3C. A total of 25 µL of the mixture containing 0.2 µg siRNA was analyzed by 1.5% agarose gel electrophoresis.

2.5. Cell Transfection

For standard transfection experiments, the cells were seeded at a density of 35,000 cells per well of a 24 well plate in 0.5 mL fully supplemented medium. The next day, the cells were transfected with polyplexes containing 30 pmol/0.4 µg siRNA per 24 well as described above in the presence of FCS and without further medium change. For siRNA targets and sequences see Table S1.

2.6. Determination of Knockdown Efficacies and Complex Uptake

Luciferase activities were determined 72 h after transfection using the Beetle-Juice Kit (PJK, Kleinblittersdorf, Germany). The medium was aspirated and the cells were lysed with 300 µL Luciferase Cell Culture Lysis Reagent (Promega, Mannheim, Germany) for 30 min at RT. In a test tube,

10 µL lysate was mixed with 25 µL substrate and the luminescence was immediately measured in a luminometer (Berthold, Bad Wildbad, Germany).

The EGFP expression was determined by flow cytometry after 72 h. The cells were trypsinized, centrifuged for 3 min at 3000 rpm, and resuspended in 0.5 mL PBS, 1% BSA. The cells were measured in an Attune® Acoustic Focusing Cytometer (Applied Biosystems, Foster City, CA, USA). Finally, 20,000 events in the vital gate were analyzed using the Attune® software (V2.1.0).

For uptake experiments, complexes were prepared as described above (Section 2.4), but using a fluorophore-labeled siRNA-Atto488. PC3 wildtype cells were transfected, after 24 h prepared as described above with an additional PBS washing step and analyzed by flow cytometry.

To visualize the complex uptake by confocal microscopy, PC3 wildtype cells were seeded at a density of 200,000 cells onto glass coverslips in a 6 well plate. The next day, the cells were transfected with complexes of the different tyrosine-modified PEIs containing Alexa Fluor ® 647-labeled siRNA (2 µg siRNA/well). After 36 h, the siRNA uptake and intracellular distribution was analyzed by confocal microscopy (TCS SP8, Leica, Wetzlar, Germany).

2.7. Cell Proliferation and Viability Assays

For proliferation assays, cells were seeded at a density of 2000 cells (PC3 and Saos-2) or 1000 cells (MV3) per well of a 96 well plate in 100 µL medium on the day before transfection. For endpoint cell viability assays, PC3 or G55T2 cells were seeded at a density of 7000 cells per 96 well in 100 µL medium. The number of metabolically active cells after transfection was determined by using a colorimetric assay (WST-8 Cell Counting Kit-8; Dojindo Molecular Technologies EU, Munich, Germany). Briefly, after aspirating the medium, 50 µL of a 1:10 dilution of WST-8 in serum-free medium was added to the cells and incubated at 37 °C for 1 h. The absorbance was measured at 450/620 nm in a plate reader.

Acute cell damage caused by the polyplexes was determined by measuring the extent of lactate dehydrogenase (LDH) release, using the Cytotoxicity Detection Kit (Roche, Mannheim, Germany) according to the manufacturer's manual. Briefly, conditioned medium from transfection experiments (negative control siRNA) was collected after 24 h. For the determination of the maximum LDH release, cells were lysed with Triton X-100 at a final concentration of 2%, and conditioned medium from untreated cells served as negative control. In a 96 well plate, 50 µL sample medium was mixed with 50 µL reagent mix and incubated for 30 min in the dark. The reaction was stopped with 50 µL 1 M acetic acid and the absorption at 490/620 nm was measured using a plate reader. For blank value correction, fresh fully supplemented medium was mixed with the reagent and subtracted from all values.

2.8. RNA Preparation and Quantitative RT-PCR (RT-qPCR)

Total RNA was isolated using a combined TRI reagent and silica column protocol. Per 24 well, cells were lysed in 500 µL TRI reagent (TriFast, VWR, Darmstadt, Germany) and incubated for 5 min at RT. The lysate was transferred into a 1.5 mL tube and 200 µL chloroform was added, mixed well by shaking and incubated for 5 min at RT. The samples were centrifuged at 12,000 g for 15 min and the upper aqueous phase (~300 µL) was pipetted into a new 1.5 mL tube containing 300 µL 100% ethanol. After mixing, the sample was loaded onto the column (Zymo-Spin IC, Zymo Research, Freiburg, Germany), prior to centrifugation at 8000 g for 1 min. The flow-through was discarded. The column was washed twice with 450 µL 3 M sodium acetate pH 5.2, and once with 70% ethanol by centrifugation at 8000 g for 1 min; the collection tube was emptied after each step. For the drying step, the collection tube was replaced by a new one, and the columns were centrifuged at 12,000 g for 2 min. For RNA elution, 15 µL DEPC-water, pre-warmed to 65 °C, was added onto the column and incubated for 2 min, before finally eluting the RNA by centrifugation at 8000 g for 2 min. RNA concentrations and purities were measured in a NanoDrop 2000c (Thermo Fisher, Schwerte, Germany).

The total RNA was reverse transcribed with the RevertAid™ H Minus First strand cDNA synthesis Kit (Thermo Fisher, Waltham, MA, USA). In brief, 1 µL random hexamer primer was added to 1 µg RNA diluted in 10 µL DEPC-treated water, followed by an incubation step for 5 min at 65 °C and cooling to 4 °C. Then, 4 µL 5× reaction buffer, 2 µL 10 mM dNTP mix, 2.5 µL DEPC-treated ddH_2O, and 0.5 µL RevertAid™ H Minus M-MuLV Reverse Transcriptase (200 U/µL) were added. The cDNA synthesis mixture was incubated at 25 °C for 10 min, 42 °C for 60 min, and heat denatured at 70 °C for 10 min.

For quantitative real time PCR, a StepOnePLUS Real-Time PCR System (Applied Biosystems, Foster City, CA, USA) was used, applying the ΔΔCt method [54]. The cDNA was 1:10 diluted with DEPC-water and 4 µL were mixed with 5 µL 2x PerfeCTa SYBR® Green FastMix ROX (Quantabio, Beverly, MA, USA) and 1 µL 5 µM forward and reverse primer mix (see Table S2 for primer sequences). The qPCR were run with a pre-incubation at 95 °C for 2 min, followed by 45 amplification cycles (95 °C for 15 s, 55 °C for 15 s, 72 °C 15 s).

2.9. *Hemolysis*

To determine the hemolytic activity of the complexes, whole blood from healthy mice was diluted in Ringer's solution and erythrocytes were purified by several centrifugation and washing steps at 5000 rpm for 5 min, until the supernatant became clear. After the final washing step, the cells were taken up into physiological NaCl solution. Then, 1×10^6 cells in 50 µL were mixed with 50 µL complexes containing different siRNA amounts and incubated for 1 h at 37 °C. For absorption measurements, 25 µL of each sample were transferred into a 96 well plate in triplicates. Erythrocytes incubated with buffer served as negative control and erythrocytes treated with Triton X-100 to a final concentration of 1% served as positive control (= 100%). The absorbance of the samples was measured at 550 nm using a plate reader.

To evaluate erythrocyte aggregation, 50 µL of the purified cells (~1×10^6 cells/mL) were mixed with 50 µL aqueous solution containing 7.5 µg P5Y/3 µg siCtrl, or 750 kDa branched PEI (1 and 3 µg) as positive control. After incubation for 2 h at 37 °C, the samples were mounted onto glass slides and examined microscopically.

2.10. *In Vivo Tumor Therapy*

Athymic nude mice (Foxn1nu, Charles River Laboratories, Sulzfeld, Germany) were kept at 23 °C in a humidified atmosphere, 12 h light/dark cycle, with standard rodent chow and water ad libitum. Animal studies were performed according to the national regulations and approved by the local authorities (Landesdirektion Sachsen, approval NO. TVV 38/16, date: 20 January 2017). Tumor xenografts were established by injecting 3×10^6 PC3 cells in 150 µL PBS subcutaneously (s.c.) into both flanks of mice. When tumors reached a size of ~100 mm^3, the mice were randomized into different treatment groups (6–9 tumors/group). The polyplexes were prepared as described above and amounts corresponding to 10 µg siRNA were i.p. injected every 2–3 days over 14 days.

For in vivo luciferase knockdown experiments, 3×10^6 HCT116-Luc cells were s.c. injected for the induction of tumor xenografts described above. Mice were treated five times every 2–3 days with P5Y/siRNA complexes (siLuc2 = siCtrl and siLuc3 = Luciferase specific siRNA). Tumors were excised and lysed with Luciferase Cell Culture Lysis Reagent (app. 100 mg tumor tissue/1 mL buffer), prior to homogenization using an ULTRA-TURRAX®. Homogenates were repeatedly centrifuged at 13,000 rpm for 5 min and the supernatants were transferred into fresh tubes until the lysate became clear. Luminescence was determined as described above. Relative light units (RLU) were normalized for total protein concentration of the lysates using the BCA assay (Pierce Thermo Fisher, Schwerte, Germany) according to the manufacturer's protocol.

For the determination of blood serum markers, healthy nude mice were i.p. injected with P5Y/siLuc3 complexes containing 10 µg siRNA every 2–3 days, with a total of four times over 8 days. Three hours after the last injection, the blood was collected. Untreated mice served as negative control. The serum was diluted 1:20 with water and serum levels of various analytes were determined using an AU480 (Beckman Coulter, Krefeld, Germany).

For the analysis of the immunostimulatory cytokines TNF-α and INF-γ, P5Y/siLuc3 complexes (10 µg siRNA) were i.v. injected twice within 24 h into immunocompetent C57BL/6 mice. Four hours after the last injection, the blood was collected. Mice treated with lipopolysaccharides (LPS) 50 µg in 150 µL (single injection) served as positive control and untreated mice served as negative control. The serum levels of TNF-α and INF-γ were measured using ELISA kits (PreproTech, Hamburg, Germany) following the manufacturer's instructions.

2.11. Statistics

Statistical analyses were performed by Student's t-test or One-way ANOVA, and significance levels are * = $p < 0.05$, ** = $p < 0.01$, *** = $p < 0.001$, and # = not significant, with at least $n = 3$.

3. Results

3.1. Identification of Optimal Complexes for In Vitro Transfection

Based on the superior siRNA complexation and transfection efficacy of 10 kDa PEI upon its tyrosine-modification, we analyzed the performance of even smaller PEIs, which had been shown previously to be inactive [51], upon tyrosine engraftment. We hypothesized that even in the case of 5 kDa or 2 kDa PEIs, the tyrosine modification may result in polymers capable of efficient siRNA complexation and delivery, thus leading to target gene knockdown and RNAi-mediated tumor cell-inhibitory effects in various cellular assays. The tyrosine was covalently coupled onto branched PEIs by using standard NHS/EDC coupling chemistry as outlined in Figure 1A. The degree of tyrosine modification was ~30% compared to ethylenimine monomers, determined by ^{1}H-NMR analysis as described ([50,51]; see Figure S1). Transfection experiments with complexes based on the tyrosine-modified 5 kDa PEI (P5Y) revealed >90% knockdown of serine/threonine-protein kinase PLK1 (polo-like kinase 1; PLK-1) when transfecting a specific siPLK1 as compared to a negative control siRNA (siCtrl; Figure 1B, left). Complexes based on P10Y or P5Y were even more efficient than their higher molecular weight 25 kDa counterpart (P25Y; data not shown), while P2Y/siRNA complexes comprising the very low molecular weight 2 kDa PEI were less efficient. Similar results were obtained after transfection of an siRNA targeting the anti-apoptotic protein survivin, with P5Y/siRNA and P10Y/siRNA complexes again resulting in a 80–90% knockdown (Figure 1B, right) and thus performing better than their P25Y/siRNA counterparts (not shown). P2Y-based nanoparticles showed somewhat reduced activity, even when using higher N/P ratios. The knockdown of the oncogenes/proto-oncogenes PLK-1 and survivin also exerted profound tumor cell-inhibitory effects in anchorage-dependent proliferation assays (Figure 1C). When using P5Y or P10Y, the transfection of 6 pmol/well siRNA was sufficient to largely abolish cell proliferation. In contrast, in the case of P2Y/siRNA complexes, even double amounts (12 pmol) were incapable of inhibiting cell growth. Only the transfection of a very potent ubiquitin siRNA, which essentially abolished tumor cell viabilities in the P5Y and P10Y transfection groups, was strong enough to partially inhibit cell growth when complexed with P2Y. For the very efficient P10Y and P5Y, the siRNA concentration could be further reduced to 3 pmol siRNA with still showing strong inhibitory effects (Figure S2A). In addition, this reduction revealed differences in the potencies of the siRNAs against different target genes.

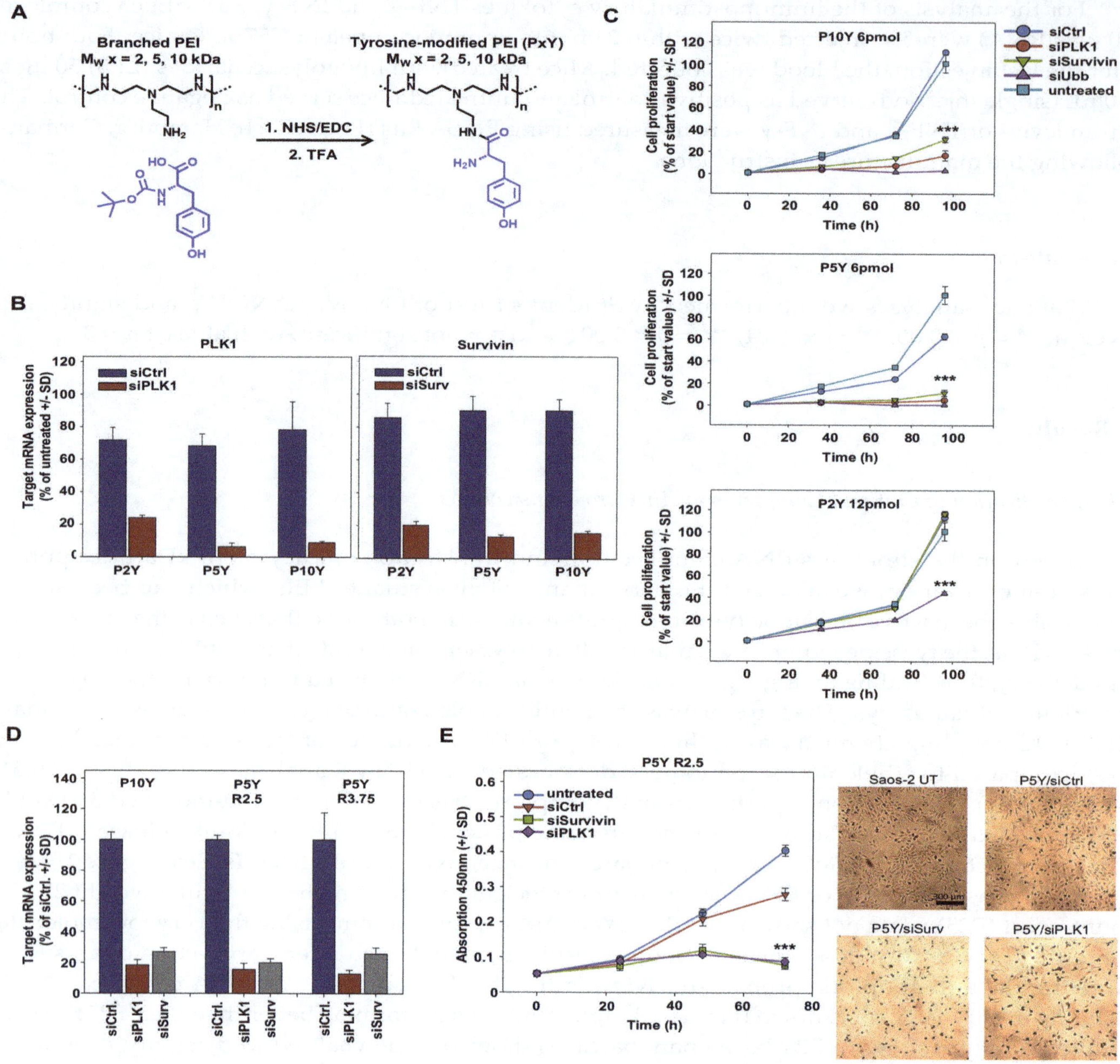

Figure 1. (**A**) Reaction scheme of tyrosine-coupling onto branched polyethylenimines (PEIs). Abbreviations: TFA, Trifluoroacetic acid; NHS, *N*-Hydroxysuccinimid; EDC, 1-Ethyl-3-(3-dimethylaminopropyl) carbodiimid (**B**) Knockdown efficacies of various tyrosine-modified PEI/siRNA complexes in PC3 cells targeting the oncogenes polo-like kinase 1 (PLK1) (left) or survivin (right), quantitated by RT-qPCR. (**C**) Determination of anchorage-dependent proliferation of PC3 cells upon transfection with the tyrosine-modified PEI/siRNA complexes using different anti-proliferative siRNAs at the amounts indicated in the figures. SiRNA-mediated cell inhibition is compared to negative-control transfected or untreated cells. (**D**) Knockdown upon transfecting Saos-2 cells with siRNAs against PLK1 or survivin, as determined by RT-qPCR. Increasing mass ratios from 2.5 to 3.75 does not further improve the knockdown efficacy. (**E**) Determination of anchorage-dependent proliferation of Saos-2 cells upon transfection with P5Y/siRNA complexes targeting PLK1 or survivin. The statistical significance indicates the difference to negative-control transfected cells. Left: quantitation based on WST-8 measurements; right: original pictures.

To further analyze possible reasons for these observed differences in biological activity, we determined intracellular levels of fluorophore-labeled siRNAs upon transfection of PC3 cells complexed with the different tyrosine-modified PEIs. The comparison of P5Y/atto488-siRNA complexes with their P10Y counterparts used for transfection in the presence of fetal calf serum (FCS) revealed a ~30% decrease in siRNA fluorescence when switching from P5Y to P10Y, while siRNA delivery in P2Y complexes was poor (Figure S3A). This was also confirmed in confocal microscopy, demonstrating atto488-siRNA signals to be largely absent upon transfection with P2Y (Figure S3B, upper panel). In contrast, profound fluorescence was observed in the case of P5Y and P10Y, with somewhat stronger signals in the case of P5Y/siRNA complexes (Figure S3B, center and lower panels). Beyond complex uptake, these differences may be based on variations in complex stabilities. Interestingly, a heparin displacement assay revealed even enhanced P5Y/siRNA complex stability in the presence vs. in the absence of serum, as indicated by the shift towards higher heparin concentrations required for siRNA release from the complex upon its pre-incubation in FCS (Figure S3C, upper panels). Under the same conditions, siRNA release from P2Y/siRNA complexes was already observed at lower heparin concentrations, indicating poor complex stability. In stark contrast, siRNA bands from heparin displacement of P10Y/siRNA complexes were weaker, independent of the heparin concentration, and thus indicating incomplete siRNA release even under very stringent conditions. Taken together, this suggests differences in siRNA delivery, complex stability, and siRNA release as underlying reasons for molecular weight-dependent differences between the tyrosine-modified PEIs. Very high efficacies of tyrosine-modified branched PEIs were observed up to as low as 5 kDa (P5Y), while only an even further reduction of the molecular weight (P2Y) eventually led to reduced transfection efficacies. This prompted us to focus in particular on P5Y as the tyrosine-modified PEI with the lowest molecular weight and highest activity, which was even slightly above P10Y.

The very profound siRNA transfection efficacies of P5Y were also confirmed in other cell lines like Saos-2 osteosarcoma cells (Figure 1D). A 1.5-fold increase of the polymer/siRNA mass ratio did not lead to enhanced knockdown, indicating that the very low polymer/siRNA mass ratio of 2.5 was already sufficient for maximum complex activity (Figure 1D). In contrast, knockdown efficacies were found to be dependent on the selection of the siRNA and the target gene, as indicated by the particularly profound >90% knockdown in the case of an siRNA targeting glyceraldehyde-3-phosphate dehydrogenase (GAPDH). As before in PC3 cells, an almost complete abolishment of cell proliferation was observed upon transfecting Saos-2 cells with P5Y/siPLK-1 or P5Y/siSurv complexes (Figure 1E). The microscopic evaluation of the wells also revealed a complete (siSurv) or almost complete (siPLK-1) loss of viable cells after 72 h (Figure 1E, right panel). In all experiments, P5Y-complexed negative control siRNA (siCtrl) was transfected in parallel, with the comparison to untransfected cells indicating non-specific transfection effects to be largely absent. As seen before in PC3 cells, an increase in the polymer/siRNA ratio by 1.5-fold did not further enhance biological efficacies. However, the P5Y/siCtrl curve indicated some non-specific inhibitory effects at this ratio due to excess polymer (Figure S2B). Specific growth inhibition upon P5Y/siRNA-mediated survivin knockdown was also observed in MV3 melanoma cells (Figure S2C), and GAPDH target gene reduction similar to the results shown above were also found in other cell lines (H441 lung adenocarcinoma cells, PC3 prostate carcinoma cells, and G55T2 glioblastoma cells; Figure S2D).

3.2. *Characterization of P5Y/siRNA Complex Properties*

For physicochemical characterization, complexes with different polymer/siRNA mass ratios were subjected to Zetasizer and Nanosight measurements. The hydrodynamic diameters determined by dynamic light scattering (DLS) were around 200–400 nm, with a slight trend towards smaller complexes with lower P5Y/siRNA mass ratios (Figure 2A).

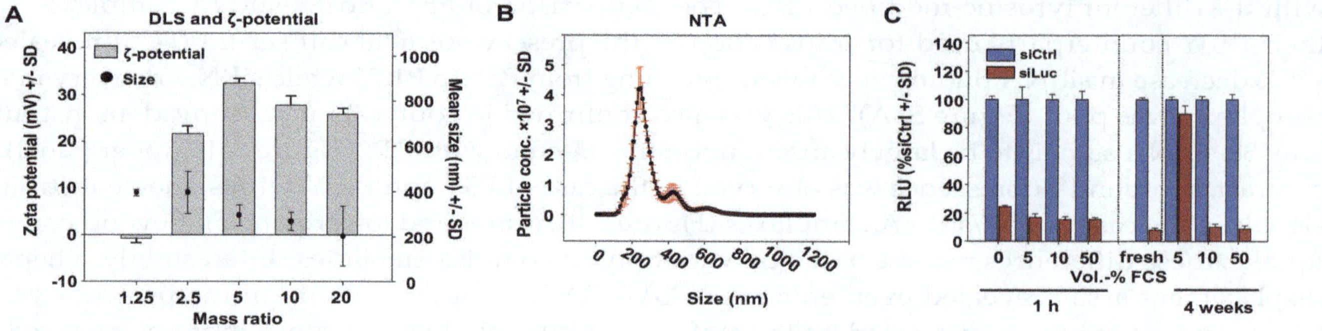

Figure 2. (**A**) Determination of the hydrodynamic diameters and zeta potentials of P5Y/siRNA complexes at different mass ratios as indicated in the figure. (**B**) Size measurement of P5Y/siRNA complexes by nanoparticle tracking (NTA) at the optimal mass ratio of 2.5. (**C**) Luciferase knockdown efficacies in H441-Luc cells for P5Y/siRNA complexes pre-incubated with increasing amounts of FCS (*v/v*) prior to transfection for 1 h (left) or upon storage for 4 weeks at 4 °C.

The diameter for the optimal mass ratio of 2.5 was additionally characterized by nanoparticle tracking (NTA) of which the main peak was at 200 nm and a second small peak at 400 nm (Figure 2B). The measurement of the zeta potentials revealed a slightly negative value for the lowest mass ratio of 1.25 indicating non complexed siRNA, and strongly increased to +20 mV for the mass ratio 2.5. The zeta potential further increased to ~30 mV at mass ratio 5 and reached a plateau of ~25 mV for mass ratios above 10. In many nanoparticle formulations, serum stability has been identified as one major issue limiting biological activity. Our transfection experiments, however, were exclusively performed in serum-containing media (10% FCS). Moreover, the presence of serum even proved beneficial: While PEI-based complexes tend to readily aggregate in aqueous solutions [42], our P5Y/siRNA complexes could be stored over weeks in the presence of 10% or even 50% FCS without losing activity, while 5% FCS was insufficient (Figure 2C).

3.3. High Biocompatibility/Absence of Toxicity of P5Y/siRNA Complexes

High biological activity may well be associated with increased cytotoxicity or other adverse effects, which were therefore assessed next. Lactate dehydrogenase (LDH) release assays, however, revealed no increase of LDH levels over background (untransfected cells). This was true for both, P5Y/siRNA and P10Y/siRNA complexes and was found in two reporter cell lines (PC3-Luc-EGFP and G55T2-Luc-EGFP cells; Figure 3A,D).

Again, the transfection led to profound target gene knockdown, indicated by 80–90% decreased EGFP activities upon siEGFP transfection as determined in flow cytometry (Figure 3B,E). Concomitantly, cell viabilities remained unaffected by P5Y/siRNA or P10Y/siRNA transfection, even after 48 h and independent of siRNA amounts, which could be increased from 4 pmol to 12 pmol without appreciable decrease in metabolic activity (Figure 3C,F). In line with the absence of adverse effects on cell membrane integrity (LDH release assay), a hemoglobin release assay in erythrocytes revealed no adverse effects. Within an almost 10-fold range of different complex amounts, no hemoglobin release over background was observed (Figure 3G). Similarly, the P5Y/siRNA complexes were tested for their erythrocyte aggregation potential. Identical complex amounts were incubated with red blood cells and analyzed under the microscope (Figure 3H). While the positive control a 750 kDa PEI led to strong aggregates at 1 μg, the P5Y complexes did not damage the red blood cells up to 3 μg complexed siRNA.

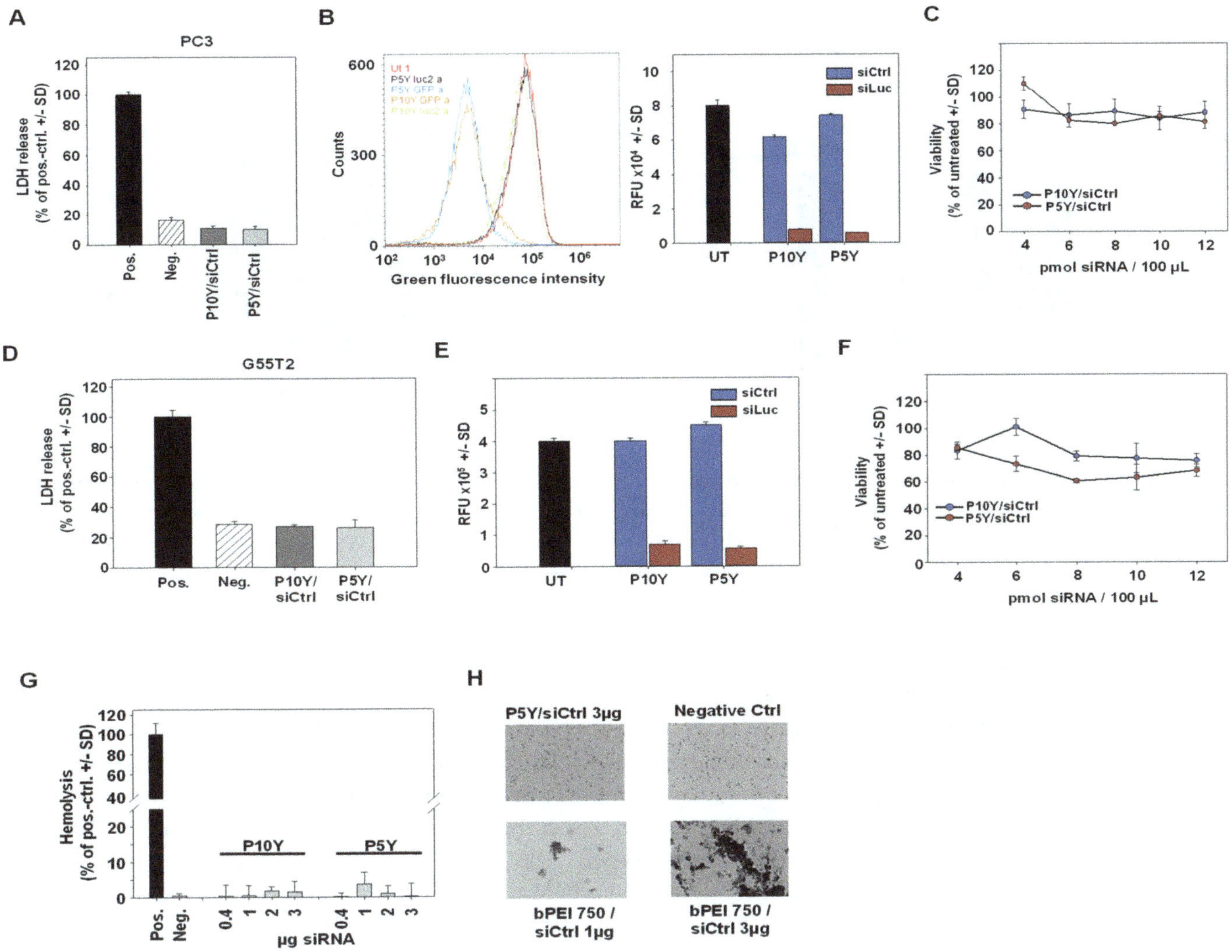

Figure 3. (**A**,**D**) Absence of early cytotoxic effects, as determined in lactate dehydrogenase (LDH) release assays for P10Y/siCtrl and P5Y/siCtrl complexes in PC3 (**A**) and G55T2 (**D**) cells. LDH release was quantitated 24 h after transfection of 30 pmol siCtrl/polymer per 24 well. (**B**,**E**) Knockdown of the Enhanced Green Fluorescent Protein (EGFP) reporter gene in stably expressing PC3-EGFP/Luc (**B**) and G55T2-EGFP/Luc (**E**) cells. Cells were transfected with P10Y and P5Y siRNA complexes and analyzed after 72 h by flow cytometry. (**C**,**F**) Cell viabilities of PC3 cells (**C**) and G55T2 cells (**F**) 48 h after transfection of P10Y/siCtrl and P5Y/siCtrl complexes at mass ratio 2.5 with increasing siRNA-concentrations. (**G**) Hemolysis assay for P5Y/siRNA complexes, demonstrating the absence of erythrocyte damage over a wider range of different concentrations. (**H**) Erythrocyte aggregation assay, further confirming the biocompatibility of P5Y/siRNA complexes as shown for 3 µg complexed siRNA (upper left; all lens magnifications: 4×). A total of 750 kDa bPEI complexes served as positive control, which led to a dose-dependent, profound aggregation of the red blood cells.

3.4. Therapeutic In Vivo Application of P5Y/siRNA Complexes Leads to Profound Anti-Tumor Effects

Pivotal in the development of nanoparticles for siRNA delivery is their applicability in vivo. In previous biodistribution assays, we showed that PEI/siRNA or P10Y/siRNA complexes become systemically available upon i.p. injection, and thus are able to reach organs/tissues remote from the injection site including tumors [50,55]. These studies were now extended towards P5Y/siRNA complexes. In a first experiment, P5Y/siRNA complexes were tested for reporter gene knockdown in mice bearing s.c. HCT116-Luc tumor xenografts. Prior to the in vivo application, the P5Y complexes were first evaluated in vitro for their potential to transfect this cell line. The luciferase expression was decreased to 60% at the lowest siRNA concentration of 15 pmol and further to 25% of control levels at 30 pmol siRNA (Figure 4A).

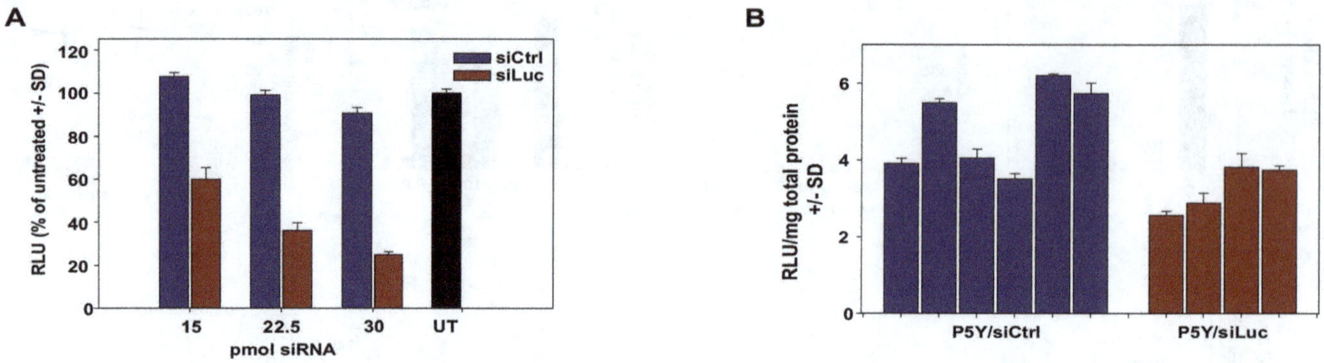

Figure 4. (**A**) Evaluation of luciferase knockdown efficacies of P5Y/siRNA complexes for in vivo use, in stably expressing HCT116-Luc cells over a range of different siRNA concentrations as indicated in the figure. (**B**) Luciferase activity of lysed HCT116-Luc tumors after in vivo treatment with P5Y/siRNA complexes. Bars represent the luciferase activities normalized for total protein concentrations from individual tumors of siCtrl-treated (blue) and siLuc-treated (red) mice.

Next, mice were injected with 5×10^6 tumor cells and, upon establishment of tumor xenografts, treated by repeated systemic application of 10 μg P5Y-complexed siRNA (3× every second day, intraperitoneal injection). Upon termination of the experiment at day 6 after treatment start, tumors were harvested and luciferase activities were analyzed from tumor lysates. Some variations were found between individual samples, especially in the negative control group. Still, the comparison of luciferase activities between the specific (P5Y/siLuc3) and the non-specific negative control (P5Y/siCtrl) group revealed a ~25% reduction of luciferase expression already after three injections (Figure 4B), and thus confirm that the treatment of mice with P5Y/siRNA complexes leads indeed to the knockdown of a given target gene in the tumors.

Switching to a more relevant therapy model, PC3 cells were s.c. injected into mice. Upon establishment of tumor xenografts of ~100 mm^3 in size and with clear growth kinetics, mice were randomized into different groups. Specific treatment relied on the P5Y-complexed siRNAs targeting the oncogenic proteins PLK-1 or survivin. For P10Y complexation, only PLK1 was selected as specific siRNA, while untreated mice or mice treated with siCtrl-containing complexes served as negative controls. The comparison of the latter groups revealed the absence of non-specific effects of repeated treatments (3×/week), as indicated by identical tumor growth curves (Figure 5A,B). In contrast, the treatment with the P5Y/siPLK-1 or P5Y/siSurv (Figure 5A) or P10Y/siSurv complexes (Figure 5B) led to profound antitumor effects.

During the experiment and upon its termination, mice were also screened and tested for possible adverse effects due to the repeated i.p. administration of P5Y/siRNA complexes. Mice showed no alterations in behavior, no obvious weight loss, and no other signs of adverse effects. In addition, possible toxic effects were determined by measuring important serum parameters. Healthy mice were repeatedly i.p. injected with P5Y complexes comprising 10 μg siCtrl four times over eight days. The serum analyses revealed no increase in liver enzymes (ASAT, ALAT), blood glucose (Gluc), urea, albumin, or LDH (Figure 6A). Other side effects may include the unwanted stimulation of the innate immune system. To test for this, immunocompetent mice were treated twice within 24 h with P5Y/siCtrl complexes. In this experiment, i.v. injection was preferred over i.p. administration to achieve instantaneous 100% bioavailability, and serum levels were analyzed at 4 h after the last injection, as described previously [50]. As shown in Figure 6B, no increase in TNFα or IFNγ levels were observed. We thus conclude that P5Y/siRNA complexes are efficient and safe in vitro and in vivo.

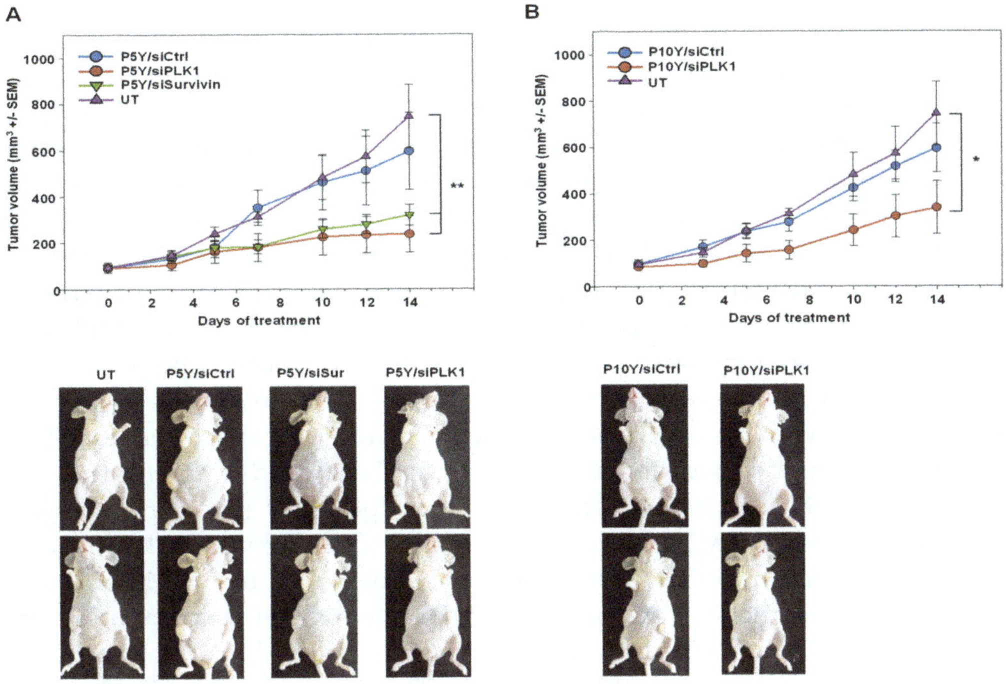

Figure 5. Therapy studies in PC3 tumor bearing mice using P5Y/siRNA (**A**) or P10Y/siRNA (**B**) complexes targeting either the oncogenes PLK1 or survivin. Mice were intraperitoneally treated with the complexes equivalent to 10 μg siRNA every 2–3 days. Tumor growth curves (upper panels) demonstrate the growth inhibiting effects of the specifically treated groups as compared to a negative control treated or untreated group. Lower panels: representative examples of mice.

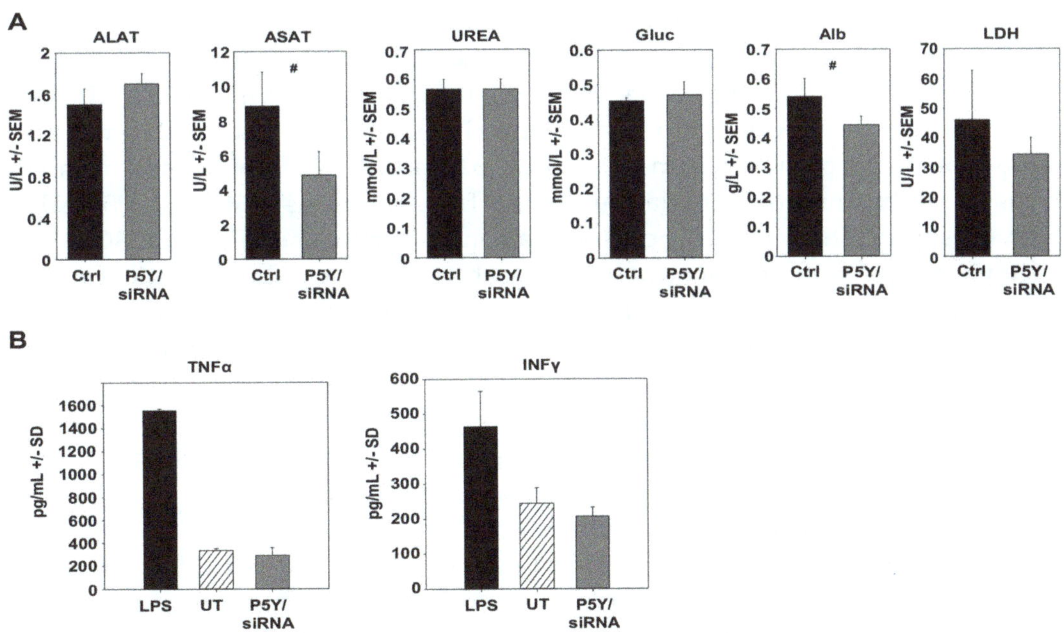

Figure 6. (**A**) Determination of blood serum markers for hepatotoxicity, cardiac or skeletal muscle damage, and kidney dysfunction. Healthy mice were repeatedly i.p. injected with P5Y/siCtrl complexes and blood serum levels were compared to untreated mice. ALAT: Alanine aminotransferase; ASAT: Aspartate aminotransferase; Gluc: Glucose; Alb: Albumin; LDH: Lactate deghydrogenase. (**B**) Absence of immunostimulation of P5Y/siCtrl complexes. Complexes were i.v. injected into immunocompetent mice twice within 24 h and blood was collected 4 h after the last injection. Treatment with lipopolysaccharides (LPS) served as positive control. #, not significant.

4. Discussion

PEIs and other cationic polymers are promising with regard to nucleic acid delivery, but they are often associated with toxicity. This is particularly true for higher molecular weight PEIs, while their lower molecular weight counterparts suffer from poor efficacy [21–23]. The toxicity of high molecular weight PEIs occurs at later stages. An early toxic effect is largely due to a disturbance of the cell membrane after contact with the complexes, leading to increased LDH release and induction of necrosis [56]. The late-stage cytotoxicity was reported to be caused by a damage of the mitochondrial membrane and subsequent activation of caspases and cytochrome C release [57–59]. While the latter findings have been frequently reported, the genotoxic potential of PEI is controversially discussed. Both, the presence and absence of DNA-damaging potential has been reported [60–63] and, possibly explaining these discrepancies, may be dependent on the tested concentrations and selected cell lines.

The fact that PEIs offer relatively easy access to chemical modification is a particularly attractive approach for further improvement of physicochemical and biological properties of the polymer and its complexes. Tyrosine may be considered as among the best candidate amino acids for chemical modification, due to its ability to balance between hydrophilicity (primary amines necessary for nucleic acid complexation) and hydrophobicity (favoring cellular internalization and endosomal escape [44,46]). Many chemical modifications of low molecular weight PEIs in order to increase their bioactivity rely on the cross-linking to create larger PEI derivatives, the coupling of lipidic groups to facilitate micellar structures for improved nucleic acid binding, or modifications with cationic groups to increase the electrostatic interactions (see Introduction). The aromatic amino acid tyrosine plays a key role in protein/DNA interactions. Several studies have reported that tyrosine is essential for the binding to nucleic acids by hydrogen bonding and by π–π-stacking [64,65], which can provide an explanation for the substantial increase in very low molecular weight PEI bioactivity upon tyrosine modification. Generally, phenol-containing molecules are an interesting motif to positively affect a given nucleic acid delivery system. For example, the pre-incubation of siRNA with EGCG, a polyphenol from green tea, and subsequent complexation with low molecular weight polyamines $\leq$5 kDa (PEI, PLL, PAMAM) strongly increased the knockdown efficacy [22].

Serum stability is an important factor for nucleic acid delivery systems, and we demonstrate high serum compatibility of our complexes based on tyrosine-modified PEIs (see Results and [50]). This may be attributed to the hydroxyl group of tyrosine. In contrast to phenylalanine, tyrosine shows negligible interactions with bovine serum albumin (BSA), as shown previously by the incubation of thymine-dityrosine or thymine-diphenylalanine with BSA solutions [66]. Still, P5Y/siRNA complex stability was even slightly enhanced upon incubation in serum (see Figure S3C). The stabilizing effect of hydroxyl groups was demonstrated in another study, by the modification of PEI with a hydroxyl-containing cyclic carbonate (EHDO). This modification improved serum-tolerance and reduced cytotoxicity as compared to the parent 25 kDa bPEI [67]. Similar results were reported for the Tris-modification of 25 kDa bPEI for pDNA and siRNA delivery [68].

Indeed, we could demonstrate in this study that tyrosine-modification allows for using very low, otherwise inactive PEIs. High complexation efficacies even at very low mass ratios are particularly relevant in the case of small oligonucleotides like siRNAs, considering the lack of binding cooperativity and their high rigidity [69]. Our results are in line with other studies demonstrating low toxicity and high biocompatibility of other (non-PEI) tyrosine-based polymers [70], as well as the safety of tyrosine in humans [71]. The beneficial effects of tyrosine modification thus allowed for using very small amounts of (derivatized) non-toxic low molecular weight PEIs whose bioactivity and biocompatibility critically relies on the grafting with tyrosine. Optimal complex stabilities, which need to be sufficiently high for efficient siRNA complexation/protection and sufficiently low for efficient intracellular siRNA release from the complex, are additional requirements. The potential relevance of the approach of using tyrosine-modified PEIs for translation into the clinic is emphasized by the fact that these nanoparticles were found to be efficacious also in vivo.

Author Contributions: Conceptualization, A.E. and A.A.; methodology, A.E., S.N., and M.K.; investigation, A.E., S.N., and M.K.; writing—original draft preparation, A.E. and A.A.; writing—review and editing, A.E. and A.A.; supervision, A.A.; project administration, A.A.; funding acquisition, A.A.

Acknowledgments: The authors are grateful to Markus Böhlmann and Anne-Kathrin Krause for expert mouse maintenance, the core unit "fluorescence technologies" (Kathrin Jäger) for cell sorting and Gabi Oehme for technical assistance in tissue culture experiments. Aileen Heinze is acknowledged for proofreading the manuscript.

References

1. Fire, A.; Xu, S.; Montgomery, M.K.; Kostas, S.A.; Driver, S.E.; Mello, C.C. Potent and specific genetic interference by double-stranded RNA in Caenorhabditis elegans. *Nature* **1998**, *391*, 806–811. [CrossRef] [PubMed]
2. Setten, R.L.; Rossi, J.J.; Han, S.P. The current state and future directions of RNAi-based therapeutics. *Nat. Rev.* **2019**, *18*, 421–446. [CrossRef] [PubMed]
3. Bartlett, D.W.; Davis, M.E. Insights into the kinetics of siRNA-mediated gene silencing from live-cell and live-animal bioluminescent imaging. *Nucleic Acids Res.* **2006**, *34*, 322–333. [CrossRef] [PubMed]
4. Dahlman, J.E.; Barnes, C.; Khan, O.; Thiriot, A.; Jhunjunwala, S.; Shaw, T.E.; Xing, Y.; Sager, H.B.; Sahay, G.; Speciner, L.; et al. In vivo endothelial siRNA delivery using polymeric nanoparticles with low molecular weight. *Nat. Nanotechnol.* **2014**, *9*, 648–655. [CrossRef]
5. Whitehead, K.A.; Langer, R.; Anderson, D.G. Knocking down barriers: advances in siRNA delivery. *Nat. Rev.* **2009**, *8*, 129–138.
6. Khvorova, A.; Watts, J.K. The chemical evolution of oligonucleotide therapies of clinical utility. *Nat. Biotechnol.* **2017**, *35*, 238–248. [CrossRef]
7. Miele, E.; Spinelli, G.P.; Miele, E.; Di Fabrizio, E.; Ferretti, E.; Tomao, S.; Gulino, A. Nanoparticle-based delivery of small interfering RNA: challenges for cancer therapy. *Int. J. Nanomed.* **2012**, *7*, 3637–3657.
8. Basarkar, A.; Singh, J. Nanoparticulate systems for polynucleotide delivery. *Int. J. Nanomed.* **2007**, *2*, 353–360.
9. Merdan, T.; Kopecek, J.; Kissel, T. Prospects for cationic polymers in gene and oligonucleotide therapy against cancer. *Adv. Drug Deliv. Rev.* **2002**, *54*, 715–758. [CrossRef]
10. Ojea-Jimenez, I.; Tort, O.; Lorenzo, J.; Puntes, V.F. Engineered nonviral nanocarriers for intracellular gene delivery applications. *Biomed. Mater.* **2012**, *7*, 054106. [CrossRef]
11. Balazs, D.A.; Godbey, W. Liposomes for use in gene delivery. *J. Drug Deliv.* **2011**, *2011*, 326497. [CrossRef] [PubMed]
12. Zhi, D.; Zhang, S.; Cui, S.; Zhao, Y.; Wang, Y.; Zhao, D. The headgroup evolution of cationic lipids for gene delivery. *Bioconjug. Chem.* **2013**, *24*, 487–519. [CrossRef] [PubMed]
13. Jensen, K.; Anderson, J.A.; Glass, E.J. Comparison of small interfering RNA (siRNA) delivery into bovine monocyte-derived macrophages by transfection and electroporation. *Vet. Immunol. Immunopathol.* **2014**, *158*, 224–232. [CrossRef] [PubMed]
14. Hu, B.; Weng, Y.; Xia, X.H.; Liang, X.J.; Huang, Y. Clinical advances of siRNA therapeutics. *J. Gene Med.* **2019**, *21*, e3097. [CrossRef]
15. Adams, D.; Gonzalez-Duarte, A.; O'Riordan, W.D.; Yang, C.C.; Ueda, M.; Kristen, A.V.; Tournev, I.; Schmidt, H.H.; Coelho, T.; Berk, J.L.; et al. Patisiran, an RNAi Therapeutic, for Hereditary Transthyretin Amyloidosis. *N. Engl. J. Med.* **2018**, *379*, 11–21. [CrossRef]
16. Lorenzer, C.; Dirin, M.; Winkler, A.M.; Baumann, V.; Winkler, J. Going beyond the liver: progress and challenges of targeted delivery of siRNA therapeutics. *J. Control. Release* **2015**, *203*, 1–15. [CrossRef]
17. Ulkoski, D.; Bak, A.; Wilson, J.T.; Krishnamurthy, V.R. Recent advances in polymeric materials for the delivery of RNA therapeutics. *Expert Opin. Drug Deliv.* **2019**, *16*, 1149–1167. [CrossRef]
18. Peng, L.; Wagner, E. Polymeric Carriers for Nucleic Acid Delivery: Current Designs and Future Directions. *Biomacromolecules* **2019**, *20*, 3613–3626. [CrossRef]
19. Hobel, S.; Aigner, A. Polyethylenimines for siRNA and miRNA delivery in vivo. *Wiley Interdiscip. Reviews. Nanomed. Nanobiotechnol.* **2013**, *5*, 484–501. [CrossRef]
20. Pandey, A.P.; Sawant, K.K. Polyethylenimine: A versatile, multifunctional non-viral vector for nucleic acid delivery. *Mater. Sci. Eng. Cmaterials Biol. Appl.* **2016**, *68*, 904–918. [CrossRef]
21. Kwok, A.; Hart, S.L. Comparative structural and functional studies of nanoparticle formulations for DNA and siRNA delivery. *Nanomed. Nanotechnol. Biol. Med.* **2011**, *7*, 210–219. [CrossRef] [PubMed]

22. Shen, W.; Wang, Q.; Shen, Y.; Gao, X.; Li, L.; Yan, Y.; Wang, H.; Cheng, Y. Green Tea Catechin Dramatically Promotes RNAi Mediated by Low-Molecular-Weight Polymers. *ACS Cent. Sci.* **2018**, *4*, 1326–1333. [CrossRef] [PubMed]
23. Shim, M.S.; Kwon, Y.J. Acid-responsive linear polyethylenimine for efficient, specific, and biocompatible siRNA delivery. *Bioconjug. Chem.* **2009**, *20*, 488–499. [CrossRef] [PubMed]
24. Werth, S.; Urban-Klein, B.; Dai, L.; Hobel, S.; Grzelinski, M.; Bakowsky, U.; Czubayko, F.; Aigner, A. A low molecular weight fraction of polyethylenimine (PEI) displays increased transfection efficiency of DNA and siRNA in fresh or lyophilized complexes. *J. Control. Release* **2006**, *112*, 257–270. [CrossRef] [PubMed]
25. Williford, J.M.; Archang, M.M.; Minn, I.; Ren, Y.; Wo, M.; Vandermark, J.; Fisher, P.B.; Pomper, M.G.; Mao, H.Q. Critical Length of PEG Grafts on lPEI/DNA Nanoparticles for Efficient in Vivo Delivery. *ACS Biomater. Sci. Eng.* **2016**, *2*, 567–578. [CrossRef] [PubMed]
26. Malek, A.; Czubayko, F.; Aigner, A. PEG grafting of polyethylenimine (PEI) exerts different effects on DNA transfection and siRNA-induced gene targeting efficacy. *J. Drug Target.* **2008**, *16*, 124–139. [CrossRef]
27. Malek, A.; Merkel, O.; Fink, L.; Czubayko, F.; Kissel, T.; Aigner, A. In vivo pharmacokinetics, tissue distribution and underlying mechanisms of various PEI(-PEG)/siRNA complexes. *Toxicol. Appl. Pharmacol.* **2009**, *236*, 97–108. [CrossRef]
28. Li, S.; Wang, Y.; Zhang, J.; Yang, W.H.; Dai, Z.H.; Zhu, W.; Yu, X.Q. Biodegradable cross-linked poly(amino alcohol esters) based on LMW PEI for gene delivery. *Mol. Biosyst.* **2011**, *7*, 1254–1262. [CrossRef]
29. Wang, C.; Yuan, W.; Xiao, F.; Gan, Y.; Zhao, X.; Zhai, Z.; Zhao, X.; Zhao, C.; Cui, P.; Jin, T.; et al. Biscarbamate Cross-Linked Low-Molecular-Weight Polyethylenimine for Delivering Anti-chordin siRNA into Human Mesenchymal Stem Cells for Improving Bone Regeneration. *Front. Pharmacol.* **2017**, *8*, 572. [CrossRef]
30. Bonner, D.K.; Zhao, X.; Buss, H.; Langer, R.; Hammond, P.T. Crosslinked linear polyethylenimine enhances delivery of DNA to the cytoplasm. *J. Control. Release* **2013**, *167*, 101–107. [CrossRef]
31. Breunig, M.; Hozsa, C.; Lungwitz, U.; Watanabe, K.; Umeda, I.; Kato, H.; Goepferich, A. Mechanistic investigation of poly(ethylene imine)-based siRNA delivery: disulfide bonds boost intracellular release of the cargo. *J. Control. Release* **2008**, *130*, 57–63. [CrossRef] [PubMed]
32. Jiang, H.L.; Islam, M.A.; Xing, L.; Firdous, J.; Cao, W.; He, Y.J.; Zhu, Y.; Cho, K.H.; Li, H.S.; Cho, C.S. Degradable Polyethylenimine-Based Gene Carriers for Cancer Therapy. *Top. Curr. Chem.* **2017**, *375*, 34. [CrossRef] [PubMed]
33. Feldmann, D.P.; Xie, Y.; Jones, S.K.; Yu, D.; Moszczynska, A.; Merkel, O.M. The impact of microfluidic mixing of triblock micelleplexes on in vitro / in vivo gene silencing and intracellular trafficking. *Nanotechnology* **2017**, *28*, 224001. [CrossRef]
34. Goyal, R.; Tripathi, S.K.; Vazquez, E.; Kumar, P.; Gupta, K.C. Biodegradable poly(vinyl alcohol)-polyethylenimine nanocomposites for enhanced gene expression in vitro and in vivo. *Biomacromolecules* **2012**, *13*, 73–83. [CrossRef] [PubMed]
35. Yamada, H.; Loretz, B.; Lehr, C.M. Design of starch-graft-PEI polymers: an effective and biodegradable gene delivery platform. *Biomacromolecules* **2014**, *15*, 1753–1761. [CrossRef] [PubMed]
36. Wu, P.; Luo, X.; Wu, H.; Yu, F.; Wang, K.; Sun, M.; Oupicky, D. Cholesterol Modification Enhances Antimetastatic Activity and siRNA Delivery Efficacy of Poly(ethylenimine)-Based CXCR4 Antagonists. *Macromol. Biosci.* **2018**, *18*, e1800234. [CrossRef] [PubMed]
37. Khan, O.F.; Kowalski, P.S.; Doloff, J.C.; Tsosie, J.K.; Bakthavatchalu, V.; Winn, C.B.; Haupt, J.; Jamiel, M.; Langer, R.; Anderson, D.G. Endothelial siRNA delivery in nonhuman primates using ionizable low-molecular weight polymeric nanoparticles. *Sci. Adv.* **2018**, *4*, eaar8409. [CrossRef]
38. Thapa, B.; Plianwong, S.; Remant Bahadur, K.C.; Rutherford, B.; Uludag, H. Small hydrophobe substitution on polyethylenimine for plasmid DNA delivery: Optimal substitution is critical for effective delivery. *Acta Biomater.* **2016**, *33*, 213–224. [CrossRef]
39. Schafer, J.; Hobel, S.; Bakowsky, U.; Aigner, A. Liposome-polyethylenimine complexes for enhanced DNA and siRNA delivery. *Biomaterials* **2010**, *31*, 6892–6900. [CrossRef]
40. Ewe, A.; Aigner, A. Nebulization of liposome–polyethylenimine complexes (lipopolyplexes) for DNA or siRNA delivery: Physicochemical properties and biological activity. *Eur. J. Lipid Sci. Technol.* **2014**, *116*, 1195–1204. [CrossRef]
41. Ewe, A.; Panchal, O.; Pinnapireddy, S.R.; Bakowsky, U.; Przybylski, S.; Temme, A.; Aigner, A. Liposome-polyethylenimine complexes (DPPC-PEI lipopolyplexes) for therapeutic siRNA delivery in vivo. *Nanomed. Nanotechnol. Biol. Med.* **2016**, *13*, 209–218. [CrossRef] [PubMed]

42. Ewe, A.; Schaper, A.; Barnert, S.; Schubert, R.; Temme, A.; Bakowsky, U.; Aigner, A. Storage stability of optimal liposome-polyethylenimine complexes (lipopolyplexes) for DNA or siRNA delivery. *Acta Biomater.* **2014**, *10*, 2663–2673. [CrossRef] [PubMed]
43. Navath, R.S.; Menjoge, A.R.; Wang, B.; Romero, R.; Kannan, S.; Kannan, R.M. Amino acid-functionalized dendrimers with heterobifunctional chemoselective peripheral groups for drug delivery applications. *Biomacromolecules* **2010**, *11*, 1544–1563. [CrossRef] [PubMed]
44. Wang, F.; Hu, K.; Cheng, Y. Structure-activity relationship of dendrimers engineered with twenty common amino acids in gene delivery. *Acta Biomater.* **2016**, *29*, 94–102. [CrossRef] [PubMed]
45. Wang, F.; Wang, Y.; Wang, H.; Shao, N.; Chen, Y.; Cheng, Y. Synergistic effect of amino acids modified on dendrimer surface in gene delivery. *Biomaterials* **2014**, *35*, 9187–9198. [CrossRef]
46. Creusat, G.; Zuber, G. Self-assembling polyethylenimine derivatives mediate efficient siRNA delivery in mammalian cells. *Chembiochem A Eur. J. Chem. Biol.* **2008**, *9*, 2787–2789. [CrossRef]
47. Yu, W.; Zheng, Y.; Yang, Z.; Fei, H.; Wang, Y.; Hou, X.; Sun, X.; Shen, Y. N-AC-l-Leu-PEI-mediated miR-34a delivery improves osteogenic differentiation under orthodontic force. *Oncotarget* **2017**, *8*, 110460–110473. [CrossRef]
48. He, D.; Muller, K.; Krhac Levacic, A.; Kos, P.; Lachelt, U.; Wagner, E. Combinatorial Optimization of Sequence-Defined Oligo(ethanamino)amides for Folate Receptor-Targeted pDNA and siRNA Delivery. *Bioconjug. Chem* **2016**, *27*, 647–659. [CrossRef]
49. Lee, D.J.; He, D.; Kessel, E.; Padari, K.; Kempter, S.; Lachelt, U.; Radler, J.O.; Pooga, M.; Wagner, E. Tumoral gene silencing by receptor-targeted combinatorial siRNA polyplexes. *J. Control. Release* **2016**, *244*, 280–291. [CrossRef]
50. Ewe, A.; Przybylski, S.; Burkhardt, J.; Janke, A.; Appelhans, D.; Aigner, A. A novel tyrosine-modified low molecular weight polyethylenimine (P10Y) for efficient siRNA delivery in vitro and in vivo. *J. Control. Release* **2016**, *230*, 13–25. [CrossRef]
51. Ewe, A.; Hobel, S.; Heine, C.; Merz, L.; Kallendrusch, S.; Bechmann, I.; Merz, F.; Franke, H.; Aigner, A. Optimized polyethylenimine (PEI)-based nanoparticles for siRNA delivery, analyzed in vitro and in an ex vivo tumor tissue slice culture model. *Drug Deliv. Transl. Res.* **2017**, *7*, 206–216. [CrossRef] [PubMed]
52. Beegle, J.; Lakatos, K.; Kalomoiris, S.; Stewart, H.; Isseroff, R.R.; Nolta, J.A.; Fierro, F.A. Hypoxic preconditioning of mesenchymal stromal cells induces metabolic changes, enhances survival, and promotes cell retention in vivo. *Stem. Cells* **2015**, *33*, 1818–1828. [CrossRef] [PubMed]
53. Campeau, E.; Ruhl, V.E.; Rodier, F.; Smith, C.L.; Rahmberg, B.L.; Fuss, J.O.; Campisi, J.; Yaswen, P.; Cooper, P.K.; Kaufman, P.D. A versatile viral system for expression and depletion of proteins in mammalian cells. *PLoS ONE* **2009**, *4*, e6529. [CrossRef] [PubMed]
54. Livak, K.J.; Schmittgen, T.D. Analysis of relative gene expression data using real-time quantitative PCR and the 2(-Delta Delta C(T)) Method. *Methods* **2001**, *25*, 402–408. [CrossRef]
55. Hobel, S.; Koburger, I.; John, M.; Czubayko, F.; Hadwiger, P.; Vornlocher, H.P.; Aigner, A. Polyethylenimine/small interfering RNA-mediated knockdown of vascular endothelial growth factor in vivo exerts anti-tumor effects synergistically with Bevacizumab. *J. Gene Med.* **2010**, *12*, 287–300.
56. Moghimi, S.M.; Symonds, P.; Murray, J.C.; Hunter, A.C.; Debska, G.; Szewczyk, A. A two-stage poly(ethylenimine)-mediated cytotoxicity: implications for gene transfer/therapy. *Mol. Ther.* **2005**, *11*, 990–995. [CrossRef]
57. Monnery, B.D.; Wright, M.; Cavill, R.; Hoogenboom, R.; Shaunak, S.; Steinke, J.H.G.; Thanou, M. Cytotoxicity of polycations: Relationship of molecular weight and the hydrolytic theory of the mechanism of toxicity. *Int. J. Pharm.* **2017**, *521*, 249–258. [CrossRef]
58. Hall, A.; Larsen, A.K.; Parhamifar, L.; Meyle, K.D.; Wu, L.P.; Moghimi, S.M. High resolution respirometry analysis of polyethylenimine-mediated mitochondrial energy crisis and cellular stress: Mitochondrial proton leak and inhibition of the electron transport system. *Biochim. Biophys. Acta* **2013**, *1827*, 1213–1225. [CrossRef]
59. Yamamoto, T.; Tsunoda, M.; Ozono, M.; Watanabe, A.; Kotake, K.; Hiroshima, Y.; Yamada, A.; Terada, H.; Shinohara, Y. Polyethyleneimine renders mitochondrial membranes permeable by interacting with negatively charged phospholipids in them. *Arch. Biochem. Biophys.* **2018**, *652*, 9–17. [CrossRef]
60. Gholami, L.; Sadeghnia, H.R.; Darroudi, M.; Kazemi Oskuee, R. Evaluation of genotoxicity and cytotoxicity induced by different molecular weights of polyethylenimine/DNA nanoparticles. *Turk. J. Biol.* **2014**, *38*, 380–387. [CrossRef]

61. Castan, L.; Jose da Silva, C.; Ferreira Molina, E.; Alves Dos Santos, R. Comparative study of cytotoxicity and genotoxicity of commercial Jeffamines(R) and polyethylenimine in CHO-K1 cells. *J. Biomed. Mater. Research. Part. Bapplied Biomater.* **2018**, *106*, 742–750. [CrossRef] [PubMed]
62. Beyerle, A.; Long, A.S.; White, P.A.; Kissel, T.; Stoeger, T. Poly(ethylene imine) nanocarriers do not induce mutations nor oxidative DNA damage in vitro in MutaMouse FE1 cells. *Mol. Pharm.* **2011**, *8*, 976–981. [CrossRef] [PubMed]
63. Hall, A.; Lachelt, U.; Bartek, J.; Wagner, E.; Moghimi, S.M. Polyplex Evolution: Understanding Biology, Optimizing Performance. *Mol. Ther.* **2017**, *25*, 1476–1490. [CrossRef] [PubMed]
64. Plyte, S.E.; Kneale, G.G. The role of tyrosine residues in the DNA-binding site of the Pf1 gene 5 protein. *Protein Eng.* **1991**, *4*, 553–560. [CrossRef]
65. Huang, J.; Zhao, Y.; Liu, H.; Huang, D.; Cheng, X.; Zhao, W.; Taylor, I.A.; Liu, J.; Peng, Y.L. Substitution of tryptophan 89 with tyrosine switches the DNA binding mode of PC4. *Sci. Rep.* **2015**, *5*, 8789. [CrossRef]
66. Roviello, G.N.; Oliviero, G.; Di Napoli, A.; Borbone, N.; Piccialli, G. Synthesis, self-assembly-behavior and biomolecular recognition properties of thyminyl dipeptides. *Arab J. Chem* 2018. [CrossRef]
67. Luo, X.H.; Huang, F.W.; Qin, S.Y.; Wang, H.F.; Feng, J.; Zhang, X.Z.; Zhuo, R.X. A strategy to improve serum-tolerant transfection activity of polycation vectors by surface hydroxylation. *Biomaterials* **2011**, *32*, 9925–9939. [CrossRef]
68. Dong, X.; Lin, L.; Chen, J.; Guo, Z.; Tian, H.; Li, Y.; Wei, Y.; Chen, X. A serum-tolerant hydroxyl-modified polyethylenimine as versatile carriers of pDNA/siRNA. *Macromol. Biosci.* **2013**, *13*, 512–522. [CrossRef]
69. Bolcato-Bellemin, A.L.; Bonnet, M.E.; Creusat, G.; Erbacher, P.; Behr, J.P. Sticky overhangs enhance siRNA-mediated gene silencing. *Proc. Natl. Acad. Sci. USA* **2007**, *104*, 16050–16055. [CrossRef]
70. Bourke, S.L.; Kohn, J. Polymers derived from the amino acid L-tyrosine: polycarbonates, polyarylates and copolymers with poly(ethylene glycol). *Adv. Drug Deliv. Rev.* **2003**, *55*, 447–466. [CrossRef]
71. Baldrick, P.; Richardson, D.; Wheeler, A.W. Review of L-tyrosine confirming its safe human use as an adjuvant. *J. Appl. Toxicol. Jat* **2002**, *22*, 333–344. [CrossRef] [PubMed]

5

Effects of Electrospinning on the Viability of Ten Species of Lactic Acid Bacteria in Poly(Ethylene Oxide) Nanofibers

Špela Zupančič [1,†], Katja Škrlec [2,†], Petra Kocbek [1], Julijana Kristl [1,*] and Aleš Berlec [1,2,*]

1 Faculty of Pharmacy, University of Ljubljana, Aškerčeva 7, SI-1000 Ljubljana, Slovenia; spela.zupancic@ffa.uni-lj.si (Š.Z.); petra.kocbek@ffa.uni-lj.si (P.K.)
2 Department of Biotechnology, Jožef Stefan Institute, Jamova 39, SI-1000 Ljubljana, Slovenia; katja.luzarskrlec@gmail.com
* Correspondence: julijana.kristl@ffa.uni-lj.si (J.K.); ales.berlec@ijs.si (A.B.)
† These authors contributed equally.

Abstract: Lactic acid bacteria can have beneficial health effects and be used for the treatment of various diseases. However, there remains the challenge of encapsulating probiotics into delivery systems with a high viability and encapsulation efficacy. The electrospinning of bacteria is a novel and little-studied method, and further investigation of its promising potential is needed. Here, the morphology, zeta potential, hydrophobicity, average cell mass, and growth characteristics of nine different species of *Lactobacillus* and one of *Lactococcus* are characterized. The electrospinning of polymer solutions containing ~10 log colony forming units (CFU)/mL lactic acid bacteria enabled the successful incorporation of all bacterial species tested, from the smallest (0.74 μm; *Lactococcus lactis*) to the largest (10.82 μm; *Lactobacillus delbrueckii* ssp. *bulgaricus*), into poly(ethylene oxide) nanofibers with an average diameter of ~100 nm. All of these lactobacilli were viable after incorporation into nanofibers, with 0 to 3 log CFU/mg loss in viability, depending on the species. Viability correlated with the hydrophobicity and extreme length of lactic acid bacteria, whereas a horizonal or vertical electrospinning set-up did not have any role. Therefore, electrospinning represents a promising method for the incorporation of lactic acid bacteria into solid delivery systems, while drying the bacterial dispersion at the same time.

Keywords: nanotechnology; biotechnology; probiotics; *Lactobacillus*; *Lactococcus*; electrospinning; nanofibers; drying; local delivery; viability

---

1. Introduction

Probiotics are living microbes that have beneficial health effects when administered to a host in a sufficient quantity. They most often belong to the very diverse genus of *Lactobacillus*, which includes a large number of species with a "generally recognized as safe" or "qualified presumption of safety" status [1,2]. In 2015, 175 genomes of lactobacilli were included in a comparative taxonomic study [2]. These are non-spore-forming rods or coccobacilli that are characterized by low genomic guanine and cytosine contents, the production of lactic acid, and complex nutritional requirements. They are aero-tolerant or anaerobic, aciduric, or acidophilic [1]. *Lactobacillus* spp. are particularly important in human nutrition and are also considered to be important cell factories in biotechnology, for the production of valuable chemicals. They have also been tested in several clinical trials to evaluate their efficiency for the treatment of a wide spectrum of diseases [1,3].

Lactobacillus probiotics are usually administered orally for the treatment of intestinal diseases, such as acute gastroenteritis [4], necrotizing enterocolitis [5], antibiotic-associated diarrhea [6], and inflammatory bowel disease [7], among others. Moreover, these probiotics have also shown promising potential for the treatment of extra-intestinal diseases, including urinary tract infections, periodontal disease, and bacterial vaginosis [8,9]. However, for such diseases, topical administration of the lactobacilli would appear advisable, to promote their higher efficiency.

For example, the vagina is densely colonized by microbiota (10^7–10^8 colony-forming units [CFU]/g vaginal fluid) [10,11]. Among the distinct ecological environments of the human body, the vaginal microbiota is the least diverse [12], where bacteria from the genus *Lactobacillus* predominate in the majority of healthy women (> 70%) [10,11]. A healthy vaginal microbiota includes from four to 12 different species [13], and the species that dominate individual microbiota include *Lactobacillus crispatus, Lactobacillus jensenii, Lactobacillus gasseri*, and *Lactobacillus iners* [11,14]. Their use for re-establishing the dominance of lactobacilli in vaginal dysbiosis (e.g., bacterial vaginosis and vaginal candidiasis) is therefore rational, and might even be the most justified among the different applications of these probiotics.

For successful treatments, probiotics need to be incorporated into patient-friendly delivery systems with large numbers of incorporated probiotics, which need to remain stable and survive for prolonged periods during storage [8]. Liquid and semi-solid dosage forms (e.g., hydrogels [15,16]) can have shorter residence times at the local site [10] and issues regarding probiotic stability compared to solid dosage forms. For preparations of these forms, different encapsulation and drying techniques have been used, including microencapsulation, emulsification, coacervation, spray drying, and lyophilization [17,18]. The main drawbacks of these techniques are the use of organic solvents and high temperatures [17]. Electrospinning represents a promising method for the incorporation of probiotics into nanofibers, allowing drying of the bacteria and preparation of a solid delivery system in a single step [19], and thereby offering considerable advantages over techniques such as microencapsulation and lyophilization.

Electrospinning is an established technique used to produce fibers with small diameters, in the range of several nanometers to micrometers, which are often called nanofibers. The manufacturing process is based on the drying of a thin liquid jet that is formed from a drop of polymer solution in a strong electric field [20]. The use of nanofibers has been suggested for several biomedical applications, including wound dressing, drug delivery, and tissue engineering [20]. Of these, drug delivery is the most promising, whereby its advantages include high drug loading, a high incorporation efficiency, the simultaneous delivery of diverse therapeutics, an increased surface area, a good mechanical resistance, an enhanced distribution at mucosal surfaces, ease of operation, and cost effectiveness [20–22].

To date, there have only been a few studies on the electrospinning of probiotics [23–28]. *Bifidobacterium animalis* subsp. *lactis* Bb12 has been incorporated into poly(vinyl alcohol) nanofibers [24]. Among the lactobacilli, *Lactobacillus acidophilus* was incorporated into poly(vinyl alcohol) and poly(vinyl pyrrolidone) nanofibers [25], and into agrowaste-based nanofibers [23]. *Lb. gasseri* was incorporated into poly(vinyl alcohol) nanofibers [28] and *Lb. rhamnosus* into poly(vinyl alcohol) and sodium alginate-based nanofibers [27]. Recently, we optimized the incorporation of *Lactobacillus plantarum* into poly(ethylene oxide) (PEO) nanofibers, and confirmed that their viability can be improved by the addition of lyoprotectants, such as trehalose [26].

Lactobacilli-containing nanofibers represent an innovative delivery system that would be particularly appropriate for topical administration. Due to scarce data on the influence of electrospinning on the viability of different *Lactobacillus* species, in the present study, we incorporated nine different species from the genus *Lactobacillus* and one from the genus *Lactococcus* into PEO nanofibers and assessed their viabilities following their incorporation, as a single study. To explain the higher susceptibilities of some strains to electrospinning, the morphology, zeta potential, hydrophobicity, average mass of bacterial cells, and growth characteristics of these 10 strains were also characterized.

2. Materials and Methods

2.1. Materials

Poly(ethylene oxide) (Mw, 900 kDa) and chloramphenicol were obtained from Sigma Aldrich (Steinheim, Germany). Phosphate-buffered saline (pH 7.4; osmolality: 280–315 mOsm/kg) was sourced from Gibco (Life Technologies, Carlsbad, CA, USA). De Man, Rogosa and Sharpe (MRS) and M-17 media for culturing the *Lactobacillus* spp. and *L. lactis*, respectively, were obtained from Merck (Darmstadt, Germany). Water, buffers, and growth media were sterilized by autoclaving at 2 bar and 121 °C for 20 min.

2.2. Bacterial Strains and Culturing Conditions

The *Lactobacillus* strains were grown at 37 °C in MRS medium without aeration. *L. lactis* MG1363 was grown at 30 °C in M-17 medium supplemented with 0.5% glucose (GM-17), without aeration (Table 1). For long-term storage, the bacterial strains were kept frozen at −80 °C in their corresponding growth medium with 20% (*v/v*) glycerol. For each experiment, fresh bacteria cultures were cultivated. Frozen cultures were first transferred onto an appropriate growth medium agar plate and incubated for 2 days at 37 °C (*Lactobacillus* spp.) or 30 °C (*L. lactis*). A single bacteria colony was picked, inoculated into 10 mL of the appropriate medium, and incubated at 37 °C or 30 °C for 24 h. Overnight cultures were diluted in fresh medium (1:100, *v/v*) and grown until a stationary growth phase was reached (as determined from the growth curves; see below). The cultures were centrifuged at 5000× *g* for 10 min (Sorvall Lynx 4000; ThermoFisher Scientific, Waltham, MA, USA). The cells were then washed twice with phosphate-buffered saline and resuspended in an appropriate volume of water.

Table 1. Bacterial strains used in this study, and some of their properties.

Strain	Source	Fermentation Type	Genome Size [bp]	Reference
Lactobacillus sp.				
Lb. acidophilus ATCC 4356	Infant feces	Homofermentative	1956.699	[29]
Lb. delbrueckii ssp. *bulgaricus* ATCC 11842	Yoghurt	Homofermentative	1864.998	[30]
Lb. casei ATCC 393	Cheese	Facultative heterofermentative	2924.929	[31]
Lb. gasseri ATCC 33323	Human isolate	Homofermentative	1894.360	[32]
Lb. paracasei ATCC 25302	Milk product	Facultative heterofermentative	2991.737	NCBI
Lb. plantarum ATCC 8014	n/a	Facultative heterofermentative	3254.764	NCBI
Lb. reuteri ATCC 55730	Breast milk	Heterofermentative	2036.000	[33]
Lb. rhamnosus ATCC 53103	Human intestine	Homofermentative	3005.051	[34]
Lb. salivarius ATCC 11741	Infant feces	Homofermentative	1956.699	NCBI
Lactococcus sp.				
Lactococcus lactis ssp. *cremoris* MG1363	Cheese	Homofermentative	2529.478	[35]

n/a: not available, NCBI: National Center for Biotechnology Information, ATCC: American Type Culture Collection.

2.3. Characterization of Bacterial Strains

2.3.1. Determination of Cell Surface Charge of the Bacteria

The cell-surface net charge of the bacteria (as represented by the zeta potential) was determined by laser Doppler micro-electrophoresis (Zetasizer Nano ZS; Malvern Instruments, Malvern, UK). Bacteria dispersions in 0.9% (*m/v*) NaCl with a concentration of 10.3 log CFU/mL were 200-fold diluted with deionized water, put into plastic cuvettes, and covered with the Zeta Dip Cell. The measurements of zeta potential were performed at 25 °C using an He-Ne laser, with a wavelength of 633 nm and the backscatter detector at the scattering angle of 173°. The electrophoretic mobilities measured for the bacterial cells in the applied electric field were employed to automatically calculate their zeta potential using the Smoluchowski approximation of the Henry equation. At least three measurements were performed for each bacterial strain.

2.3.2. Determination of Cell Surface Hydrophobicity of the Bacteria

The hydrophobicity of the bacteria was determined according to the method of Perez et al. [36], with some modifications. Cultures of the strains were harvested in the stationary phase by centrifugation at 12,000× *g* for 5 min at 4 °C, washed twice with 50 mM K_2HPO_4 (pH 6.5) buffer, and finally resuspended in the same buffer. The cell suspensions were adjusted to an absorbance at 560 nm (A_{560}) of 0.5. Three milliliters of bacterial suspensions was added to 0.6 mL n-hexadecane, vortexed for 120 s, and left for 30 min at room temperature, to allow separation of the two phases. The aqueous phase was carefully removed and A_{560} was measured using a spectrophotometer (Lambda Bio+; Perkin Elmer, Weltham, MA, USA). The decrease in the absorbance of the aqueous phase was taken as the measure of the cell surface hydrophobicity (H%), which was calculated as in Equation (1):

$$H\% = [(A_0\text{-}A)/A_0] \times 100 \quad (1)$$

where A_0 and A are the absorbances before and after extraction with n-hexadecane, respectively.

2.3.3. Determination of Mass of the Bacterial Cells

Bacterial dispersions in water with known numbers of cells and known dispersion volumes were frozen at −80 °C for 24 h, and then lyophilized (Beta 1-8K; Martin Christ, Osterode am Harz, Germany). The first drying phase (T_{shelf} = −5 °C; P = 0.63 mbar) was performed for 24 h, and the second drying phase (T_{shelf} = 20 °C) for 1 h. The lyophilizates obtained were weighed.

2.3.4. Growth Curves of *Lactobacillus* spp. and *L. lactis*

Overnight cultures of *Lactobacillus* spp. and *L. lactis* MG1363 were diluted (1:100) in 200 μL fresh MRS or GM-17 growth medium, respectively, in 96-well microplates. The plates were sealed with sealing film and incubated in a microplate reader (Sunrise; Tecan, Salzburg, Austria) at 37 °C (or 30 °C for *L. lactis*) for 24 h. A_{595} was measured every 2 min. The plates were shaken for 10 s before each measurement. Each culture was grown in quadruplicate. The growth rates and lag phases of the growth curves were analyzed using the DMFit 3.5 software and the model of Baranyi and Roberts [37].

2.4. *Preparation of Polymer Solutions with the Bacteria*

Overnight cultures of bacteria were diluted (1:100) in 500 mL fresh medium and grown to an optical density at 600 nm (OD_{600}) of 2.50 to 3.00. The cultures were centrifuged at 5000× *g* for 10 min, and washed twice with phosphate-buffered saline. To obtain 4% (*w/v*) PEO bacterial dispersions, the cells were dispersed in an appropriate volume of deionized water. PEO was added to the bacterial dispersions with 10.6 ± 0.8 log CFU/mL in deionized water, and stirred at room temperature for 4 h.

2.5. *Rheological Characterization of Polymer Solutions with the Bacteria*

Rotational and oscillatory tests of PEO solutions with the bacteria were performed using a rheometer (Physica MCR 301; Anton Paar, Graz, Austria) with a cone-plate measuring system (CP50-2; cone radius, 24.981 mm; cone angle, 2.001°) at a constant temperature of 25.0 ± 0.1 °C, as previously described [27,28]. The zero-gap was set to 0.209 mm. The shear rate during the rotational tests ranged from 1 /s to 100 /s, and the viscosity (η) was calculated as $\eta = \tau_c/\dot{\gamma}$, where τ_c is the shear stress and $\dot{\gamma}$ is the shear rate. The relative viscosity was calculated as the viscosity of the PEO solutions with bacteria, divided by the viscosity of the PEO solution, at a shear rate of 1 /s. Oscillatory tests were performed at a frequency from 0.2 /s to 100 /s, and an amplitude of 1%, which was within the linear viscoelastic region determined in prior amplitude-sweep experiments, to define the phase shift angle (δ). The storage (G') and loss modulus (G'') were calculated as in Equations (2) and (3), respectively:

$$G' = (\tau_a/\gamma_a) \times \cos\delta \quad (2)$$

$$G'' = (\tau_a/\gamma_a) \times \sin\delta \quad (3)$$

where τ_a is the shear stress and γ_a is the deformation. The damping factor was calculated as $\tan\delta = G''/G'$.

2.6. *Preparation of Bacteria-Loaded Nanofibers by Electrospinning*

The bacterial dispersions in 4% (*m/v*) PEO solutions were transferred into a 5 mL syringe fitted with a metallic needle of a 1 mm inner diameter and located horizontally on a syringe pump (model R-99E; RazelTM, Linari Engineering, Valpiana, Italy). The electrode of a high-voltage power supply (model HVG-P60-R-EU; Linari Engineering, Valpiana, Italy) was clamped onto the metallic needle, and the collector was grounded and covered with a piece of aluminum foil. The process was set to a flow rate of 0.4 mL/h, voltage of 15 kV, and nozzle-to-collector distance of 15 cm. Additionally, PEO solution with *Lb. delbrueckii* ssp. *bulgaricus* was electrospun in a vertical electrospinning set-up employing the same equipment and conditions as used for the horizontal electrospinning.

2.7. *Characterization of Nanofibers Loaded with the Bacteria*

2.7.1. Morphology of the Bacterial Cells and Nanofibers

Three microliters of each bacterial dispersion was pipetted onto a metal stub and air dried, and the nanofiber mats were attached to metal stubs with double-sided conductive tape. The samples were not coated prior to the imaging under scanning electron microscopy (Supra 35 VP; Carl Zeiss, Oberkochen, Jena, Germany), which was operated at an acceleration voltage of 1 kV, with a secondary detector. The length and width of at least 30 randomly selected bacteria and the diameters of 50 randomly selected nanofibers (as parts not containing any bacteria) were measured using the ImageJ 1.51j8 software (National Institutes of Health, Bethesda, MD, USA).

2.7.2. Viability of the Bacteria

The viability of the bacterial cells in the PEO solutions was determined prior to the electrospinning and after their incorporation into the nanofibers. The number of viable suspended bacteria in a known volume of bacterial dispersion was determined using the drop plate method [38]. Eight ten-fold serial dilutions of bacterial cells in PEO solutions were prepared using 50 mM phosphate buffer at pH 7.4, with each dilution in a final volume of 1 mL. Ten microliters of each dilution was pipetted onto agar plates as five replicates, and after incubation, the dilution that contained 3 to 30 colonies per single drop was counted, and replicates were averaged. These data were expressed as CFU/mL and were converted into log CFU/mL. The viability of the bacteria incorporated into the nanofibers was determined by dissolving a known mass of nanofibers in 50 mM phosphate buffer, with a pH of 7.4. Bacterial diluting and counting were performed as described above; here, the data were expressed as CFU/mg nanofibers, and were converted to log CFU/mg. The experimental bacteria loading was compared to the theoretical bacteria loading. The theoretical bacteria loading (CFU/mg) was calculated as the number of bacterial cells in the polymer solution (CFU) per dry weight of polymer and bacterial cells, in 1 mL dispersion. The dry weight of PEO was assumed to be 4 mg, while the dry weight of 1×10^{10} bacterial cells was determined as described in Section 2.3.3, and is shown in Table 2.

2.8. *Statistics*

The effects of hydrophobicity on the viability of the bacteria were analyzed by applying Mann–Whitney nonparametric tests (*, $p < 0.05$), using the GraphPad Prism 5.00 software. All of the data are presented as means ± standard deviation (SD).

3. Results

3.1. *Physical Characteristics of the Lactobacillus spp. and L. lactis*

The physical properties of the lactic acid bacteria (e.g., size, charge, and hydrophobicity) were hypothesized to affect their viability after incorporation into the nanofibers. Despite the wealth of information on lactic acid bacteria available, studies that compare physical properties and growth characteristics of multiple lactic acid bacteria are scarce; these were therefore determined in the present study for the selected pool of lactobacilli and *L. lactis* (Table 2, Figure 1). The lactobacilli differed little in terms of their average cell width. Two species had average cell lengths >2 μm, namely *Lb. gasseri* (4.68 μm) and *Lb. delbrueckii* ssp. *bulgaricus* (10.82 μm). The zeta potentials of the different species were comparable, at around −10 mV. The exceptions here were *Lactobacillus casei* and *Lactobacillus rhamnosus*, with zeta potentials of ~0 mV, and *Lactobacillus paracasei*, with the lowest zeta potential (−23.9 mV). There were considerable differences in the cell hydrophobicities, allowing division of the bacterial species into two groups: bacteria with a lower hydrophobicity (<40%; hydrophilic) and bacteria with a higher hydrophobicity (>70%; hydrophobic). Differences in mass (dry weight) of the bacteria might be attributed to the production of exopolysaccharides that differ among these different species. Exopolysaccharides can remain attached to bacteria, despite the washing step. The highest mass was determined for *Lb. rhamnosus* ATCC 53103 and *Lb. delbrueckii* ssp. *bulgaricus* ATCC 11842, which are known producers of exopolysaccharides [39,40].

Table 2. Selected physical characteristics of the bacterial species used in this study.

Bacteria Species	Average Cell Width [μm]	Average Cell Length [μm]	Zeta Potential [mV]	Hydrophobicity [%]	Mass of 1 × 10^{10} Bacterial Cells [mg]
Lb. acidophilus	0.56 ± 0.04	1.28 ± 0.26	−9.1 ± 5.0	78.6 ± 1.0	0.65
Lb. delbrueckii ssp. *bulgaricus*	0.51 ± 0.07	10.82 ± 3.31	−9.4 ± 5.5	28.5 ± 3.9	9.14
Lb. casei	0.58 ± 0.06	1.54 ± 0.36	−0.4 ± 5.5	11.3 ± 0.5	4.22
Lb. gasseri	0.65 ± 0.07	4.68 ± 1.43	−7.9 ± 4.6	92.5 ± 2.1	5.59
Lb. paracasei	0.68 ± 0.09	2.05 ± 0.49	−23.9 ± 4.4	36.4 ± 4.8	2.13
Lb. plantarum	0.52 ± 0.04	1.33 ± 0.29	−12.7 ± 4.0	74.2 ± 2.3	0.54
Lb. reuteri	0.72 ± 0.08	1.43 ± 0.37	−13.7 ± 5.7	71.9 ± 5.8	1.04
Lb. rhamnosus	0.64 ± 0.08	2.16 ± 0.51	−3.9 ± 4.4	31.5 ± 7.7	16.31
Lb. salivarius	0.70 ± 0.07	1.39 ± 0.31	−11.7 ± 4.6	90.1 ± 1.3	1.92
L. lactis	0.53 ± 0.05	0.74 ± 0.18	−12.8 ± 5.5	24.2 ± 6.3	0.48

3.2. Growth Characteristics of the Lactobacillus spp. and L. lactis

Apart from their physical properties, the bacteria also differed in their growth characteristics when cultured under the same conditions (Figure 1). *Lactobacillus salivarius* was the fastest growing *Lactobacillus* spp., with a growth rate of ~0.3 /h. *Lb. plantarum* and *Lactobacillus reuteri* had a growth rate of ~0.2 /h, while the majority of strains grew at growth rates of 0.1 /h to 0.2 /h. The slowest growers were *Lb. delbrueckii* ssp. *bulgaricus* and *Lb. casei*, with growth rates just above 0.05 /h. These last two and *Lb. paracasei* also had the longest lag times (>5 h), while the rest of the bacteria had lag times of <3 h.

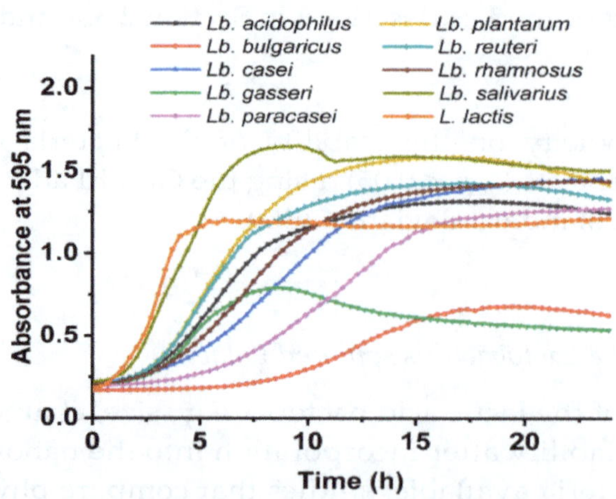

Figure 1. Representative growth curves of the *Lactobacillus spp.* and *L. lactis*.

3.3. Viscosity of Polymer Solutions with the Dispersed Bacteria

The dispersions of the bacteria in 4% (*m/v*) PEO solution increased the viscosity in comparison to 4% (*m/v*) PEO solution without the bacteria (Figure 2). The viscosity at the low shear rate (1 /s) of the PEO solution was 1.36 Pas. PEO solutions with *Lb. rhamnosus* and *Lb. salivarius* had the highest viscosities, with 2.8-fold and 2.5-fold increases, respectively, compared to the PEO solution without these bacteria. Conversely, *Lb. casei* and *Lb. plantarum* had the lowest viscosities among these bacterial dispersions, with only a 1.3-fold increase (Figure 2a). The PEO solutions and all of the PEO solutions with dispersed bacteria showed shear-thinning behavior, which was similar for all of the samples tested, with the exception of the PEO solution with *Lb. rhamnosus*, where the viscosity decreased more rapidly through an increase in the shear rate (Figure 2b). For all of the dispersions tested, the loss modulus dominated over the storage modulus (Figure 2c), and consequently, the damping factor (tan δ), as the ratio between the loss and storage modulus was >1 at all of the tested angular frequencies (Figure 2d). Therefore, in these viscoelastic dispersions, the viscous portion prevailed over the elastic one. All of these dispersions were comparable, with the exception of the PEO solution with *Lb. rhamnosus*, where the storage modulus was a lot higher (Figure 2c) and the damping factor was lower (Figure 2d). This might be attributed to the production of exopolysaccharides and the pronounced growth of *Lb. rhamnosus* as chains, as seen in Figure 3. Viscosity did not correlate with zeta potential or bacterial hydrophobicity.

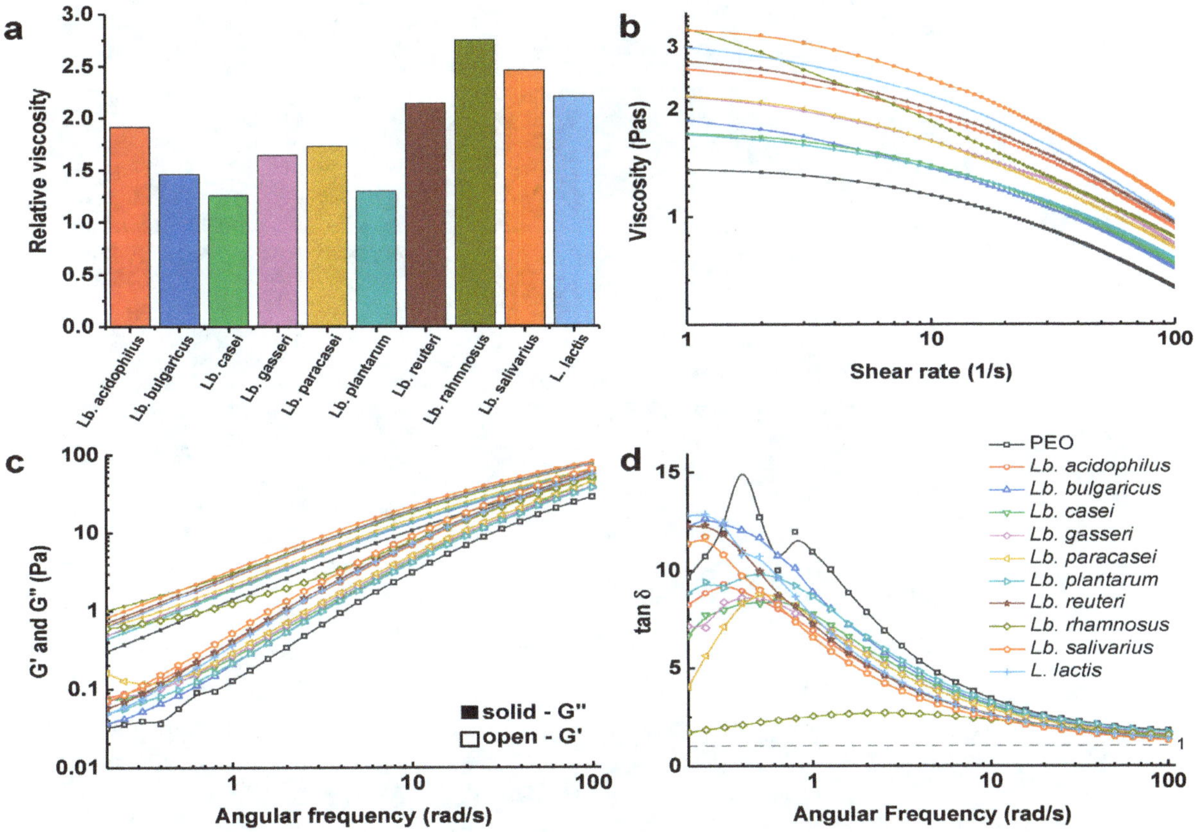

Figure 2. Rheological characterization of 4% (*m/v*) poly(ethylene oxide) (PEO) solutions without bacteria and with the dispersed *Lactobacillus* spp. or *L. lactis*. (**a**) Relative viscosity, as the ratio of the viscosity of the PEO dispersions with bacteria to that of the PEO solution, at a 1 /s shear rate. (**b**) Viscosity of the dispersions as a function of the shear rate. (**c**) Storage (G′) and loss (G″) moduli, and (**d**) tan δ as a function of the angular frequency.

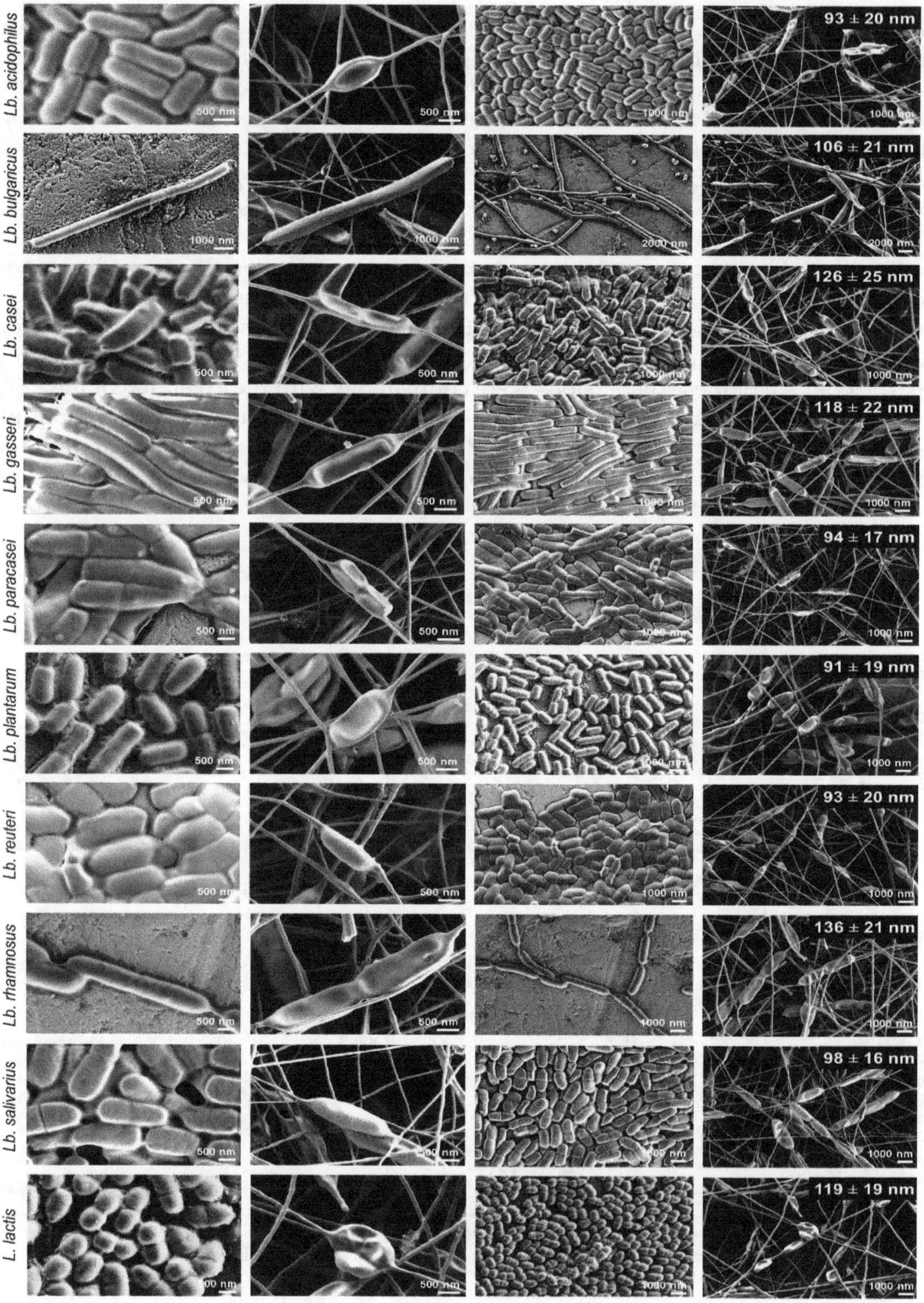

Figure 3. Scanning electron microscopy images of the lactic acid bacteria air dried from the water dispersion (columns 1, 3; under high and low magnification, respectively) and bacteria-loaded nanofibers (columns 2, 4; under high and low magnification, respectively). The numbers given in column 4 indicate the average nanofiber diameters.

3.4. Morphology of Nanofibers with the Bacteria

Under scanning electron microscopy, the thin nanofibers with a thickness of ~100 nm showed local thickenings in the shape of the bacteria, which confirmed the effective incorporation of all of these bacterial species into nanofibers (Figure 3). During SEM analysis, we did not observe any bacteria, which were not incorporated into nanofibers. The nanofiber polymer coating of the bacterial cells was thin, homogenous, and showed no cracks. Single or dividing cells were oriented along the nanofibers and evenly distributed over the nanofiber mats. These mostly retained their shape, compared to the bacteria before the incorporation; however, in some cases, the flattening of cells was seen (Figure 3). The diameters of the nanofibers with the incorporated bacteria in regions without the bacteria varied slightly among these different strains (Table 3). However, these differences did not correlate with the viscosities of the bacterial/PEO dispersions.

Table 3. Growth rates and lag times of the *Lactobacillus* spp. and *L. lactis* determined from their growth curves.

Bacterial Species	Growth Rate [/h]	Lag Time [h]
Lb. acidophilus	0.158 ± 0.005	2.31 ± 0.09
Lb. bulgaricus	0.066 ± 0.001	8.14 ± 0.15
Lb. casei	0.116 ± 0.002	3.41 ± 0.07
Lb. gasseri	0.118 ± 0.004	1.60 ± 0.15
Lb. paracasei	0.102 ± 0.010	5.50 ± 0.23
Lb. plantarum	0.199 ± 0.002	2.52 ± 0.21
Lb. reuteri	0.193 ± 0.009	1.82 ± 0.51
Lb. rhamnosus	0.125 ± 0.001	1.92 ± 0.34
Lb. salivarius	0.297 ± 0.028	1.11 ± 0.08
L. lactis	0.326 ± 0.013	0.84 ± 0.07

3.5. Viability of the Different Lactic Acid Bacteria after Electrospinning

All of the bacterial species were viable following their incorporation into the nanofibers. For five species (*Lb. acidophilus, Lb. gasseri, Lb. reuteri, Lb. salivarius*, and *L. lactis*), the survival decreased by <1 log unit, indicating a high viability. Four species (*Lb. casei, Lb. paracasei, Lb. plantarum*, and *Lb. rhamnosus*) showed a decreased survival of between 1 and 2 log units. The worst survival was for *Lb. delbrueckii* ssp. *bulgaricus*, with more than a 2 log decrease in viability (Table 4).

Table 4. Viability of the lactic acid bacteria in PEO solution before and after their incorporation into nanofibers.

Bacterial Species	Theoretical Bacteria Loading (log CFU/mg)	Experimental Bacteria Loading (log CFU/mg)	Decrease in Viability (log CFU/mg)
Lb. acidophilus	9.89 ± 0.18	9.18 ± 0.21	0.71
Lb. bulgaricus	8.74 ± 0.15	5.91 ± 0.15	2.83
Lb. casei	8.85 ± 0.21	7.33 ± 0.19	1.52
Lb. gasseri	9.30 ± 0.18	9.20 ± 0.11	0.09
Lb. paracasei	9.53 ± 0.12	8.02 ± 0.18	1.51
Lb. plantarum	9.99 ± 0.06	8.70 ± 0.38	1.29
Lb. reuteri	9.76 ± 0.13	9.32 ± 0.04	0.44
Lb. rhamnosus	8.55 ± 0.13	7.41 ± 0.16	1.14
Lb. salivarius	9.21 ± 0.06	6.75 ± 0.07	0.73
L. lactis	9.06 ± 0.14	8.19 ± 0.33	0.87

Interestingly, the loss of viability correlated with the hydrophobicity of the bacterial cells. The hydrophilic bacteria showed significantly higher decreases in viability than the hydrophobic bacteria (Figure 4). This suggests that hydrophobic molecules at the bacterial surface (e.g., including exopolysaccharides) offer better protection for the bacteria during their incorporation into nanofibers. There were no correlations between the loss of viability and viscosity of dispersion or zeta potential of cells.

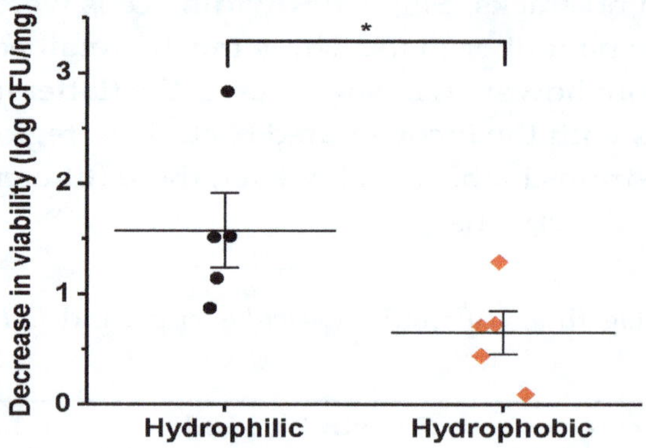

Figure 4. Bacterial cells with a lower hydrophobicity (< 40%, hydrophilic, black circles) showed larger decreases in viability after incorporation into nanofibers, in comparison to bacterial cells with a higher hydrophobicity (> 70%, hydrophobic, red diamonds). The horizontal lines indicate the means. *, $p < 0.05$ (Mann–Whitney tests).

In general, the width or length of the cells did not correlate with the viability of the bacteria. However, for *Lb. delbrueckii* ssp. *bulgaricus* in particular, the loss of viability might also be correlated with the bacterial cell size, as these bacteria had by far the longest cells and by far the highest decrease in viability. To exclude any influence of the direction of the electrospinning and possible losses of bacteria during the electrospinning due to the gravitational force, horizontal electrospinning was replaced with vertical electrospinning. The survivals here were not significantly different (Figure 5), which suggests that the direction of electrospinning has no major role in the bacterial viability.

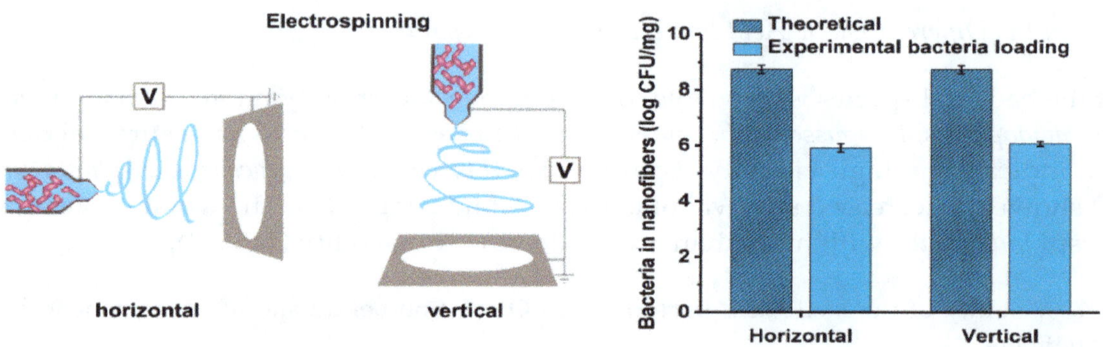

Figure 5. Theoretical and experimental loading of *Lb. delbrueckii* ssp. *bulgaricus* in nanofibers using either horizontal or vertical electrospinning.

4. Discussion

The scope of the use of probiotics can be widened by the introduction of novel delivery systems. The incorporation of probiotics into nanofibers is an emerging approach for the delivery of probiotics to body sites that require their controlled and/or sustained release. We and others have recently demonstrated the effective incorporation of lactic acid bacteria into nanofibers, and have shown that these incorporated bacteria retain their viability. However, previous studies have been limited to just five species of lactic acid bacteria: *Lb. acidophilus*, *Lb. gasseri Lb. plantarum*, *Lb. rhamnosus*, and *Bifidobacterium animalis* [19,23–28]. Different species of lactic acid bacteria can differ considerably in their properties and therapeutic effects, and therefore, it is crucial to strengthen our knowledge of the behavior of the different lactic acid bacteria during electrospinning.

We effectively incorporated nine taxonomically different species of the genus *Lactobacillus* and one species of the genus *Lactococcus* into PEO nanofibers, and have thus considerably increased our knowledge of the number of lactic acid bacteria that can be delivered using electrospun nanofibers. The dispersions of these bacteria in 4% (*m/v*) PEO solution had different rheological properties. A higher viscosity was attributed to the production of exopolysaccharides or to the pronounced chain growth phenotype. Although the bacteria in the PEO solution affected the viscosity, there was no need to change the process parameters during the electrospinning of the previously optimized electrospinning of PEO solutions without the bacteria, which enabled the production of smooth PEO nanofibers in a continuous process [26]. The previously reported mean diameter of PEO nanofibers without the incorporated bacteria was 135 ± 25 nm [26], which was similar to *Lb. rhamnosus*-loaded nanofibers here, whereas the other nanofibes were a little smaller, with the lowest mean diameter of 91 ± 19 nm for *Lb. plantarum*-loaded nanofibers. In line with previous studies, the addition of the bacteria to the PEO solutions did not only changed the viscosity, but also the dispersion conductivity. A prominent influence of conductivity over viscosity might lead to the decreased nanofiber diameters seen for the bacteria-loaded nanofibers [19,26].

While observing the bacteria-loaded nanofibers using scanning electron microscopy, we could clearly distinguish incorporated cells in nanofibers. Thus, electrospinning provided complete incorporation of the bacteria, even for the strain with the largest cells among those studied here (i.e., *Lb. delbrueckii* ssp. *bulgaricus*; cell length, 10.82 μm). As observed previously [26], although the morphology of the bacterial cells in the nanofibers was similar to their morphology obtained after air-drying the bacterial dispersions, some of the cells were flattened due to their drying and dehydration, or to the mechanical stress they had undergone [41].

All of these species of lactic acid bacteria that were incorporated survived the electrospinning; however, the theoretical and experimental bacterial loading differed. The electrospinning process results in a high incorporation efficiency of drugs [42] or bacteria [19] and here, the difference between both loadings was probably due to the decrease of bacterial viability. There were no correlations between the growth characteristics, viscosity of the dispersion, or zeta potential of the lactic acid bacteria and their survival. On the other hand, the decrease in viability of the bacteria in the nanofibers correlated with the hydrophobicities of the cells. Hydrophobicity depends on the surface structures of the bacterial cells, such as lipoteichoic acid, S-layer proteins, outer membrane proteins and lipids, surface fibrils, and various fimbriae or core oligosaccharides [43]. Considerable differences among the surface properties of lactic acid bacteria were also seen in our previous study [44]. We hypothesize that the hydrophobic surface offers better protection from the hydrophilic solution in which the bacteria are dispersed.

Another possible predictor of bacterial viability in these nanofibers is their extreme morphology. *Lb. delbrueckii* ssp. *bulgaricus* had by far the largest cells and the lowest viability, as the only species with a >2 log unit decrease in viability. This might be a consequence of the large bacteria surface per cell. The viability was not affected by the direction of electrospinning, which thus excluded gravitational effects.

To summarize, while the electrospinning process is feasible regardless of the species of lactic acid bacteria used, the prediction of viability is challenging and will require the testing of individual strains.

5. Conclusions

In the present study, we incorporated a range of safe lactic acid bacteria into PEO-based nanofibers, several of which are confirmed probiotics. All of the lactic acid bacteria remained viable after their incorporation into the nanofibers using an electrospinning procedure appropriate for PEO solutions, without the need for additional optimization. However, the survival of these lactic acid bacteria differed across two log units, and despite the determination of the physical and growth characteristics and the viscosities of the bacterial dispersions, no clear relationships were seen between the survival and the parameters measured. This suggests that the prediction of bacterial survival during the electrospinning process is challenging, and that the formulation of each particular bacterial strain will need to be optimized separately. The exceptions are the cell hydrophobicity and the extreme morphological characteristics of the bacteria (e.g., greatest size for *Lb. delbrueckii* ssp. *bulgaricus*), which offer some indications in terms of bacterial survival after their incorporation into nanofibers. The developed nanofiber-based delivery systems could be useful for the delivery of lactic acid bacteria to mucosal surfaces, such as oral, nasal, or vaginal surfaces.

Author Contributions: Conceptualization, methodology, investigation, K.Š. and Š.Z.; writing—original draft preparation, A.B., K.Š. and Š.Z.; writing—review and editing, A.B., J.K., K.Š., P.K. and Š.Z.; visualization, A.B. and Š.Z.; supervision, project administration, resources, funding acquisition, A.B. and J.K.

Acknowledgments: We thank Christopher Berrie for critical reading of the manuscript.

References

1. Salvetti, E.; Torriani, S.; Felis, G.E. The Genus Lactobacillus: A Taxonomic Update. *Probiotics Antimicrob. Proteins* **2012**, *4*, 217–226. [CrossRef] [PubMed]
2. Sun, Z.; Harris, H.M.; McCann, A.; Guo, C.; Argimon, S.; Zhang, W.; Yang, X.; Jeffery, I.B.; Cooney, J.C.; Kagawa, T.F.; et al. Expanding the biotechnology potential of lactobacilli through comparative genomics of 213 strains and associated genera. *Nat. Commun.* **2015**, *6*, 8322. [CrossRef] [PubMed]
3. Bosma, E.F.; Forster, J.; Nielsen, A.T. Lactobacilli and pediococci as versatile cell factories - Evaluation of strain properties and genetic tools. *Biotechnol. Adv.* **2017**, *35*, 419–442. [CrossRef] [PubMed]
4. Guarino, A.; Guandalini, S.; Lo Vecchio, A. Probiotics for Prevention and Treatment of Diarrhea. *J. Clin. Gastroenterol.* **2015**, *49* (Suppl. 1), S37–S45. [CrossRef]
5. AlFaleh, K.; Anabrees, J. Probiotics for prevention of necrotizing enterocolitis in preterm infants. *Cochrane Database Syst. Rev.* **2014**. [CrossRef] [PubMed]
6. Cai, J.; Zhao, C.; Du, Y.; Zhang, Y.; Zhao, M.; Zhao, Q. Comparative efficacy and tolerability of probiotics for antibiotic-associated diarrhea: Systematic review with network meta-analysis. *United Eur. Gastroenterol. J.* **2018**, *6*, 169–180. [CrossRef] [PubMed]
7. Ganji-Arjenaki, M.; Rafieian-Kopaei, M. Probiotics are a good choice in remission of inflammatory bowel diseases: A meta analysis and systematic review. *J. Cell. Physiol.* **2018**, *233*, 2091–2103. [CrossRef] [PubMed]
8. Rupa, P.; Mine, Y. Recent advances in the role of probiotics in human inflammation and gut health. *J. Agric. Food Chem.* **2012**, *60*, 8249–8256. [CrossRef] [PubMed]
9. Matsubara, V.H.; Bandara, H.M.; Ishikawa, K.H.; Mayer, M.P.; Samaranayake, L.P. The role of probiotic bacteria in managing periodontal disease: A systematic review. *Expert Rev. Anti. Infect. Ther.* **2016**, *14*, 643–655. [CrossRef]
10. Borges, S.; Barbosa, J.; Teixeira, P. Drug Delivery Systems for Vaginal Infections. *Front. Clin. Drug Res.* **2016**, *2*, 233.
11. Petrova, M.I.; Lievens, E.; Malik, S.; Imholz, N.; Lebeer, S. Lactobacillus species as biomarkers and agents that can promote various aspects of vaginal health. *Front. Physiol.* **2015**, *6*, 81. [CrossRef] [PubMed]
12. Belkaid, Y.; Naik, S. Compartmentalized and systemic control of tissue immunity by commensals. *Nat. Immunol.* **2013**, *14*, 646. [CrossRef] [PubMed]
13. Sycuro, L.K.; Fredricks, D.N. *Microbiota of the Genitourinary Tract. The Human Microbiota: How Microbial Communities Affect. Health and Disease*; John Wiley Sons: Hoboken, NJ, USA, 2013; pp. 167–210.
14. Ravel, J.; Gajer, P.; Abdo, Z.; Schneider, G.M.; Koenig, S.S.; McCulle, S.L.; Karlebach, S.; Gorle, R.; Russell, J.; Tacket, C.O.; et al. Vaginal microbiome of reproductive-age women. *Proc. Natl. Acad. Sci. USA* **2011**, *108*, 4680–4687. [CrossRef] [PubMed]
15. Gao, S.; Tang, G.; Hua, D.; Xiong, R.; Han, J.; Jiang, S.; Zhang, Q.; Huang, C. Stimuli-responsive bio-based polymeric systems and their applications. *J. Mater. Chem. B* **2019**, *7*, 709–729. [CrossRef]
16. Ding, Q.; Xu, X.; Yue, Y.; Mei, C.; Huang, C.; Jiang, S.; Wu, Q.; Han, J. Nanocellulose-Mediated Electroconductive Self-Healing Hydrogels with High Strength, Plasticity, Viscoelasticity, Stretchability, and Biocompatibility toward Multifunctional Applications. *ACS App. Mater. Inter.* **2018**, *10*, 27987–28002. [CrossRef] [PubMed]

17. Ghorani, B.; Tucker, N. Fundamentals of electrospinning as a novel delivery vehicle for bioactive compounds in food nanotechnology. *Food Hydrocolloid* **2015**, *51*, 227–240. [CrossRef]
18. Mirtič, J.; Rijavec, T.; Zupančič, S.; Zvonar Pobirk, A.; Lapanje, A.; Kristl, J. Development of probiotic-loaded microcapsules for local delivery: Physical properties, cell release and growth. *Eur. J. Pharm. Sci.* **2018**, *121*, 178–187. [CrossRef] [PubMed]
19. Zupancčič, Š.; Rijavec, T.; Lapanje, A.; Petelin, M.; Kristl, J.; Kocbek, P. Nanofibers with Incorporated Autochthonous Bacteria as Potential Probiotics for Local Treatment of Periodontal Disease. *Biomacromolecules* **2018**, *19*, 4299–4306. [CrossRef]
20. Hu, X.; Liu, S.; Zhou, G.; Huang, Y.; Xie, Z.; Jing, X. Electrospinning of polymeric nanofibers for drug delivery applications. *J. Control. Release* **2014**, *185*, 12–21. [CrossRef]
21. Chou, S.F.; Carson, D.; Woodrow, K.A. Current strategies for sustaining drug release from electrospun nanofibers. *J. Control. Release* **2015**, *220*, 584–591. [CrossRef]
22. Zupančič, Š. Core-shell nanofibers as drug delivery systems. *Acta Pharm.* **2019**, *69*, 131–153. [CrossRef] [PubMed]
23. Fung, W.Y.; Yuen, K.H.; Liong, M.T. Agrowaste-based nanofibers as a probiotic encapsulant: Fabrication and characterization. *J. Agric. Food Chem.* **2011**, *59*, 8140–8147. [CrossRef] [PubMed]
24. Lopez-Rubio, A.; Sanchez, E.; Wilkanowicz, S.; Sanz, Y.; Lagaron, J.M. Electrospinning as a useful technique for the encapsulation of living bifidobacteria in food hydrocolloids. *Food Hydrocolloid* **2012**, *28*, 159–167. [CrossRef]
25. Nagy, Z.K.; Wagner, I.; Suhajda, A.; Tobak, T.; Harasztos, A.H.; Vigh, T.; Soti, P.L.; Pataki, H.; Molnar, K.; Marosi, G. Nanofibrous solid dosage form of living bacteria prepared by electrospinning. *Express Polym. Lett.* **2014**, *8*, 352–361. [CrossRef]
26. Skrlec, K.; Zupancic, S.; Prpar Mihevc, S.; Kocbek, P.; Kristl, J.; Berlec, A. Development of electrospun nanofibers that enable high loading and long-term viability of probiotics. *Eur. J. Pharm. Biopharm.* **2019**, *136*, 108–119. [CrossRef] [PubMed]
27. Ceylan, Z.; Meral, R.; Karakaş, C.Y.; Dertli, E.; Yilmaz, M.T. A novel strategy for probiotic bacteria: Ensuring microbial stability of fish fillets using characterized probiotic bacteria-loaded nanofibers. *Innov. Food Sci. Emerg. Technol.* **2018**, *48*, 212–218. [CrossRef]
28. Amna, T.; Hassan, M.S.; Pandeya, D.R.; Khil, M.S.; Hwang, I.H. Classy non-wovens based on animate L. gasseri-inanimate poly(vinyl alcohol): Upstream application in food engineering. *Appl. Microbiol. Biotechnol.* **2013**, *97*, 4523–4531. [CrossRef] [PubMed]
29. Palomino, M.M.; Allievi, M.C.; Fina Martin, J.; Waehner, P.M.; Prado Acosta, M.; Sanchez Rivas, C.; Ruzal, S.M. Draft Genome Sequence of the Probiotic Strain Lactobacillus acidophilus ATCC 4356. *Genome Announc.* **2015**, *3*. [CrossRef] [PubMed]
30. van de Guchte, M.; Penaud, S.; Grimaldi, C.; Barbe, V.; Bryson, K.; Nicolas, P.; Robert, C.; Oztas, S.; Mangenot, S.; Couloux, A.; et al. The complete genome sequence of Lactobacillus bulgaricus reveals extensive and ongoing reductive evolution. *Proc. Natl. Acad. Sci. USA* **2006**, *103*, 9274–9279. [CrossRef] [PubMed]
31. Toh, H.; Oshima, K.; Nakano, A.; Takahata, M.; Murakami, M.; Takaki, T.; Nishiyama, H.; Igimi, S.; Hattori, M.; Morita, H. Genomic adaptation of the Lactobacillus casei group. *PLoS ONE* **2013**, *8*, e75073. [CrossRef] [PubMed]
32. Azcarate-Peril, M.A.; Altermann, E.; Goh, Y.J.; Tallon, R.; Sanozky-Dawes, R.B.; Pfeiler, E.A.; O'Flaherty, S.; Buck, B.L.; Dobson, A.; Duong, T.; et al. Analysis of the genome sequence of Lactobacillus gasseri ATCC 33323 reveals the molecular basis of an autochthonous intestinal organism. *Appl. Environ. Microbiol.* **2008**, *74*, 4610–4625. [CrossRef] [PubMed]
33. Saulnier, D.M.; Santos, F.; Roos, S.; Mistretta, T.A.; Spinler, J.K.; Molenaar, D.; Teusink, B.; Versalovic, J. Exploring metabolic pathway reconstruction and genome-wide expression profiling in Lactobacillus reuteri to define functional probiotic features. *PLoS ONE* **2011**, *6*, e18783. [CrossRef] [PubMed]
34. Morita, H.; Toh, H.; Oshima, K.; Murakami, M.; Taylor, T.D.; Igimi, S.; Hattori, M. Complete genome sequence of the probiotic Lactobacillus rhamnosus ATCC 53103. *J. Bacteriol.* **2009**, *191*, 7630–7631. [CrossRef] [PubMed]
35. Linares, D.M.; Kok, J.; Poolman, B. Genome sequences of Lactococcus lactis MG1363 (revised) and NZ9000 and comparative physiological studies. *J. Bacteriol.* **2010**, *192*, 5806–5812. [CrossRef] [PubMed]
36. Perez, P.F.; Minnaard, Y.; Disalvo, E.A.; De Antoni, G.L. Surface properties of bifidobacterial strains of human origin. *Appl. Environ. Microbiol.* **1998**, *64*, 21–26. [PubMed]

37. Baranyi, J.; Roberts, T.A. A dynamic approach to predicting bacterial growth in food. *Int. J. Food Microbiol.* **1994**, *23*, 277–294. [CrossRef]
38. Herigstad, B.; Hamilton, M.; Heersink, J. How to optimize the drop plate method for enumerating bacteria. *J. Microbiol. Methods* **2001**, *44*, 121–129. [CrossRef]
39. Lebeer, S.; Verhoeven, T.L.; Francius, G.; Schoofs, G.; Lambrichts, I.; Dufrene, Y.; Vanderleyden, J.; De Keersmaecker, S.C. Identification of a Gene Cluster for the Biosynthesis of a Long, Galactose-Rich Exopolysaccharide in Lactobacillus rhamnosus GG and Functional Analysis of the Priming Glycosyltransferase. *Appl. Environ. Microbiol.* **2009**, *75*, 3554–3563. [CrossRef]
40. Zeidan, A.A.; Poulsen, V.K.; Janzen, T.; Buldo, P.; Derkx, P.M.F.; Oregaard, G.; Neves, A.R. Polysaccharide production by lactic acid bacteria: From genes to industrial applications. *FEMS Microbiol. Rev.* **2017**, *41*, S168–S200. [CrossRef]
41. Reznik, S.N.; Yarin, A.L.; Zussman, E.; Bercovici, L. Evolution of a compound droplet attached to a core-shell nozzle under the action of a strong electric field. *Phys. Fluids* **2006**, *18*, 062101. [CrossRef]
42. Kajdič, S.; Vrečer, F.; Kocbek, P. Preparation of poloxamer-based nanofibers for enhanced dissolution of carvedilol. *Eur. J. Pharm. Sci.* **2018**, *117*, 331–340. [CrossRef] [PubMed]
43. Krasowska, A.; Sigler, K. How microorganisms use hydrophobicity and what does this mean for human needs? *Front. Cell Infect. Microbiol.* **2014**, *4*, 112. [CrossRef] [PubMed]
44. Zadravec, P.; Štrukelj, B.; Berlec, A. Improvement of LysM-mediated surface display of designed ankyrin repeat proteins (DARPins) in recombinant and nonrecombinant strains of Lactococcus lactis and Lactobacillus Species. *Appl. Environ. Microbiol.* **2015**, *81*, 2098–2106. [CrossRef] [PubMed]

6

Development and In Vitro-In Vivo Evaluation of a Novel Sustained-Release Loxoprofen Pellet with Double Coating Layer

Dongwei Wan [1], Min Zhao [1], Jingjing Zhang [1] and Libiao Luan [2,*]

[1] College of Pharmacy, China Pharmaceutical University, No. 639 Longmian Road, Nanjing 211100, China; 710176323@163.com (D.W.); 19850856528@163.com (M.Z.); 15651915012@163.com (J.Z.)

[2] College of Pharmacy, China Pharmaceutical University, Xuanwumen Campus, No. 24 Tongjiaxiang, Nanjing 210009, China

* Correspondence: luanlibiao@126.com;

Abstract: This study aimed to develop a novel sustained release pellet of loxoprofen sodium (LXP) by coating a dissolution-rate controlling sub-layer containing hydroxypropyl methyl cellulose (HPMC) and citric acid, and a second diffusion-rate controlling layer containing aqueous dispersion of ethyl cellulose (ADEC) on the surface of a LXP conventional pellet, and to compare its performance in vivo with an immediate release tablet (Loxinon®). A three-level, three-factor Box-Behnken design and the response surface model (RSM) were used to investigate and optimize the effects of the citric acid content in the sub-layer, the sub-layer coating level, and the outer ADEC coating level on the in vitro release profiles of LXP sustained release pellets. The pharmacokinetic studies of the optimal sustained release pellets were performed in fasted beagle dogs using an immediate release tablet as a reference. The results illustrated that both the citric acid (CA) and ADEC as the dissolution- and diffusion-rate controlling materials significantly decreased the drug release rate. The optimal formulation showed a pH-independent drug release in media at pH above 4.5 and a slightly slow release in acid medium. The pharmacokinetic studies revealed that a more stable and prolonged plasma drug concentration profile of the optimal pellets was achieved, with a relative bioavaibility of 87.16% compared with the conventional tablets. This article provided a novel concept of two-step control of the release rate of LXP, which showed a sustained release both in vitro and in vivo.

Keywords: sustained release pellets; double coating layer; loxoprofen; citric acid; pharmacokinetic studies

---

1. Introduction

Pellets, as multiple unit preparations, offer a lot of clinical benefits compared with single unit dosage forms, such as reduced intra- and inter-subject variability on drug plasma, decreased local irritations, less dose dumping risk, and stable plasma concentrations [1,2]. To prepare sustained release pellets, film coating is an ideal method. With the development of aqueous-based dispersion systems, film coating technologies have shifted from organic-based polymeric solutions to aqueous-based polymeric dispersion systems [3]. As one of the aqueous ethyl cellulose dispersions, Surelease® (ADEC) could be used alone or combined with other polymers to obtain satisfactory release profiles [4–7]. Additionally, most of these release profiles showed a diffusion-controlled release mechanism, which meant a predictable release pattern could be achieved by altering the ADEC coating weight gain [8,9].

Loxoprofen sodium (LXP), as a 2-phenylpropinate non-steroidal anti-inflammatory drug (NSAD), was first introduced by Sankyo Company in Japan. It has been widely used for the treatment of osteoarthritis, scapulohumeral periarthritis, rheumatoid arthritis, arthritis, toothache, and post-operation pain [10]. As a pro-drug, LXP is converted to its active metabolite (trans-OH LXP) in vivo to inhibit the activity of cycloosygenase (COX), which mediates the production of inflammatory prostaglandins [11]. Due to the short elimination half-life of approximately 65 min [12], the commercial tablet of LXP has to be administrated three times a day to maintain the therapeutic concentration in plasma, which might cause high risks of gastrointestinal (GI) lesions and systemic side effects [13,14]. Several studies have been reported on the preparation of LXP sustained release dosage forms [15–17]. However, due to its high solubility, most of the preparations, especially for the matrix-based formulations, showed a burst release (drug release >30%) during the first 2 h [18], which could cause unexpected GI mucosal injury for patients. Therefore, a sustained release dosage form with decreased initial release would be necessary.

As a weakly acidic drug, loxoprofen shows good solubility at high pH, while poor solubility at low pH. Several strategies have been developed to prepare sustained release formulations of the pH-sensitive drugs [19–22]. Among them, incorporation of pH-modifiers into the preparation was a common approach in matrix or coating systems. These pH modifiers could significantly modify the micro-environmental pH (pH_M) inside the systems, and result in a decrease or increase of the drug solubility, leading to a modified drug dissolution rate [22–24]. In addition, their extent and duration played an important role on the drug release rate [25]. Approaches like using coated pH-modifier as the starting core [23], blending pH-modifier with drugs into the core with a subsequent coating [26], or incorporating pH-modifiers into the matrix formulations [20], have been proposed and studied to achieve the sustained release of pH-sensitive drugs. However, for the maintenance of an appropriate pH_M inside the dosage forms, more than 20% pH-modifiers in the preparations were often needed [20,23,26], which might cause undesired GI irritations, especially for patients with GI ulcers. In order to reduce the usage of pH-modifiers and maintain an appropriate pH_M in the dosage form, citric acid (CA) as the pH-modifier was first proposed to be incorporated into the dissolution-rate controlling layer to decrease the dissolution rate of LXP.

Drug delivery systems (DDS), based on their system design or rate-controlling mechanism, can be divided into models such as dissolution, diffusion, erosion, osmosis, and swelling [27]. As for the film coating systems, the diffusion or osmosis mechanisms were often applied to elucidate the drug release profiles [5,28–30], while the influence of drug dissolution rate was often omitted or just attributed to the drug diffusion rate [27]. In the most common cases, only one of these mechanisms was applied to control the drug release rate in DDS, except for the bio-erodible or hydrogel matrix systems, where the drug release rate was controlled by two or three of these release mechanisms [31,32]. Although theoretical approaches regarding the dissolution-diffusion mechanism have been extensively reported [33,34], a combination of the dissolution and diffusion release mechanisms as a rate-controlling strategy was seldom reported.

In this study, a novel concept of two-step control of the drug release rate is proposed. A schematic diagram of this hypothesis is illustrated in Figure 1. In this system, the first-step control was to reduce the dissolution rate of LXP by creating a sub-coating layer containing pH-modifier CA, while the second-step control was to decrease the diffusion rate of LXP by creating a non-soluble polymeric film. Furthermore, a three-level, three-factor Box-Behnken experiments design was conducted to optimize and evaluate the effects of different parameters on the drug release. Additionally, the pharmacokinetic studies of the optimal formulation were performed in fasted beagles to compare its in vivo performance with the conventional tablet.

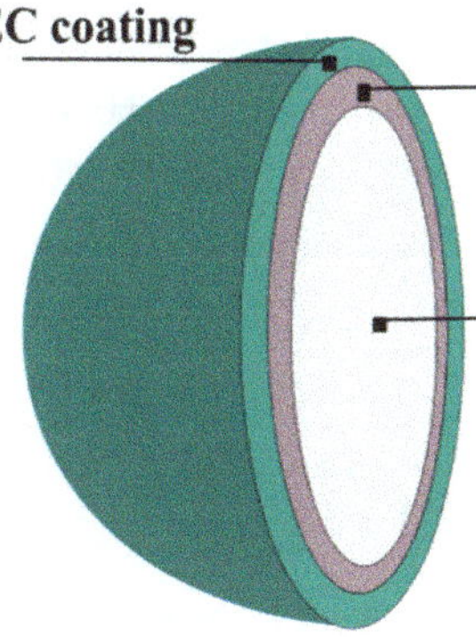

Figure 1. Schematic diagram of the sustained release pellets.

2. Materials and Methods

2.1. Materials

LXP dihydrate was purchased from Fujian Hui Tian biological Pharmaceutical Co., Ltd. (99.1% purity, China). Loxonin® tablets were purchased from Daiichi Sankyo Co., Ltd. (Tokyo, Japan). Ketoprofen was purchased from Sigma (St. Louis, MO, USA). Microcrystalline cellulose SH-101 and corn starch were supplied by Sunhere Pharmaceutical Co., Ltd. (Huainan, China). Hydroxypropylmethyl cellulose (Methocel E5LV) and Surelease® E-7-7050 (aqueous ethyl cellulose dispersion) were supplied by Colorcon Ltd. (Dartford, Kent, UK). Hard gelatin capsules were from Suzhou Capsugel Ltd. (Suzhou, China). Other chemicals were of reagent grade or higher grades.

2.2. HPLC-Assay for LXP and CA Contents

HPLC methods were used for the determination of LXP and CA. Chromatograph was carried out on Shimadzu LC-2030 (Shimadzu, Japan), equipped with an autosampler and an SPD-20A UV detector. The mobile phase used for the determination of LXP consisted of a mixture of methanol-water-acetic acid-triethylamine (600:400:1:1, *v/v*). Separation was achieved by applying an Inertsil C18 column (5 μm, 4.6 × 150 mm, Shimadzu, Japan), and the chromatogram was recorded at 223 nm. The limit of determination (LOD) and limit of quantitation (LOQ) for LXP were 0.03 and 0.1 μg/mL respectively. The mobile phase performed for the determination of CA was carried out with one part isopropanol and 999 parts 0.018 M phosphate buffer, adjusted to pH 2.5 with phosphoric acid. An Inertsil C18 column (5 μm, 4.6 × 150 mm, Shimadzu, Japan) was employed to separate the CA content. The flow rate was 1 mL/min, and the column temperature was controlled at 40 °C with the UV detection at 210 nm. The LOD and LOQ for CA were 0.2 and 0.6 μg/mL respectively. In addition, the calibration curve over the concentration range of 0.6–60 μg/mL had a regression coefficient of 0.9996.

2.3. Solubility/pH Profiles of LXP

Solubilities of LXP in different pH media were determined by adding excess of LXP to different buffer solutions: hydrochloric acid solutions (pH 1.2, 2.2), phosphate buffers (pH 3.0, 3.5, 4.0, 4.5 and 6.8). After vibrated at 25 °C for 24 h in a constant-temperature shaker (SHZ-82, Guohua Co., Ltd., Changzhou, China), 2 mL of the saturated solution was filtered through a membrane filter, and was diluted to avoid crystallization. Sample was determined by HPLC method.

2.4. Preparation of Drug-Loaded Pellets

The core consisted of loxoprofen sodium (37.1%, *w/w*), microcrystalline cellulose (41.9%, *w/w*), corn starch (19.9%, *w/w*), and talc (1.1%, *w/w*). Briefly, the mixture was blended in an ERWEKA mixer (Type AR YB5, Heusenstamm, Germany) at a speed of 40 rpm for 30 min. Then it was kneaded with the ethanol water solution (30%, *v/v*) in a laboratory kneader (Type LK5, Heusenstamm, Germany) for 10 min. The obtained moist mass was extruded at a speed of 500 rpm through a stainless steel barrel with a die of 0.8 mm diameter. Then, 300 g of the extrudates were processed in a 23 cm radial cut plate of spheronizer (JBZ-300, Liaoning New Drug Research Institute, China) at 1000 rpm for 10 min. The obtained pellets were collected on a Teflon tray and were dried in a hot oven at 60 °C for 24 h to remove the residual water and ethanol. Pellets with fraction size between 800 and 1250 μm were used for the following procedure.

2.5. Preparation of Sustained-Release Pellets

2.5.1. Preparation of the Dissolution-Rate Controlling Layer

Methocel E5 LV was added to purified water to achieve a hydroxypropylmethyl cellulose concentration of 4% (*w/w*). Then the solution was mixed with critic acid, with a concentration range from 0% to 6% (*w/w*), and was plasticized with PEG 6000 (0.5%, *w/w*) for 40 min [9]. Then, talc was added to the polymer mixture at a concentration of 2.5% (*w/w*). The aqueous suspension was stirred during the coating process. Using bottom spray with a Wurster insert, 50 g pellets were coated in a laboratory-scale fluid bed coater (Hanse, Changzhou, China). The process parameters were as follows: inlet temperature 50 °C, material temperature 40 °C, atomization pressure 0.15 MPa, spray rate 0.8 mL/min, and air flow rate 35 m^3/h.

2.5.2. Preparation of the Diffusion-Rate Controlling Layer

ADEC was separately used as the diffusion-rate controlling layer. Mainly, aqueous dispersion of Surelease® was diluted in purified water to achieve a solid content of 15% (*w/w*), and was stirred for 45 min before coating. Then the aqueous dispersion was sprayed on pellets sub-coated with the dissolution-rate controlling layer in the same equipment. The process parameters for ADEC coating were as follows: inlet temperature 54 °C, material temperature 42 °C, atomization pressure 0.18 MPa, spray rate 1.0 mL/min and air flow rate 40 m^3/h. After the coating process, pellets were cured in a hot oven at 60 °C for 16 h.

2.6. Experimental Design

A three-factor, three-level Box-Behnken experiment design was applied to evaluate the effects of different parameters on drug release rate. Briefly, the design is equal to the three replicated centre points and the set of points lying at the midpoint of each surface of the three-dimensional cube that defines the region of interest of each parameter. The three independent variables (X_1, X_2 or X_3) were the concentration of CA in the sub-coating aqueous dispersion (X_1), the sub-coating weight gain based on the dry uncoated pellet mass (X_2), and the ADEC coating weight gain based on the sub coated pellets mass (X_3). Each variable was coded to be in the range of −1, 0, 1, which represented different variable levels. Levels of the factors and constraints for the in vitro drug release based on preliminary pharmacokinetic study are listed in Table 1. The design required 15 experimental formulations. The independent variables of each formulation and their responses are listed in Table 2. The response surface model generated by the design is given as Equation (1):

$$Y = a_0 + a_{1\times1} + a_2X_2 + a_3X_3 + a_4X_1X_2 + a_5X_2X_3 + a_6X_1X_3 + a_7X_1{}^2 + a_8X_2{}^2 + a_9X_3{}^2 \quad (1)$$

where Y is the response parameter, X_1, X_2, and X_3 are the independent parameters, a_0 is the intercept, $a_1 - a_3$ are the main effect coefficients, $a_4 - a_9$ are coefficients of parameters with interaction or quadratic effects. Statistical analysis of the model was performed in Design-Expert software (V.8.0.6, Stat-Ease Inc., Minneapolis, MN, USA). The regression models of Y_1, Y_2, and Y_3 were evaluated in terms of statistically significant coefficients using analysis of variance (ANOVA) and r^2 values. Only coefficients with p values less than 0.05 were constructed in the models. In addition, response surface plots were performed to visualize the effect of parameters and their interactions on the responses. Design space, which was determined from the common region of successful operating ranges for the responses, was established following the obtained response surface to clarify the optimal formulation.

Table 1. The factors and responses of the Box-Behnken design.

Independent Variables	Levels Used		
	−1	0	1
X_1 = citric acid concentration (%)	1	2	3
X_2 = subcoating weight (%)	6	8	10
X_3 = ADEC coating weight (%)	10	13	16
Responses		Constraints	
Y_1 = the drug release within 2 h		<30%	
Y_2 = the drug release within 6 h		50–70%	
Y_3 = the drug release within 12 h		>90%	

Table 2. Independent variables and observed responses of the Box-Behnken design.

Formulations	Factors (%)			Responses (%)		
	X_1	X_2	X_3	Y_1	Y_2	Y_3
1	2.0	10.0	10.0	21.5	71.2	93.8
2	3.0	10.0	13.0	8.4	46.0	78.5
3	2.0	6.0	16.0	7.4	40.9	68.9
4	2.0	8.0	13.0	17.1	54.8	87.0
5	3.0	6.0	13.0	13.1	53.8	81.0
6	1.0	6.0	13.0	31.4	75.0	91.0
7	1.0	8.0	16.0	21.0	58.0	86.0
8	2.0	8.0	13.0	17.7	59.7	89.0
9	1.0	10.0	13.0	27.8	75.5	92.6
10	3.0	8.0	16.0	13.6	33.1	57.7
11	1.0	8.0	10.0	56.0	88.0	99.0
12	2.0	10.0	16.0	8.6	40.2	68.3
13	3.0	8.0	10.0	20.5	60.2	91.0
14	2.0	6.0	10.0	38.2	81.6	90.0
15	2.0	8.0	13.0	13.9	60.7	89.0

2.7. *In Vitro Release of LXP and CA*

A dissolution test was carried out at 37 °C in 900 mL water, using a dissolution apparatus (78X-6A, Huanghai medicine inspecting institute, China) with the basket rotation speed of 100 rpm, which is specified in China Pharmacopoeia. The prepared sustained-release pellets containing 90 mg of anhydrous LXP were added to the dissolution apparatus. At pre-determined intervals, 5 mL of the sample was withdrawn and replaced with fresh medium. Then the samples were analyzed by HPLC.

In order to better understand the impact of CA on the drug release rate, simultaneous release profiles of CA and LXP in formulations with different CA concentrations were conducted. Additionally, the impact of dissolution media on the release of CA and LXP were investigated by performing the dissolution tests in the following media: pH 1.0 HCl, pH 4.5 and 6.8 phosphate buffers, and water. The contents of CA and LXP in the formulations were determined by HPLC.

2.8. *Release Mechanism Studies*

The in vitro release mechanisms of LXP were analyzed by seven kinetics models. As shown in Table 3, Q_t is the release amount of LXP at time t, Q_0 is the initial amount of LXP in the pellets, k_0 is the zero order release constant and k_1 is the first order release constant, k_H is the Higuchi dissolution constant, n is exponent constant characterizing different release mechanisms, a is a time scale parameter and b is a shape parameter that characterizes the curves of the release profiles. The dissolution data of LXP were fitted to these models by linear or non-linear least-squares fitting methods. The correlation coefficients calculated by regression analysis were used to evaluate the goodness of fit for each model.

Table 3. Models for drug release.

Model Name	Equation
Zero-order model	$Q_t = k_0 t$
First-order model	$ln(Q_0 - Q_t) = -k_1 t + Q_0$
Higuchi diffusion model	$Q_t = k_H t^{1/2}$
Ritger–Peppas model	$lnQ_t = n\ lnt + k$
Weibull distribution model	$log[-ln(1 - Q_t)] = b\ logt - loga$
Hixson–Crowell model	$(1 - Q_t)^{1/3} = 1 - kt$
Baker–Lonsdale model	$3/2\ [\ 1 - (1 - Q_t)^{2/3}] - Q_t = kt$

2.9. Morphology Study

Scanning electron microscopy (S-8000; Hitachi High-Technologies Europe, Krefeld, Germany) was used to evaluate the morphology of the surface and cross-section of coating pellets. Samples were fitted on the copper sample holder with a double sided adhesive tape, sputter coated with a 10-nm thick gold layer under argon atmosphere.

2.10. The Pharmacokinetic Studies

2.10.1. Administration Programme

All animal treatments were performed in accordance with the Regulations of the Administration of Affairs Concerning Experimental Animals and the study protocol was admitted by the Ethics Committee of China Pharmaceutical University (Approval No. 2018-0315). An open label, randomized, two-period crossover experiment design with one week wash-out period was used in this study. Six male beagle dogs (weight 8.7 ± 1.1 kg), fasted but free access to water for 12 h prior to the experiment, were used in the study. Pellets of the optimal formulation were filled into hard gelatin capsules. The immediate release tablet (Loxonin®, 60 mg anhydrous LXP) and the capsule of the optimal formulation (90 mg anhydrous LXP) were administered to beagles in the morning with 100 mL water. Then, 6 h after dosing, dogs were provided with standard food.

A total of 2 mL of the blood samples were withdrawn before and then 0.5, 1.0, 2.0, 3.0, 4.0, 5.0, 6.0, 8.0, 10.0, and 12.0 h after dosing via cannulated needle from front legs. Plasma was obtained by centrifuging the blood at 4000 rpm for 15 min, and was kept frozen at −20 °C before analysis.

2.10.2. Determination of LXP in Plasma

A stable and selective HPLC method, modified by previous papers [12,35], was applied for the analysis of LXP in dog plasma. Pretreatment was carried out by adding 50 μL of internal standard (100 μg/mL ketoprofen in acetonitrile), 50 μL of zinc sulfate solution (10%, *w/w*) and 750 μL acetonitrile into 500 μL plasma sample. After vortex-mixing for 1 min, sample was centrifuged at 8000 rmp for 15 min. Then 10 μL of the supernatant was injected into the HPLC system. The separation was performed on an Inertsil C18-ODS column (5 μm, 4.6 × 150 mm, Shimadzu, Japan) with a guard column (4.6 × 10 mm, 5 μm particle size, ANPEL Laboratory Technologies Inc, Shanghai, China) at a flow rate of 1 mL/min. Additionally, the mobile phase was a mixture of acetonitrile and 0.05 M monopotassium phosphate (35:65, *v/v*), adjusted to pH 3.0 with phosphoric acid. Chromatograms were recorded at 223 nm with a Shimadzu-SPD detector. The linear range of this method was 0.1–20.0 μg/mL with an r^2 value of not less than 0.999. The lower limit of quantification (LLOQ) was 100 ng/mL and the extraction recoveries of high, middle, and low concentrations of LXP were 102.5 ± 2.0%, 97.1 ± 2.5%

and 97.1 ± 5.9%, respectively. The R.S.D.s reflecting the intra-day and inter-day precision of LXP were less than 11.77%.

2.10.3. Bioavailability Study

Non-compartmental pharmacokinetic analysis was applied to calculate parameters such as T_{max}, C_{max}, AUC_{0-t}, and $AUC_{0-\infty}$ from the plasma concentration-time curve data using WinNonlin software (version 1.5, Pharsight Corp. Mountain View, CA, USA). The relative bioavailability of the optimal formulation to the commercial tablet (reference) was calculated using the following Equation (2):

$$\text{Relative.bioavaibility} = \frac{AUC_{T0-\infty} \times X_R}{AUC_{R0-\infty} \times X_T} \times 100\% \quad (2)$$

where X_R and X_T were the administered dose of the reference and test respectively. Results were presented as means ± standard deviation. A one-way ANOVA (SPSS, version 19) with $p < 0.05$ as a level of significance was applied to examine the differences of C_{max} and $AUC_{0-\infty}$ between the test and reference.

3. Results and Discussions

3.1. Impact of CA on Drug Release

Formulations with different concentrations of CA in the sub-layer were developed to evaluate the effect of pH-modifier on the drug release rate, while the dissolution-controlling layer and ADEC coating levels were kept at 8% and 11% respectively. The results in Figure 2 illustrated that formulation without CA showed a fast release of LXP (>80% within 2 h), while the drug release within 2 h was decreased to 40% at a CA concentration of 1%. Additionally, the release rate continued to decrease with the increase of CA concentration, which showed 16.37%, 11.34%, and 7.77% of LXP release within the first 2 h. At the CA concentration of 1%, a completed drug release was finished within 6 h. While at higher CA concentrations, there were still 21.80% (2.5% CA) and 32.43% (4.0% CA) of the initial drug amount released after 6 h.

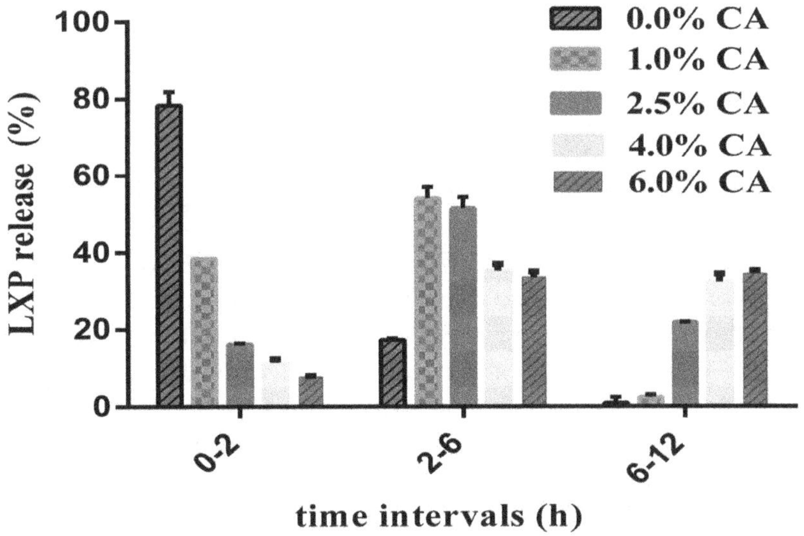

Figure 2. Effect of citric acid concentration on the drug release within different intervals.

As a pH modifier, CA was aimed to modulate the pH_M inside the systems. For pH-sensitive compound, its solubility is more appropriate to be described as the solubility in the diffusion layer at the surface of the dissolving particles [25]. Therefore, according to the Noyes–Whitney theory, the dissolution rate of LXP was much more dependent on the solubility in the low pH_M beneath the diffusion-controlling layer, other than the dissolution media. Theoretically, drug release rate from a coherent film coating system is controlled by both the coating level and the drug concentration gradient across the coating film, which obeyed the Fick's diffusion law. As the film coating level was kept constant, drug release rate was predominantly controlled by the drug concentration gradient, which was determined by the dissolution rate of LXP inside the pellets. Therefore, as the drug release was significantly decreased with the increase of CA concentrations (Figure 2), the first step of developing a dissolution-rate controlling layer proved to work.

Furthermore, simultaneous release profiles in Figure 3 were constructed to investigate the impact of dynamic release process of CA on the drug release rate. In formulations with lower CA concentrations, with the release of CA during the dissolution period, pH_M could be changed from 0.4 (the saturated solution pH of CA) to the approximate equilibrium pH of the dissolution medium [36]. As the solubility of LXP changed approximately 300 times within this pH range (Supplementary Materials Figure S1), the drug dissolution rate was significantly dependent on the amount of CA left inside the pellets. Therefore, matching release profiles of LXP and CA were observed at low concentrations of CA.

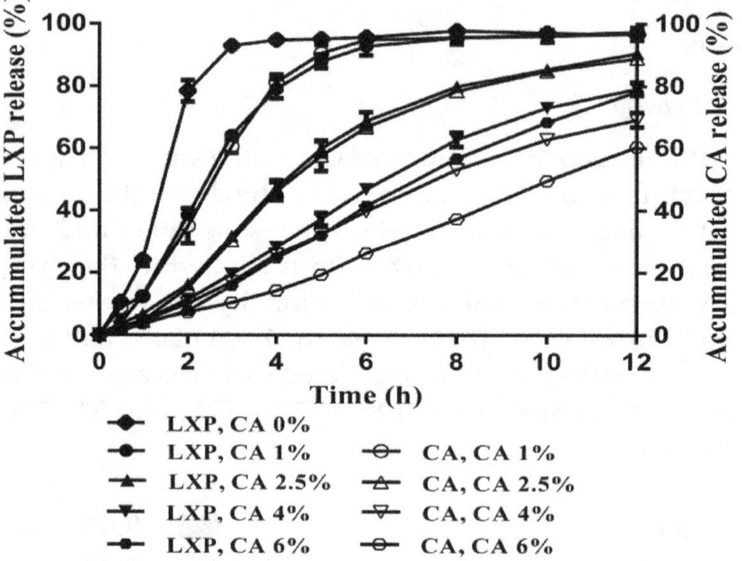

Figure 3. The simultaneous release profiles of citric acid and loxoprofen from sustained release pellets at different concentrations of citric acid (n = 3).

While in formulations with higher CA concentrations, as a sufficient amount of CA remained inside the pellets at the end of the dissolution period, e.g., 30% or 40% of the initial CA amount left at the concentration of 4% or 6% respectively, a constant and effective pH_M was achieved inside the pellets, which resulted in no further decrease of the drug release rate (Figure 3). A similar phenomenon was observed in a matrix tablet containing dipyridamole, due to a constant and effective pH_M maintained by fumaric acid inside the dosage form, no further enhancement of the dipyridamole release was observed after increasing the fumaric acid concentration to 40% [37]. Therefore, a discrepancy of the release profiles between CA and LXP was observed in formulations with higher CA concentrations.

3.2. Release Experiments and Statistical Evaluation

3.2.1. Testing of Drug Release

Experimental variables and observed responses of all the 15 formulations were listed in Table 2. And their drug dissolution profiles were displayed in Figure 4. At a low level of CA concentration, most of the formulations (Formulation Nos. 6, 9, 11) showed a fast drug release except Formulation No. 7, which had a high coating level of ADEC. The fast release in Formulation Nos. 6, 9, 11 was attributed to an inefficient pH_M inside the pellets and the short diffusion pathway of ADEC coating, which could be identified as the failure of the first- and second-step control. As a prolonged diffusion pathway was developed in Formulation No. 7, the release rate of LXP was significantly decreased. While at a low coating level of ADEC, most of the formulations (Formulation Nos. 1, 11, 14) showed a fast drug release rate, expect Formulation No. 13, which was incorporated with a high concentration of CA. The fast release in Formulation Nos. 1, 11, 14 could be explained by a failure of the second-step control, as a short diffusion pathway created by the low coating level of ADEC was unable to retard the release rate of LXP. However, when 3% of the CA concentration was applied in Formulation No. 13, the effective control of the drug dissolution-rate could compensate for the failure of the diffusion-rate control to achieve a sustained release of LXP.

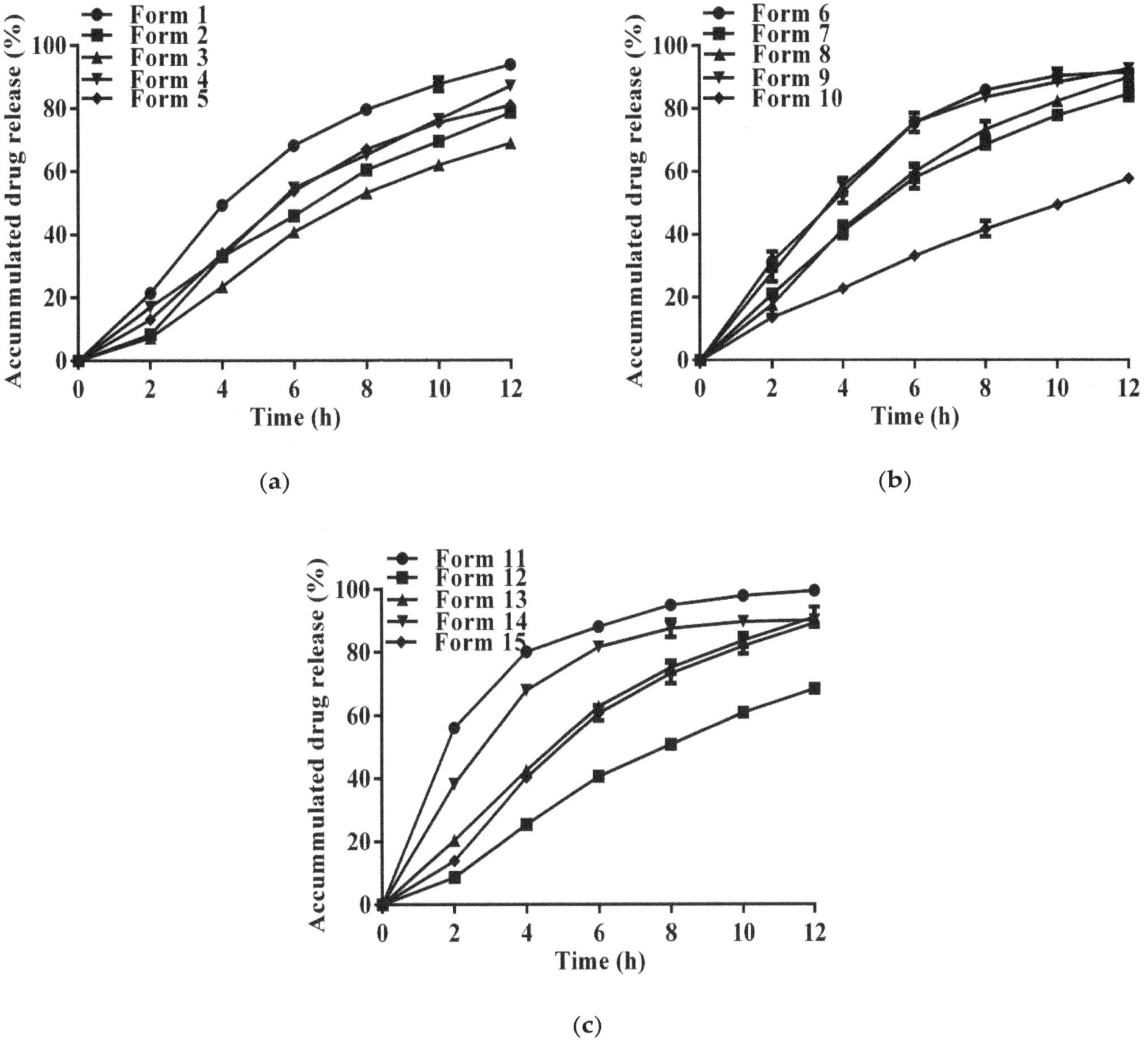

Figure 4. Dissolution profiles of loxoprofen in formulations prepared by the Box-Behnken design experiments (**a**) Formulation Nos. 1–5, (**b**) Formulation Nos. 6–10, (**c**) Formulation Nos. 11–15.

3.2.2. Regression Equations

Based on the experiment data, the coefficients and their p-values of the fitted full quadratic equations calculated by Expert-Design 8.0.6 (Stat-Ease Inc., Minneapolis, MN, USA) are listed in Table 4.

The final equations consisted of only statistically significant coefficients. It is clear that the citric acid concentration (X_1) and ADEC coating weight gain (X_3) showed significant effects on the drug release rate throughout the dissolution period, while the weight gain of the dissolution-rate controlling layer (X_2) showed only a weak effect during the dissolution period. The impact of X_1 on the drug release rate verified the effectiveness of the first-step control on the drug release rate, which could be explained by its impact on the pH_M, as extensively reported in the literature [36,37]. The effect of X_3 on the drug release rate could be attributed to its control on the drug diffusion rate, which was considered as the second-step control [38]. Besides, an interaction effect of X_1 and X_3 was observed on the response of Y_1 and Y_3, which might be explained by a speculation that X_3 also showed an effect on the release rate of citric acid. Additionally, it seemed that X_3 played a more dominant role on the final drug release, as high coefficients of the main, interaction, and quadratic effects of X_3 were observed in Y_3. From the statistic results in Table 4, we could conclude that both the dissolution-rate and diffusion-rate controlling steps have significant effects on the drug release rate.

Table 4. Regression coefficients and associated *p*-values of the fitted models.

Term	Drug Release Within 2 h (Y_1)		Drug Release Within 6 h (Y_2)		Drug Release Within 12 h (Y_3)	
	Cofficient	*p*-Value	Cofficient	*p*-Value	Cofficient	*p*-Value
Constant	16.23	0.000	58.40	0.000	88.33	0.000 *
X_1	−10.08	0.001 *	−12.91	0.001 *	−7.38	0.000 *
X_2	−2.98	0.007 *	−2.30	0.091	0.29	0.697
X_3	−10.70	0.001 *	−16.11	0.001 *	−11.79	0.000 *
X_1*X_2	−0.27	0.787	−2.07	0.240	−1.02	0.347
X_2*X_3	4.47	0.006 *	2.42	0.180	−1.10	0.316
X_1*X_3	7.03	0.000 *	0.70	0.672	−4.72	0.005 *
X_1*X_1	6.40	0.001 *	2.78	0.148	0.13	0.902
X_2*X_2	−2.45	0.058	1.40	0.427	2.69	0.047 *
X_3*X_3	5.15	0.004 *	−1.33	0.451	5.39	0.003 *
Regression equation	$Y_1 = 16.23 - 10.08X_1 - 2.98X_2 - 10.7X_3 - 4.47X_2X_3 + 7.03X_1X_3 + 6.4X_1^2 + 5.15X_3^2$		$Y_2 = 58.40 - 12.91X_1 - 16.11X_3$		$Y_3 = 88.33 - 7.38X_1 - 11.79X_3 - 4.72X_1X_3 - 2.69X_2^2 - 5.39X_3^2$	
R-Squared	0.9921		0.9865		0.9891	

* *p*-value < 0.05.

3.2.3. Response Surface Plots

The relationship between the dependent and independent variables was further elucidated using a 3D response surface plot, which is useful to see the effect of two factors on the response at one time while the third factor is kept at a constant level. The effects and interactions between concentration of citric acid (X_1), the sub coating weight gain (X_2), and ADEC coating weight gain (X_3) on the finial drug release (Y_3) are given in Figure 5. The similar impacts of the three factors on the other responses (Y_1 and Y_2) can be seen in Supplementary Materials Figures S2 and S3. As illustrated in Figure 5a,b, it was clear to see that X_2 showed little effect on Y_3 irrespective of the levels of other two factors. This was attributed to the fact that the dissolution-rate controlling layer is made up of aqueous polymer, which was dissolved before 12 h.

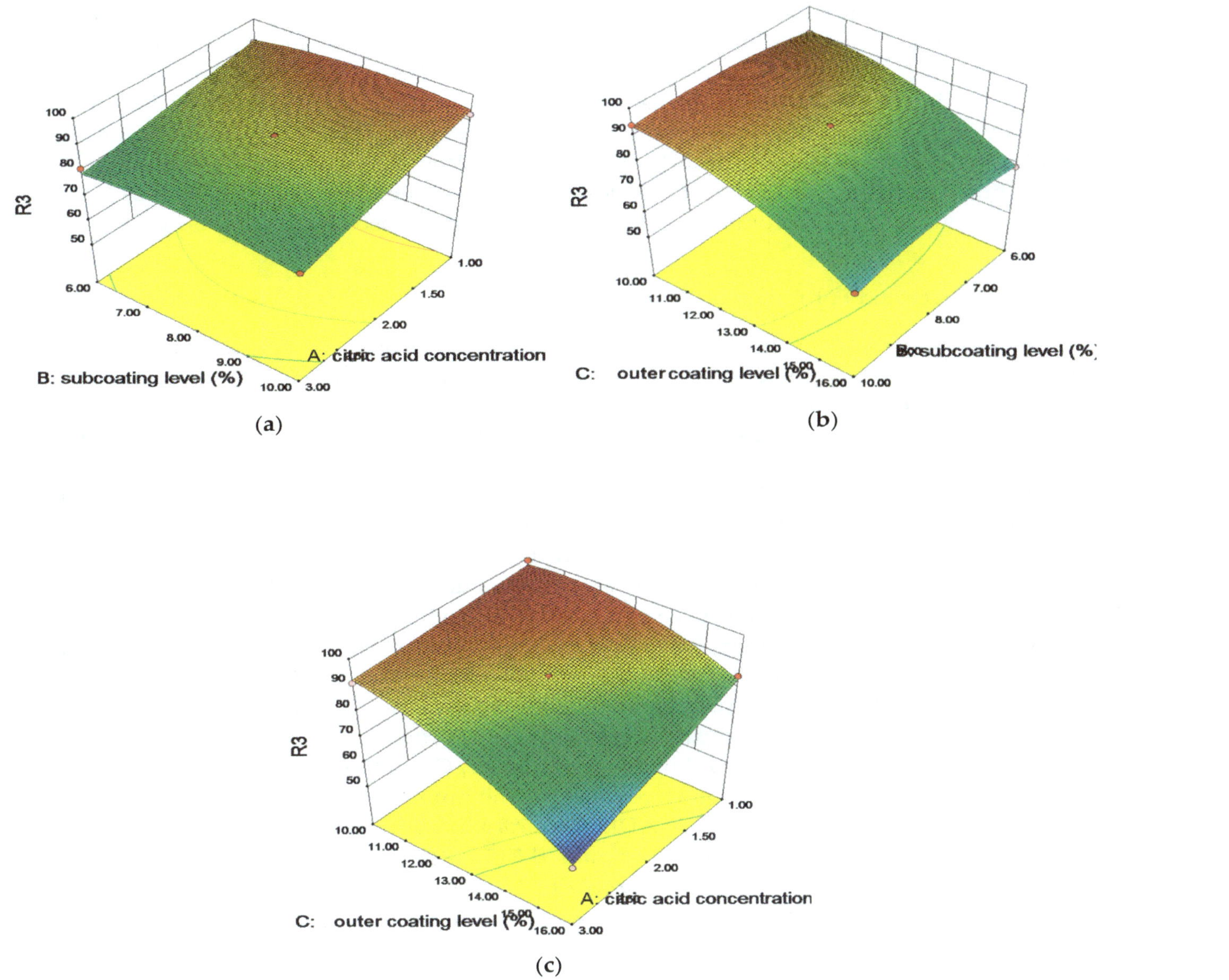

Figure 5. Contour plots showing the effects of (**a**) X_1 and X_2, (**b**) X_2 and X_3, and (**c**) X_1 and X_3 on the response Y_3.

The effects of citric acid concentration (X_1) and the ADEC coating weight gain (X_3) on Y_3 are depicted in Figure 5c. While X_3 was kept at low level, the increase of X_1 from 1% to 3% showed no effect on Y_3, which kept nearly constant at above 90%. While at a high level of X_3, the increase of X_1 from 1% to 3% resulted in a significant decrease of Y_3 from 85% to 60%. The result indicated that an interaction effect of the two factors existed on the drug release rate, as mentioned in Section 3.2.2. At a high level of X_3, an effective diffusion barrier was formed on the surface of the pellets [38], which significantly reduced the diffusion rate of loxoprofen. However, the release rate of loxoprofen was not solely controlled by the diffusion-controlling layer. For example, a nearly complete release of loxoprofen (>85%) was observed at a high level of X_3 (Figure 5c), when X_1 was kept at a low level of 1%. Therefore, the release rate of loxoprofen was a combined result of the two controlling steps. At a low level of X_3, the citric acid was soon released regardless of its concentrations, which resulted in a quick increase of the pH_M and a fast drug release rate. When the concentration of citric acid and ADEC coating weight gain were kept at high levels, both the drug dissolution and diffusion rate were reduced, which resulted in a prominent decrease of the drug release rate.

3.2.4. Design Space and Formulation Parameters Optimization

Design space was defined by the ICH Q8 as the relationship between the process inputs (material attributes and process parameters) and the critical quality attributes that have been demonstrated to provide assurance of quality [39]. The wider the design space is, the more robust and flexible the process is to resist variations [40]. As the response surface models of the output parameters as a function of selected variables were given, design space of X_1, X_2, and X_3 was determined by applying constraints on Y_1 (<30%), Y_2 (50–70%), and Y_3 (>90%). The yellow overlap region of ranges for the three responses in Figure 6a–c show the proposed design space of the citric acid concentration X_1 and the ADEC coating weight gain X_3 at three different levels of the sub-coating weight gain X_2. As shown in Figure 6a, there was no design space of X_1 and X_3 at the low level of X_2. Additionally, Figure 6c depicted a narrow design space of X_1 and X_3 at high level of X_2, which would increase the difficulty of the operation process since an accurate coating load of ADEC must be achieved during the manufacturing process. While at the medium level of X_2 (Figure 6b), the design space was expanded, which showed a less strict field of ADEC coating level. As the design space depicted the ranges of the formulation parameters for achieving the desired quality of product, the levels of the three factors for the optimal formulation must be set within the design space. Considering the robustness and flexibility, parameters of the optimal formulation were set at the medium level of sub coating weight gain with the CA concentration and coating level of ADEC at 2.5% and 11.0% respectively. The model predicted a release profile of 19.87% at 2 h, 64.48% at 6 h, and 91.71% at 12 h. To verify these values, a new batch of the optimal formulation was prepared. The obtained release data of the optimal formulation were in close agreement with the predicted values with a maximum percentage error of 11.73% at the initial release (data not showed).

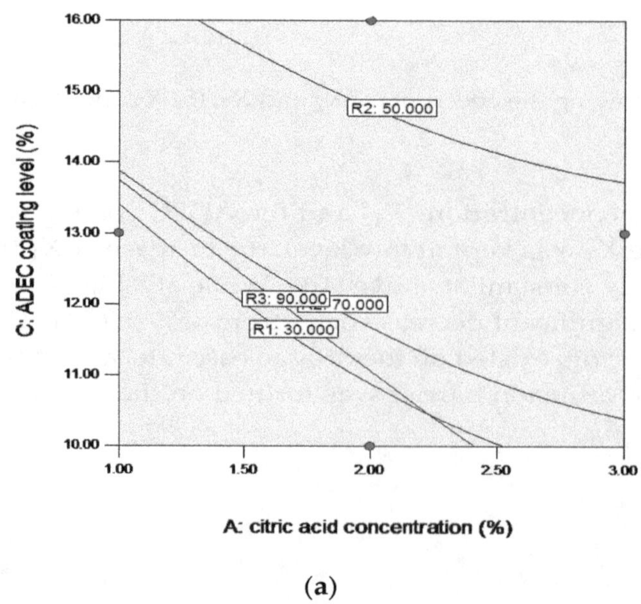

(a)

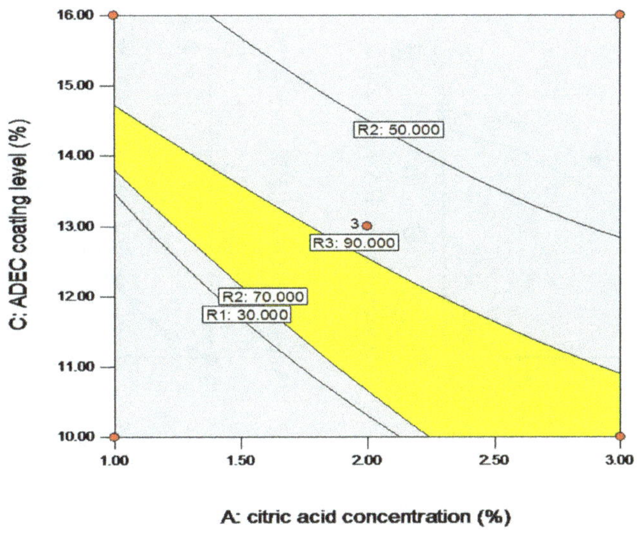

(b)

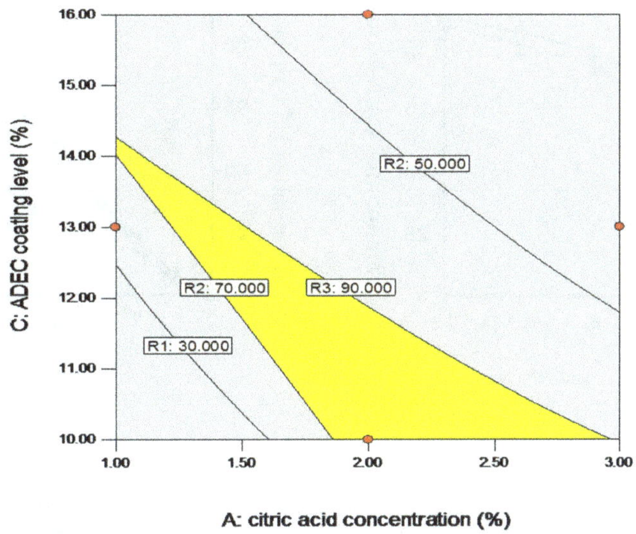

(c)

Figure 6. Design space of operating variables of the citric acid (CA) concentration and aqueous dispersion of ethyl cellulose (ADEC) coating level (**a**) at the low level of the sub-layer coating weight gain, (**b**) at the medium level of the sub-layer coating weight gain, and (**c**) at the high level of the sub-layer coating weight gain (yellow zone: design space; grey zone: failure space).

3.3. Simultaneous Release of CA and LXP from the Optimal Formulation in Different Dissolution Media

In order to evaluate the effect of pH on drug release, various media simulating different physiology pH values were applied. As shown in Figure 7, dissolution tests were performed in pH 1.0 HCl, pH 4.5 and pH 6.8 phosphate buffer solutions and water. Furthermore, the release profiles of CA were also investigated in these media. As illustrated in Figure 7, drug release profiles were pH-independent at pH above 4.5, and showed similar release profiles to that of CA.

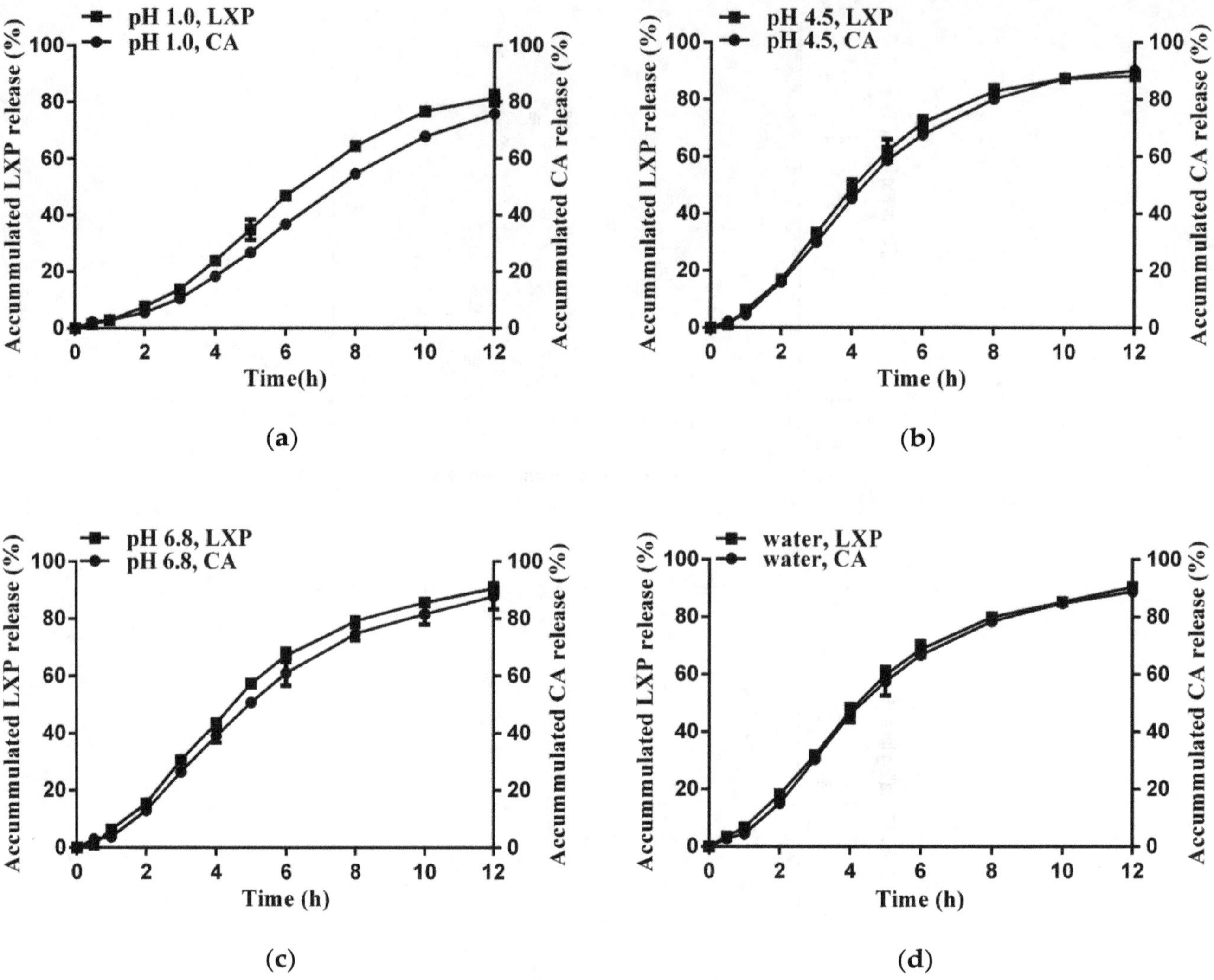

Figure 7. Loxoprofen and citric acid released from sustained release pellets in different dissolution media. (**a**) pH 1.0 HCl (**b**) pH 4.5 phosphate buffer (**c**) pH 6.8 phosphate buffer (**d**) water (means ± SD, $n = 3$).

Although the solubility of LXP was pH-independent in media with pH above 4.5 (Supplementary Materials Figure S1), it seemed that the dissolution media were not the reason for this pH-independent release behavior. As the drug showed a completed release within 3 h without the incorporation of CA inside the pellets (Figure 3, formulation with the CA concentration of 0%), it should exhibit a similar release for the optimal formulation as the dissolution media were also above 4.5. In the contrast, the optimal formulation showed sustained release for almost 12 h. It was the pH_M created by CA, which showed similar release profiles at pH above 4.5, that accounted for the pH-independent release profiles of LXP (Figure 7). As mentioned before, the saturated solution pH of CA was 0.4 [36], which was much lower than that of the dissolution media except the pH 1.0 HCl. However, with the release of CA during the dissolution period, the amount of CA left inside the optimal pellets was insufficient to maintain a constant pH_M inside the pellets. The pH_M was gradually increased, which resulted in a consistent enhancement of the drug solubility. In addition, matching sustained release profiles of LXP and CA were achieved in Figure 7.

While at pH 1.0, it was the dissolution media that showed a major effect on the drug release rate. With the decrease of CA, the pH_M would soon be increased up to above 1.0. However, the dissolution media that penetrated into the pellets provided a stable pH_M inside the pellets, which in turn resulted in a different release profile to the other three. In conclusion, the dissolution media and the incorporated CA played a combined effect on the drug release rate. In media with high pH values, the CA showed a greater effect on the drug release rate. While in media with low pH values, it was the dissolution media that dominated the drug release rate.

3.4. Release Mechanism Studies

In order to elucidate the transport mechanism of LXP in the optimal formulation, different mathematical models were applied to analyze the kinetics of the release data. As shown in Table 5, the incorporation of CA into the sub-layer resulted in abnormal release kinetics of this ADEC coating system, as the n value for Ritger–Peppas was 0.7422, which is between 0.45 and 0.89, indicating a non-Fick diffusion [41]. Additionally, a general empirical equation of Weibull distribution model with r^2 of 0.9944 was more appropriate to describe the release process of the optimal formulation. In the model, the derived estimate of b value was calculated to be 1.38, which represented a sigmoid shape curve ($b > 1$) for the release profile [41]. The initial slow release representing the starting part of the sigmoid curve was a result of several factors. As reported previously, the permeability of water through the EC coating is much faster than the permeability of the compound [38], which might contribute to the initial slow release of LXP. Besides, the decreased dissolution rate created by the initial low pH_M inside the pellets also played an important role on the initial slow release. Furthermore, the hydration of the hydroxypropyl methyl cellulose (HPMC) inside the pellets during the initial dissolution period could also inhibit the initial drug release rate. Thereafter, due to the saturation of water inside the pellets and the disruption of the dissolution-rate controlling layer, the drug release rate was dominated by the dissolution- and diffusion-rate control, which resulted in a sustained release profile.

Table 5. Models simulated for the drug release profiles of the optimal formulation.

Content	Model	Equation	r^2
loxoprofen	Zero-order model	$Q_t = 0.0833t + 0.0238$	0.9288
	First-order model	$ln(Q_0 - Q_t) - lnQ_0 = -0.1787t + 0.0814$	0.9794
	Higuchi diffusion model	$Q_t = 0.3126t^{1/2} - 0.1496$	0.9454
	Ritger–Peppas model	$lnQ_t = 0.7422\ lnt + 2.7562$	0.9597
	Weibull distribution model	$log[-ln(1 - Q_t)] = 1.3840\ logt - 1.0449$	0.9944
	Hixson–Crowell model	$(1 - Q_t)^{1/3} = -0.0514t + 1.0167$	0.9874

3.5. Scanning Electron Photomicrographs

Figure 8 shows the scanning electron photomicrographs of the optimal pellets. The surface of pellets were smooth (Figure 8a,b), and no crack could be seen. Besides, layers of the dissolution-rate controlling layer and the diffusion-rate controlling layer were clearly seen in the cross-section of the coating pellets (Figure 8c,d). These results indicated that a successful procedure had been developed for manufacturing the sustained release pellets.

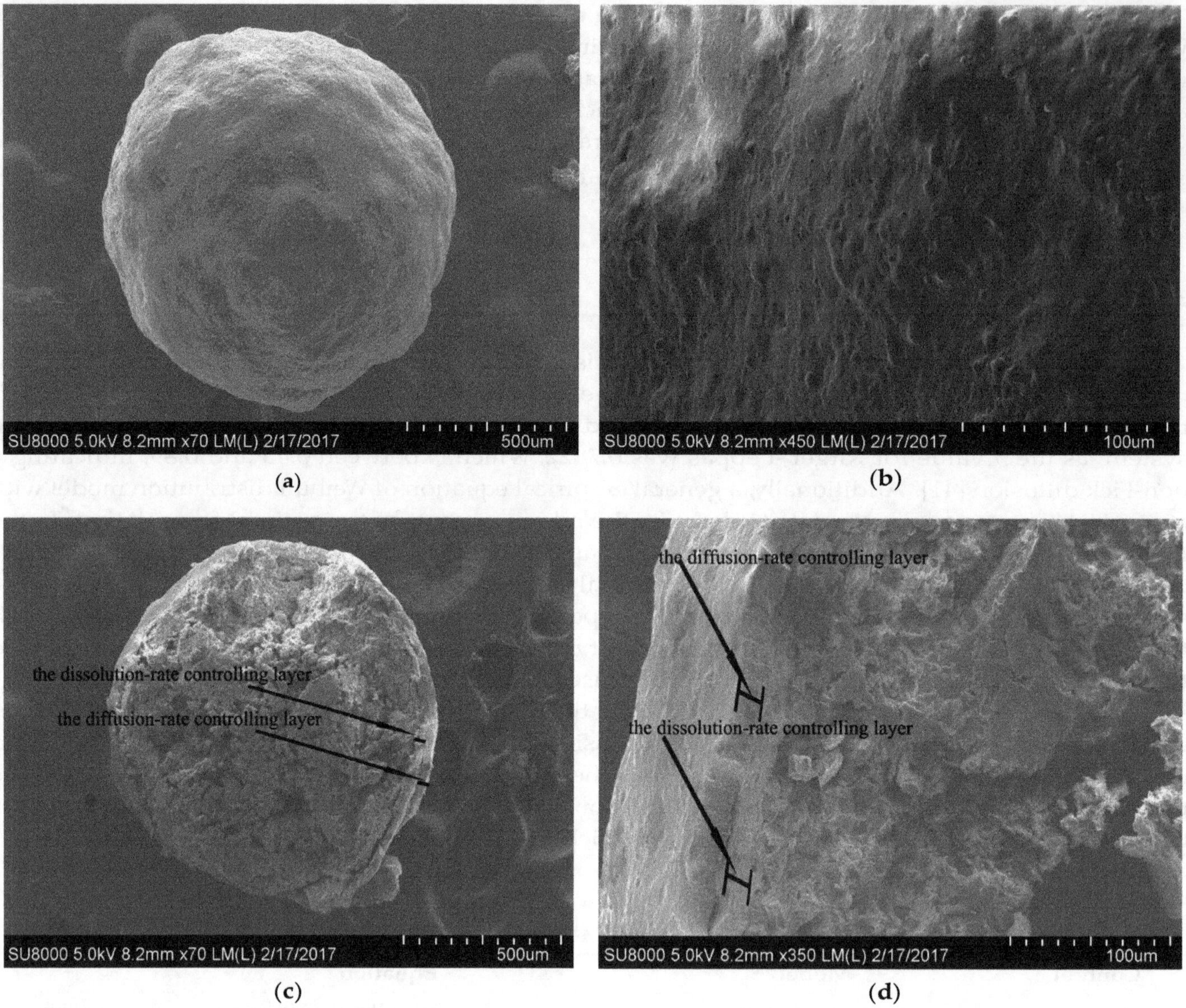

Figure 8. SEM photographs of pellets with double coating layers: (**a**) Surface of sustained release pellets with 70 magnifications, (**b**) surface of sustained release pellets with 450 magnifications, (**c**) cross-section of sustained release pellets with 70 magnifications, (**d**) cross-section of sustained release pellets with 350 magnifications.

3.6. Pharmacokinetic Studies

The pharmacokinetic studies of the optimal pellets and the commercial tablets were investigated on fasted beagles. The profile of mean plasma concentrations of LXP versus time is shown in Figure 9. The main pharmacokinetic parameters are summarized in Table 6. As shown in Figure 9, the plasma concentration of the commercial tablet quickly increased and reached the peak concentration of 5.16 μg/mL at 0.5 h after administration. Then it dropped down and was only 0.2 μg/mL at 6 h. This was attributed to the short half-life ($t_{1/2}$ = 64.46 min) of LXP [12], which resulted in a quick elimination of the drug in vivo. The optimal formulation reached the maximum plasma concentration of 2.40 μg/mL at 5 h after administration, and the drug concentration fell slowly even at 12 h, when the drug concentration was 0.15 μg/mL, in contrast with the undetectable drug concentration in plasma for the commercial tablet 8 h after administration.

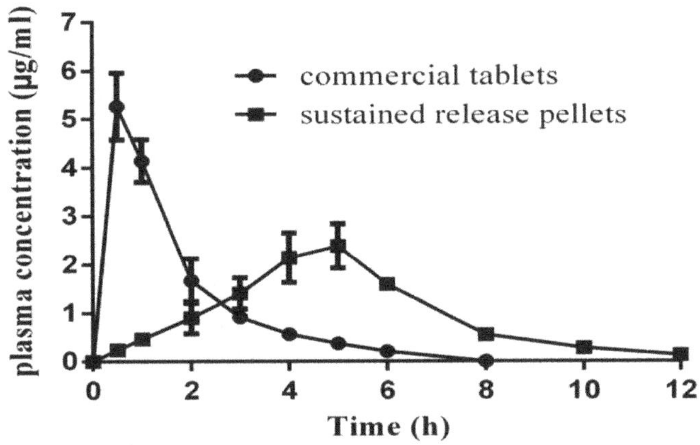

Figure 9. Plasma drug concentrations vs. time after oral administration of conventional tablets (60 mg) and sustained release pellets (90 mg).

Table 6. The pharmacokinetic parameters of loxoprofen after oral administration of the optimal sustained release pellets and commercial tablets in beagle dogs (n = 6).

Pharmacokinetic Parameters	C_{max} (μg/mL)	T_{max} (h)	AUC_{0-12} (μg h/mL)	$AUC_{0-\infty}$ (μg h/mL)	Relative Bioavailability (%)
Optimal pellets (90 mg)	2.60 ± 0.23	4.80 ± 0.57	12.77 ± 0.88	13.48 ± 0.94	87.16 ± 0.07
Commercial tablets (60 mg)	5.16 ± 0.60	0.60 ± 0.22	9.73 ± 0.61	10.31 ± 0.45	-

As a pro-drug, LXP inhibits the activities of cyclooxygenase-1 and -2 (COX-1 and COX-2) by its active metabolite trans-OH LXP, of which the IC_{50} values for COX-1 and COX-2 were 0.38 and 0.12 μM, respectively [42]. It has been reported that the concentration of trans-OH LXP, which was the major metabolite of LXP, was equal to more than half of the LXP concentration detected in plasma [12]. As the LXP concentration range in plasma of the optimal pellets was 0.6–10.0 μM, we can deduce that the concentration of trans-alcohol LXP after administration of the optimal pellet would be higher than the IC_{50} of the trans-OH LXP. Therefore, a therapy concentration of trans-OH LXP in plasma after administration of the optimal pellets would be maintained for almost 12 h. As the frequency of dosage of the optimal formulation was reduced to two times a day, the patient's compliance would be better improved. It has been reported that the incidence of gastric lesions after administration of LXP in rats showed a dose-dependent manner. Additionally, the amount of PGE_2, which has a strong protective effect on the GI mucosa, also decreased in a concentration-dependent manner after treatment of LXP within the concentration range of 1.0 μM to 1.0 M [14,43]. Therefore, the risk of GI lesions would be significantly decreased, since the initial burst release disappeared in vivo and the C_{max} of LXP was significantly decreased from 20 to 10 μM after administration of the optimal formulation. Besides, a less fluctuant drug concentration in plasma was achieved for the optimal pellets in Figure 9. The significant difference ($p < 0.05$) of $AUC_{0-\infty}$/dose between the test formulation and conventional tablet might be caused by the limited GI absorption site of LXP, which would need further investigation. The relative bioavailability of the test formulation was 87.16% compared with the reference, and it would be improved in patients as a prolonged GI transit time has been reported in humans [44].

4. Conclusions

In conclusion, this article provided a novel concept of two-step control of the release rate of pH-sensitive drugs. Additionally, the results of the drug in vitro release profiles proved that both the dissolution-rate controlling step created by the sub-layer containing CA and the diffusion-rate controlling step developed by the ADEC coating showed significant effects on the release rate of LXP. In addition, the amount of the acid modifier in the optimal formulation, which accounted for only approximately 3% of the total preparation weight, was dramatically decreased compared with other formulations containing acidic modifiers. The in vivo studies revealed that this novel two-step control system could achieve a more stable and sustained release plasma concentration of LXP compared with the immediate release tablet.

Author Contributions: Conceptualization, D.W. and L.L.; methodology, D.W., M.Z., J.Z.; and L.L.; formal analysis, L.L.; investigation, D.W.; writing—original draft preparation, D.W. and M.Z, writing—review and editing, D.W. and M.Z.

Acknowledgments: We are thankful to Colorcon Coating School® for technical and excipient supports.

References

1. Peter, J.C. Tramadol SR formulations: Pharmacokinetic comparison of a multiple-units dose (capsule) versus a single-unit dose (tablet). *Clin. Drug Investig.* **2005**, *7*, 435–443.
2. Chen, T.; Li, J.; Chen, T.; Sun, C.C.; Zheng, Y. Tablets of multi-unit pellet system for controlled drug delivery. *J. Control. Release* **2017**, *262*, 222–231. [CrossRef] [PubMed]
3. Felton, L.A. Mechanisms of polymeric film formation. *Int. J. Pharm.* **2013**, *457*, 423–427. [CrossRef] [PubMed]
4. Howick, K.; Alam, R.; Chruscicka, B.; Kandil, D.; Fitzpatrick, D.; Ryan, A.M.; Cryan, J.F.; Schellekens, H.; Griffin, B.T. Sustained-release multiparticulates for oral delivery of a novel peptidic ghrelin agonist: Formulation design and in vitro characterization. *Int. J. Pharm.* **2018**, *536*, 63–72. [CrossRef] [PubMed]
5. Thapa, P.; Thapa, R.; Choi, D.H.; Jeong, S.H. Effects of pharmaceutical processes on the quality of ethylcellulose coated pellets: Quality by design approach. *Powder Technol.* **2018**, *339*, 25–38. [CrossRef]
6. López, E.V.; Luzardo Álvarez, A.; Blanco Méndez, J.; Otero Espinar, F.J. Cellulose-polysaccharide film-coating of cyclodextrin based pellets for controlled drug release. *J. Drug Deliv. Sci. Technol.* **2017**, *42*, 273–283. [CrossRef]
7. Dekyndt, B.; Verin, J.; Neut, C.; Siepmann, F.; Siepmann, J. How to easily provide zero order release of freely soluble drugs from coated pellets. *Int. J. Pharm.* **2015**, *478*, 31–38. [CrossRef] [PubMed]
8. Muschert, S.; Siepmann, F.; Leclercq, B.; Carlin, B.; Siepmann, J. Prediction of drug release from ethylcellulose coated pellets. *J. Control. Release* **2009**, *135*, 71–79. [CrossRef] [PubMed]
9. Sadeghi, F.; Ford, J.L.; Rajabi-Siahboomi, A. The influence of drug type on the release profiles from Surelease-coated pellets. *Int. J. Pharm.* **2003**, *254*, 123–135. [CrossRef]
10. Terada, A.; Naruto, S.; Wachi, K.; Tanaka, S.; Iizuka, Y.; Misaka, E. Synthesis and antiinflammatory activity of [(cycloalkylmethyl)phenyl]acetic acids and related compounds. *J. Med. Chem.* **1984**, *27*, 212–216. [CrossRef] [PubMed]
11. Mu, R.; Bao, C.D.; Chen, Z.W.; Zheng, Y.; Wang, G.C.; Zhao, D.B.; Hu, S.X.; Li, Y.J.; Shao, Z.W.; Zhang, Z.Y. Efficacy and safety of loxoprofen hydrogel patch versus loxoprofen tablet in patients with knee osteoarthritis: A randomized controlled non-inferiority trial. *Clin. Rheumatol.* **2016**, *35*, 165–173. [CrossRef] [PubMed]
12. Cho, H.Y.; Park, C.H.; Lee, Y.B. Direct and simultaneous analysis of loxoprofen and its diastereometric alcohol metabolites in human serum by on-line column switching liquid chromatography and its application to a pharmacokinetic study. *J. Chromatogr. B Analyt. Technol. Biomed. Life Sci.* **2006**, *835*, 27–34. [CrossRef] [PubMed]
13. Mizukami, K.; Murakami, K.; Yamauchi, M.; Matsunari, O.; Ogawa, R.; Nakagawa, Y.; Okimoto, T.; Kodama, M.; Fujioka, T. Evaluation of selective cyclooxygenase-2 inhibitor-induced small bowel injury: Randomized cross-over study compared with loxoprofen in healthy subjects. *Dig. Endosc.* **2013**, *25*, 288–294. [CrossRef] [PubMed]
14. Yamakawa, N.; Suemasu, S.; Matoyama, M.; Kimoto, A.; Takeda, M.; Tanaka, K.; Ishihara, T.; Katsu, T.; Okamoto, Y.; Otsuka, M.; et al. Properties and synthesis of 2-{2-fluoro (or bromo)-4-[(2-oxocyclopentyl)methyl]phenyl}propanoic acid: Nonsteroidal anti-inflammatory drugs with low membrane permeabilizing and gastric lesion-producing activities. *J. Med. Chem.* **2010**, *53*, 7879–7882. [CrossRef]

15. Tak, J.W.; Gupta, B.; Thapa, R.K.; Woo, K.B.; Kim, S.Y.; Go, T.G.; Choi, Y.; Choi, J.Y.; Jeong, J.H.; Choi, H.G.; et al. Preparation and optimization of immediate release/sustained release bilayered tablets of loxoprofen using box-behnken design. *AAPS PharmSciTech* **2017**, *18*, 1125–1134. [CrossRef]
16. Venkatesan, P.; Manavalan, R.; Valliappan, K. Preparation and evaluation of sustained release loxoprofen loaded microspheres. *J. Basic. Clin. Pharm.* **2011**, *2*, 159–162.
17. Zaman, M.; Rasool, S.; Ali, M.Y.; Qureshi, J.; Adnan, S.; Hanif, M.; Sarfraz, R.M.; Ijaz, H.; Mahmood, A. Fabrication and analysis of hydroxypropylmethyl cellulose and pectin-based controlled release matrix tablets loaded with loxoprofen sodium. *Adv. Polym. Technol.* **2015**, *34*, 1624–1631. [CrossRef]
18. Khanum, H.; Ullah, K.; Murtaza, G.; Khan, S.A. Fabrication and in vitro characterization of HPMC-g-poly(AMPS) hydrogels loaded with loxoprofen sodium. *Int. J. Biol. Macromol.* **2018**, *120*, 1624–1631. [CrossRef]
19. Sonawane, R.O.; Patil, S.D. Fabrication and statistical optimization of starch-kappa-carrageenan cross-linked hydrogel composite for extended release pellets of zaltoprofen. *Int. J. Biol. Macromol.* **2018**, *120*, 2324–2334. [CrossRef]
20. Patil, H.; Tiwari, R.V.; Upadhye, S.B.; Vladyka, R.S.; Repka, M.A. Formulation and development of pH-independent/dependent sustained release matrix tablets of ondansetron HCl by a continuous twin-screw melt granulation process. *Int. J. Pharm.* **2015**, *496*, 33–41. [CrossRef]
21. Kasashima, Y.; Uchida, S.; Yoshihara, K.; Yasuji, T.; Sako, K.; Namiki, N. Oral sustained-release suspension based on a lauryl sulfate salt/complex. *Int. J. Pharm.* **2016**, *515*, 677–683. [CrossRef] [PubMed]
22. Kang, W.H.; Nguyen, H.V.; Park, C.; Choi, Y.W.; Lee, B.J. Modulation of microenvironmental pH for dual release and reduced in vivo gastrointestinal bleeding of aceclofenac using hydroxypropyl methylcellulose-based bilayered matrix tablet. *Eur. J. Pharm. Sci.* **2017**, *102*, 85–93. [CrossRef] [PubMed]
23. Ploen, J.; Andersch, J.; Heschel, M.; Leopold, C.S. Citric acid as a pH-modifying additive in an extended release pellet formulation containing a weakly basic drug. *Drug Dev. Ind. Pharm.* **2009**, *35*, 1210–1218. [CrossRef] [PubMed]
24. Healy, A.M.; Corrigan, O.I. Predicting the dissolution rate of ibuprofen-acidic excipient compressed mixtures in reactive media. *Int. J. Pharm.* **1992**, *84*, 167–173. [CrossRef]
25. Badawy, S.I.; Hussain, M.A. Microenvironmental pH modulation in solid dosage forms. *J. Pharm. Sci.* **2007**, *96*, 948–959. [CrossRef] [PubMed]
26. Xu, L.; Luo, Y.; Feng, J.; Xu, M.; Tao, X.; He, H.; Tang, X. Preparation and in vitro–in vivo evaluation of none gastric resident dipyridamole (DIP) sustained-release pellets with enhanced bioavailability. *Int. J. Pharm.* **2012**, *422*, 9–16. [CrossRef]
27. Frenning, G. Modelling drug release from inert matrix systems: From moving-boundary to continuous-field descriptions. *Int. J. Pharm.* **2011**, *418*, 88–99. [CrossRef] [PubMed]
28. Cuppok, Y.; Muschert, S.; Marucci, M.; Hjaertstam, J.; Siepmann, F.; Axelsson, A.; Siepmann, J. Drug release mechanisms from Kollicoat SR: Eudragit NE coated pellets. *Int. J. Pharm.* **2011**, *409*, 30–37. [CrossRef]
29. Marucci, M.; Ragnarsson, G.; Nilsson, B.; Axelsson, A. Osmotic pumping release from ethyl-hydroxypropyl-cellulose-coated pellets: A new mechanistic model. *J. Control. Release* **2010**, *142*, 53–60. [CrossRef]
30. Marucci, M.; Ragnarsson, G.; Axelsson, A. Evaluation of osmotic effects on coated pellets using a mechanistic model. *Int. J. Pharm.* **2007**, *336*, 67–74. [CrossRef]
31. Ferrero, C.; Massuelle, D.; Doelker, E. Towards elucidation of the drug release mechanism from compressed hydrophilic matrices made of cellulose ethers. II. Evaluation of a possible swelling-controlled drug release mechanism using dimensionless analysis. *J. Control. Release* **2010**, *141*, 223–233. [CrossRef] [PubMed]
32. Siepmann, J.; Kranz, H.; Bodmeier, R.; Peppas, N.A. HPMC-matrices for controlled drug delivery: A new model combining diffusion, swelling, and dissolution mechanisms and predicting the release kinetics. *Pharm. Res.* **1999**, *16*, 1748–1756. [CrossRef] [PubMed]
33. Xiang, A.; Mchugh, A.J. A generalized diffusion–dissolution model for drug release from rigid polymer membrane matrices. *J. Membr. Sci.* **2011**, *366*, 104–115. [CrossRef]
34. Cabrera, M.I.; Luna, J.A.; Grau, R.J.A. Modeling of dissolution-diffusion controlled drug release from planar polymeric systems with finite dissolution rate and arbitrary drug loading. *J. Membr. Sci.* **2006**, *280*, 693–704. [CrossRef]
35. Choo, K.; Kim, I.; Jung, J.; Suh, Y.; Chung, S.; Lee, M.; Shim, C. Simultaneous determination of loxoprofen

and its diastereomeric alcohol metabolites in human plasma and urine by a simple HPLC-UV detection method. *J. Pharm. Biomed. Anal.* **2001**, *25*, 639–650. [CrossRef]

36. Badawy, S.I.; Williams, R.C.; Gilbert, D.L. Effect of different acids on solid-state stability of an ester prodrug of a IIb/IIIa glycoprotein receptor antagonist. *Pharm. Dev. Technol.* **1999**, *4*, 325–331. [CrossRef] [PubMed]
37. Siepe, S.; Lueckel, B.; Kramer, A.; Ries, A.; Gurny, R. Strategies for the design of hydrophilic matrix tablets with controlled microenvironmental pH. *Int. J. Pharm.* **2006**, *316*, 14–20. [CrossRef] [PubMed]
38. Kazlauske, J.; Cafaro, M.M.; Caccavo, D.; Marucci, M.; Lamberti, G.; Barba, A.A.; Larsson, A. Determination of the release mechanism of Theophylline from pellets coated with Surelease(R)-A water dispersion of ethyl cellulose. *Int. J. Pharm.* **2017**, *528*, 345–353. [CrossRef] [PubMed]
39. Food and Drug Administration CDER. Guidance for Industry Q8 (R2) Pharmaceutical Development International Conference on Harmonisation of Techniccal Requirements for Registration of Pharmaceuticals for Human Use. 2009; pp. 1–19. Available online: https://www.ich.org/fileadmin/Public_Web_Site/ICH_Products/Guidelines/Quality/Q8_R1/Step4/Q8_R2_Guideline.pdf (accessed on 6 May 2019).
40. Charoo, N.A.; Shamsher, A.A.; Zidan, A.S.; Rahman, Z. Quality by design approach for formulation development: A case study of dispersible tablets. *Int. J. Pharm.* **2012**, *423*, 167–178. [CrossRef]
41. Costa, P.; Lobo, J.M.S. Modeling and comparison of dissolution profiles. *Eur. J. Pharm. Sci.* **2001**, *13*, 123–133. [CrossRef]
42. Kawai, S.; Nishida, S.; Kato, M.; Furumaya, Y.; Okamoto, R.; Koshino, T.; Mizushima, Y. Comparison of cyclooxygenase-1 and -2 inhibitory activities of various nonsteroidal anti-inflammatory drugs using human platelets and synovial cells. *Eur. J. Pharmacol.* **1998**, *347*, 87–94. [CrossRef]
43. Yamakawa, N.; Suemasu, S.; Kimoto, A.; Ishihara, T.; Yokomizo, K.; Okamoto, Y.; Otsuka, M. Low Direct Cytotoxicity of Loxoprofen on Gastric Mucosal Cells. *Biol. Pharm. Bull.* **2010**, *33*, 398. [CrossRef] [PubMed]
44. Hatton, G.B.; Yadav, V.; Basit, A.W.; Merchant, H.A. Animal farm: Considerations in animal gastrointestinal physiology and relevance to drug delivery in humans. *J. Pharm. Sci.* **2015**, *104*, 2747–2776. [CrossRef] [PubMed]

7

Release Profile of Gentamicin Sulfate from Polylactide-*co*-Polycaprolactone Electrospun Nanofiber Matrices

Silvia Pisani [1], Rossella Dorati [1,2,*], Enrica Chiesa [1], Ida Genta [1], Tiziana Modena [1,2], Giovanna Bruni [3], Pietro Grisoli [1] and Bice Conti [1,2]

1 Department of Drug Sciences, University of Pavia, Viale Taramelli 12/14, 27100 Pavia, Italy; silvia.pisani01@universitadipavia.it (S.P.); enrica.chiesa01@universitadipavia.it (E.C.); ida.genta@unipv.it (I.G.); tiziana.modena@unipv.it (T.M.); pietro.grisoli@unipv.it (P.G.); bice.conti@unipv.it (B.C.)
2 Polymerix S.r.l., Via Taramelli 24, 27100 Pavia, Italy
3 Department of Chemistry, University of Pavia, Viale Taramelli 12/14, 27100 Pavia, Italy; giovanna.bruni@unipv.it
* Correspondence: rossella.dorati@unipv.it

Abstract: The advent and growth of resistance phenomena to antibiotics has reached critical levels, invalidating the action of a majority of antibiotic drugs currently used in the clinical field. Several innovative techniques, such as the nanotechnology, can be applied for creating innovative drug delivery systems designed to modify drug release itself and/or drug administration route; moreover, they have proved suitable for overcoming the phenomenon of antibiotic resistance. Electrospun nanofibers, due to their useful structural properties, are showing promising results as antibiotic release devices for preventing bacteria biofilm formation after surgical operation and for limiting resistance phenomena. In this work gentamicin sulfate (GS) was loaded into polylactide-*co*-polycaprolactone (PLA-PCL) electrospun nanofibers; quantification and in vitro drug release profiles in static and dynamic conditions were investigated; GS kinetic release from nanofibers was studied using mathematical models. A preliminary microbiological test was carried out towards *Staphylococcus aureus* and *Escherichia coli* bacteria.

Keywords: electrospinning; gentamicin sulfate; polylactide-*co*-polycaprolactone; drug release kinetics

---

1. Introduction

Electrospinning is a straightforward method of producing polymeric matrices made of ultrafine entangled polymeric fibers with micro- to nano-meter range diameters and controlled surface morphology. The ultrafine fibers are generated by application of a strong electric field on a polymer solution or melt; fibers are stretched and collected on a metallic surface (plate or mandrel). During fiber formation, solvent must evaporate in order to achieve dry and homogeneous fibers. Electrospinning process parameters have been extensively studied and reviewed in the literature in the recent years [1,2].

In these years, the electrospinning technique raised tremendous interest in the pharmaceutical field, as an emerging processing technique of drug delivery systems. Different kinds of drug delivery systems have been investigated to improve the therapeutic effect and to reduce the toxicity of conventional dosage forms. Nanoscale formulations, such as liposomes, polymeric micelles, complexes, and nanofibers, attracted special attention during the last decade. Compared with other formulations, electrospinning affords great flexibility in selecting and combining materials and drugs. Drug molecule encapsulation into electrospun polymer nanofibers, promotes intimate drug to polymer contact, also modifying drug apparent solubility [3–11]. As far as electrospun materials are concerned, the ability of reaching high encapsulation efficiencies, simultaneous delivery of diverse drugs, and drug release modification are recognized as significant advantages. Moreover, the electrospinning process itself has notable advantages, such as ease of operation, cost-effectiveness, reproducibility, and easy up-scalability [1,12,13]. The use of electrospun nanofibers as drug carriers is promising in diverse pathologies, such as postoperative local chemotherapy administration wound dressing [14,15].

Several studies can be found in the literature concerning drug release from drug loaded electrospun matrices, either reporting drug release behavior or drug release kinetic evaluation. The latter is an important parameter to be investigated since drug release kinetic gives an indication of drug release mechanism. While a zero-order kinetic with constant release rate is preferred, drug release from polymeric drug delivery systems, such as electrospun nanofibers, in many cases shows initial burst release followed by a more controlled release of the drug over a longer duration.

The behavior depends on the drug dispersion state in the polymer fibers (i.e., molecular dispersion (obtained starting from drug/polymer solution) or solid dispersion (obtained starting from a drug suspension into polymer solution)). Therefore, in order to attain successful encapsulation of a drug into the electrospun nanofibers, the physicochemical properties of polymers, as well as their interaction with the drug molecules, must be precisely considered, as they significantly affect drug-encapsulation efficiency, drug distribution inside the fibers, and, ultimately, drug release from the nanofibers.

Various carrier materials, including natural and synthetic (biodegradable and non-degradable) polymers and a blend of both, were used and are being studied for electrospinning. The drugs investigated for electrospinning belong to different therapeutic classes, such as anticancer drugs, antibiotics and anti-infective, proteins, cardiovascular, DNA, and RNA [9,16–25].

The aim of this work was to prepare electrospun matrices loaded with GS and to in vitro evaluate the drug kinetic profile and its microbiologic activity. In vitro release profiles were attained through conventional static in vitro release test, and through an innovative dynamic bioreactor system that was tested in this work and compared to the conventional in vitro drug release test. The data were elaborated by kinetic release equation models [26]. The GS-loaded electrospun matrices could be used for local controlled drug delivery for treating infected skin and gum or during bone surgery in order to prevent or arrest infection.

Rationale for GS local administration resides in its poor oral bioavailability, and the high occurrence of side effects, such as ototoxicity and toxicity in the kidney, when the drug is administered by intravenous or intramuscular routes, which are the preferential administration routes for Gentamicin. Moreover, topical administration of GS is required with infected burns, excoriations, acne, and impetigo, and in these cases local delivery through a polymer nano-fibrous matrix promoting controlled drug release and prolonged therapeutic effect could be of interest.

2. Materials

Copolymer poly-L-lactide-poly-ε-caprolactone (PLA-PCL) 70:30 molar ratio (Resomer LC 703 S – M_w 160,000 Da), freely soluble in methylene chloride (MC), soluble in *N,N*-dimethylformamide (DMF), was obtained from Evonik Industries (Evonik Nutrition and Care GmbH, 64275 Damstadt, Germany). Analytical grade MC and DMF were supplied by Carlo Erba, with no further purification. Gentamicin sulfate, GS (Gentamicin C_1, $C_{21}H_{43}N_5O_7$, M_w 477.6 g/mol, Gentamicin C_2, $C_{20}H_{41}N_5O_7$, M_w 463.6 g/mol, Gentamicin C_{1a}, $C_{19}H_{39}N_5O_7$, M_w 449.5 g/mol), water solubility 100 mg/mL, insoluble in MC, slightly soluble in DMF (1% *w/w*), and ninhydrin (NH), M_w 178,14 g/mol; purity grade ≥ 95% were from Sigma Aldrich, Milano, Italy.

3. Methods

3.1. Preparation of Polymeric Electrospun Fibers Loaded with GS

GS powder (3.3% *w/w*) was first dissolved in DMF and then it was added to PLA-PCL solution (20% *w/w*, solubilized in MC) and maintained under magnetic stirring at 300 rpm for 2 h, until formation of creaming homogeneous yellowish system. The final PLA-PCL/GS solution, whose composition was 1% *w/w* GS and 14% *w/w* PLA-PCL, was sonicated to eliminate air bubbles.

The polymer solubility in MC:DMF 70:30 ratio was previously evaluated. The process parameter, set up in a previous work of the research group, were as follows: flow rate 1 mL/h, voltage 20 k/V, needle Gauge 18 [27]. A metallic plate collector covered with aluminum foil was used for avoiding any fiber damage during recovering; syringe distance from collector plate was maintained at 15 cm. The electrospinning process was performed at room temperature (25 °C) and controlled humidity value (~50%). Electrospinning time was 30 min in order to achieve nanofiber matrices with suitable GS loading.

3.2. UV Quantification of GS

GS quantification was carried out by NH test. Briefly, NH test is a colorimetric assay for quantitative assessment of GS. It is based on the reaction of NH with the primary and secondary gentamicin amino groups leading to the formation of purple compound. The color intensity is directly proportional to gentamicin concentration [28,29]. GS was extracted from electrospun matrices (either the whole matrices or their portions) with the following protocol.

For GS recovery, the whole electrospun matrix was solubilized in 3 mL MC and then Phosphate Buffer Saline PBS (4 mL, pH 7.4) were added for extracting GS. The system was maintained under magnetic stirring at 1000 rpm for 1 h to promote GS extraction. The MC/PBS mixture were centrifuged (16,000 rpm, 10 min) in order to separate organic and aqueous phases and recover GS in the aqueous phase. The extraction of GS in the aqueous phase was guarantee by the high affinity of gentamicin for aqueous phase, the poor solubility of PLA-PCL in the aqueous phase, and the partial miscibility organic (MC) and aqueous phases (PBS). After centrifugation, the supernatant containing GS was recovered, and GS quantified by NH assay. A schematic representation of extraction protocol is represented in Figure 1. The extraction protocol was validated and extraction yield was confirmed to be 95 ± 3.0%.

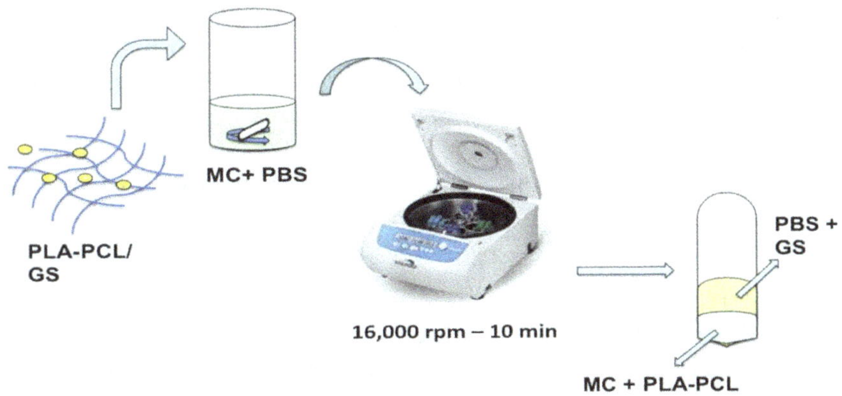

Figure 1. Schematic representation of Gentamicin (GS) extraction from polylactide-co-polycaprolactone (PLA-PCL) electrospun matrices.

A total of 500 μL of NH solution (5 mg/mL concentration), previously solubilized in PBS was added to 500 μL of supernatant. The final solution was vortexed to ensure complete mixing and subsequently heated to 95 °C for 15 min in order to induce reaction between gentamicin and NH molecules. After 15 min, the solution was stored in water/ice bath for 10 min to stop the reaction. Each sample was analyzed at UV spectrophotometer at 418 nm wavelength, using quartz cuvettes (UV-1601, UV-visible spectrophotometer, Shimadzu, ON, Canada).

PBS solution containing 1% *w/w* GS and placebo electrospun matrices were used as controls. All samples underwent the same extraction protocol as GS electrospun matrices before analysis with NH assay.

A six-points calibration curve was obtained with GS standard solutions at concentrations between 0.001 and 0.5 mg/mL. The instrument was calibrated using a blank made of 500 µL of NH solution (0.5% *w/v*) added to 500 µL of PBS at pH 7.4.

In order to evaluate drug loading uniformity, all electrospun matrices were cut in a spherical mold. The spherical mold was chosen because when electrospun fibers are collected on a plate collector, they form a circular film that widens as long as fiber deposition is prolonged over time. The reduction and/or prevention in further deposition of fibers could be due to the forming of insulator layer, which depend on electrospun membrane thickness. The mechanism of fiber formation makes that the core of circular film is made of fibers collected from the beginning of the process, while the crown of circular film is made of fiber later collected. Considering no significant differences of drug loading between the core and crown section, it is reasonable to postulate that GS feeding solution was stable during the electrospinning process.

GS extraction and quantification were performed following the protocol reported above. Each electrospun matrix, whose diameter was 7 ± 0.5 cm, was cut in two concentric parts as shown in Figure 2. Part 1 (identified as crown) having 1.75 cm external circle radius, and part 2 (identified as core) having 3.5 cm diameter. GS was extracted, and in both electrospun matrix molds was quantified.

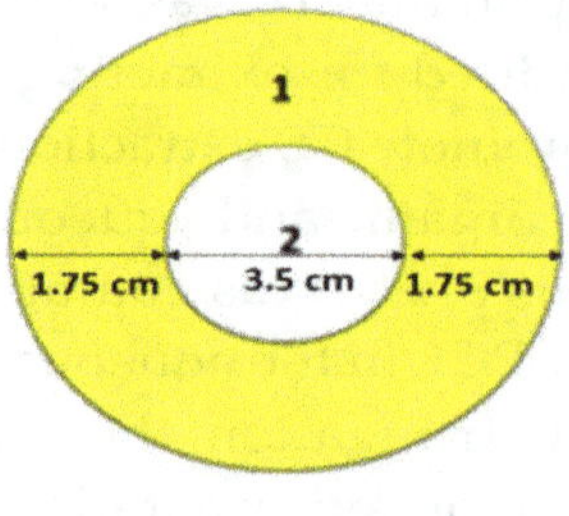

Figure 2. Representation of the two cut concentric portions of electrospun matrices: (1) crown, (2) core.

Each analysis was performed in triplicate, and average values and standard deviations (sd) were calculated. The reference for GS content percentage determination was the theoretical amount of GS loaded in the matrix calculated as follows:

$$\text{GS content (\%)} = \text{mg GS in matrix/mg GS in the electrospun polymer solution} \times 100$$

3.3. *Morphology Characterization by Scanning Electron Microscopy (SEM)*

SEM analysis was carried out on placebo and GS-loaded electrospun matrices in order to characterize their morphology in term of nanofiber size, shape, and orientation. Zeiss EVO MA10 apparatus (Carl Zeiss, Oberkochen, Germany) was used with 5000× magnification. Nanofiber size was determined by digital elaboration of SEM images with ImageJ software (National Institutes of Health (NIH) open source image processing program).

3.4. *In Vitro GS Release Test*

In vitro drug release tests were performed at 37 °C, both in static and dynamic conditions, in order to evaluate how medium flow rate and its direction affect drug release profile. The tests were carried out on both the whole electrospun matrices and on portions of the electrospun matrices that were cut as explained above.

3.4.1. In Vitro GS Release Test in Static Conditions

Each sample was placed in Erlenmeyer flasks and soaked in 10 mL of PBS (pH 7.4) at 37 °C in a thermostatic chamber. Medium was withdrawn (1 mL) at scheduled times up to GS complete release; PBS was restored with fresh buffer at each withdrawal.

3.4.2. In Vitro GS Release Test in Dynamic Conditions

In vitro release tests in dynamic conditions were performed using IVTech Livebox1 (LB1) and Livebox2 (LB2) combined with a peristaltic pump (IPC4 - ISMATEC), as shown in Figure 3. IVTech LiveBox 1 is a bioreactor made of a transparent silicon cell with a capacity of 1.5 mL and tangential flow perfusion of the incubation medium, (Figure 3A). The cell is delimitated both on the upper side and on the lower side by little glass disks (Ø 20 mm), and the locking system guarantees closure and endurance during the test. IVTech LiveBox2 (LB2) has the same structural characteristics of LB1 but with vertical perfusion flow configuration (down–top), (Figure 3B).

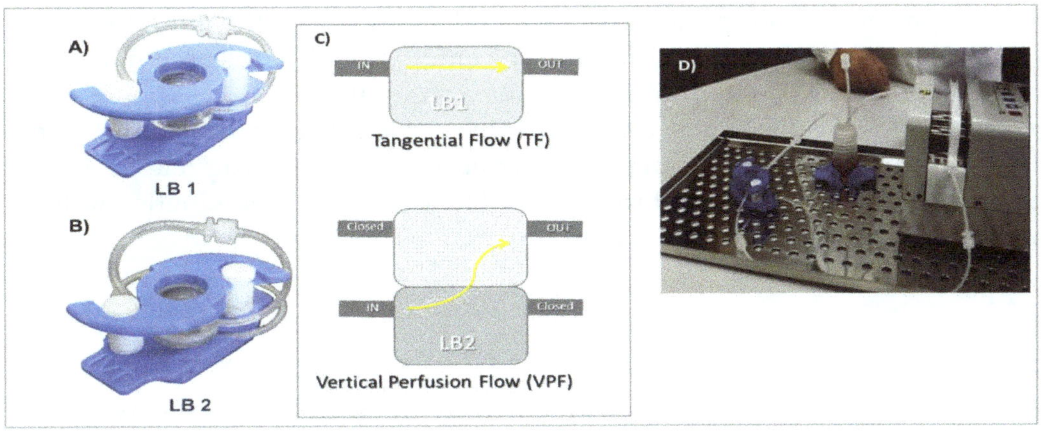

Figure 3. (**A**) Live Box1 (from IVTech website); (**B**) Live Box 2 (from IVTech website); (**C**) IVTech live Box 1 and scheme and flow configuration: Tangential Flow (TF) and Vertical Perfusion Flow (VPF); and (**D**) IVTech system equipped with pump and tubing systems.

The PBS buffer (10 mL, pH 7.4) was continuously recirculated from the reservoir vial (see Figure 3C) at two different flow rates: 0.3 mL/min and 0.6 mL/min maintaining temperature at 37 °C. IVTech LiveBox has peculiar characteristics; the sample is in contact with a small volume of incubation medium simulating the most physiologic condition of implantation into the human body. The flow through the cell creates dynamic conditions; the flow rate can be selected in the range 0.1–0.4 mL/min for LiveBox 1 (TF), and up to 0.5 mL/min in apical or basal compartments for LiveBox 2 (VPF). Flow direction can be either tangential or vertical perfusion.

In vitro release test was performed on small portions of electrospun matrix sections (1 and 2) because of the limited IVTech LiveBox chamber size. The final data were expressed as averages of the two small parts. All data were normalized against their weight in order to make them comparable with data obtained for whole matrices.

3.4.3. Kinetic Release Equations

Most common kinetic profiles considered to describe drug release are zero-order, first-order, Higuchi model, or Korsmeyer-Peppas [27–31]. The in vitro release data were elaborated using the following kinetic release equation models:

Zero-order model

$$Q_t = Q_0 + K_0 t \quad (1)$$

where Q_t is the amount of drug determined in the incubation medium at the fixed times, t is the time spans, and K_0 is the zero-order release constant expressed in units of concentration/time. The model fits drug release from dosage forms that do not disaggregate and where drug release rate is independent of its concentration. The model is used to describe drug dissolution from several types of modified release pharmaceutical dosage forms.

First-order release model

$$\text{Log } Q_t = \text{Log} Q_0 - k_1\, t/2.303 \tag{2}$$

where Q_t and Q_0 are the amounts of drug released at time t and at time zero respectively, K_1 is the first order release constant, and t is time. Drug release rate depends on its concentration; this model can be used to describe drug dissolution in pharmaceutical dosage forms containing water-soluble drugs in porous matrices.

Higuchi model

$$Q = K^{H}\, t^{1/2} \tag{3}$$

Equation (3) represent the simplified Higuchi model where Q is the amount of drug released in time t and K_H is the Higuchi dissolution constant. The amount of drug released in the fixed time spans, represented as function of the square root of time, fits a straight line.

The Higuchi model is suitable as model for drug release from thin films, containing finely dispersed drugs into perfect sink conditions; this model suggests that drug release is by diffusion, and it takes into account matrix porosity and tortuosity. The premise of the kinetic model is that perfect sink conditions are attained in the release environment.

Korsmeyer-Peppas model

$$M_t/M = k\, t^n \tag{4}$$

where M_t and M are the amount of drug at time t and loaded into the drug delivery system respectively, k is the kinetic constant related to the delivery system and encapsulated substance properties. n is release exponent and depends on the type of transport, geometry, and polydispersity of solute; it illustrates the solute transport mechanism as follows: (i) $n < 0.5$ corresponds to a pseudo-Fickian behavior of diffusion; (ii) $n = 0.5$ suggests Fickian behaviour; (iii) $0.5 < n < 1$ indicates an anomalous diffusion; (iv) $n = 1$ shows non-Fickian diffusion. The amount of drug released in the fixed time spans is represented on a log–log basis.

3.5. *In Vitro Degradation Study: Mass Loss Analysis*

Degradation study, evaluated on gravimetric basis: mass loss % (ML %) in the dissolution medium, was monitored on a parallel set of samples along all in vitro release test times, and it was determined with the following protocol. The initial mass of the matrix (M_0) was determined by weighing the lyophilized samples with an analytical balance (Mettler Toledo, AG245 mod, Milano, Italy) before being subjected to in vitro degradation tests (time zero).

The samples were incubated in PBS pH 7.4 at 37 °C, the same conditions as for the in vitro release test were followed. Each sample was taken from the buffer, at the sampling times fixed for the degradation test (3, 5, 14, 21, and 28 days), it was washed with distilled water to remove the water-soluble oligomers that can form due to copolymer degradation, and lyophilized (Lio 5P) at −48 °C at 0.4 mbar for 12 h to eliminate all water traces. The lyophilized samples were subsequently weighed (M_x). Mass loss was calculated using the following equation:

$$\textit{Mass Loss}\ (\%) = M_0 - Mx/M_0 \times 100$$

3.6. *Antibacterial Activity Measurements*

The antimicrobial activity of GS-loaded electrospun matrices (EL-GS) was evaluated against the following reference bacterial strains: *Staphylococcus aureus* ATCC 6538 and *Escherichia coli* ATCC 10356. Before testing, bacteria were grown overnight in Tryptone Soya Broth (TSA, Oxoid, Basingstoke, UK) at 37 °C. The cultures were centrifuged at 224 g for 20 min, in order to separate the microorganisms from the culture broth, and then washed with purified water. Washed cells were further suspended in Dulbecco's PBS (phosphate buffered saline, Sigma-Aldrich, Milan, Italy) and optical density (OD) was adjusted to 0.3, corresponding approximately to 1×10^8 colony forming units (CFU)/mL at 650 nm wavelength.

The antimicrobial activity was evaluated in the presence of the EL-GS, or a placebo to be used as a control. Viable microbial counts were evaluated after contact for scheduled time with EL-GS and with placebo samples (electrospun matrices without GS); bacterial colonies were enumerated in TSA after incubation at 37 °C for 24 h. The microbicidal effect (ME value) was calculated for each test organisms and contact times according to the following Equation [32]:

$$ME = \log Nc - \log Nd \qquad (5)$$

where Nc is the number of CFU of the control microbial suspension and Nd is the number of CFU of the microbial suspension in presence of patches.

4. Results

4.1. *Preparation of Polymeric Electrospun Fibers Loaded with GS*

The GS-loaded electrospun matrices, obtained after 30 min electrospinning, were round matrices whose diameter was 7 ± 0.5 cm and with average weight value of 58 ± 2.9 mg, as determined on six replications obtained in the same experimental conditions reported in the method section.

4.2. *UV Quantification of GS*

The results of GS quantification in the whole electrospun matrices are reported in Figure 4.

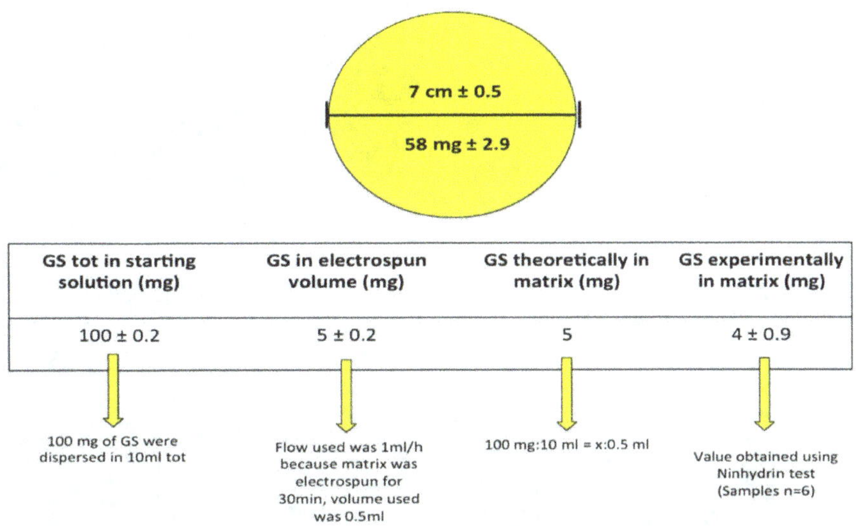

Figure 4. GS quantification in electrospun PLA-PCL matrices. The figure refers to GS amount in the whole electrospun matrix.

The amount of GS experimentally determined in the electrospun matrices, expressed as relative mass ratio of the loaded drug to the fiber, was 6.8 *w/w*%, and corresponded to the GS theoretically calculated amount. Slight loss of GS micrograms was due to the cleaning step during the electrospinning process. The results of GS determination in the matrix's portions are reported in Figure 5. GS content result was uniform compared to weight, in the two sections considered. This confirmed GS was uniformly dispersed in the polymer solution during the electrospinning process.

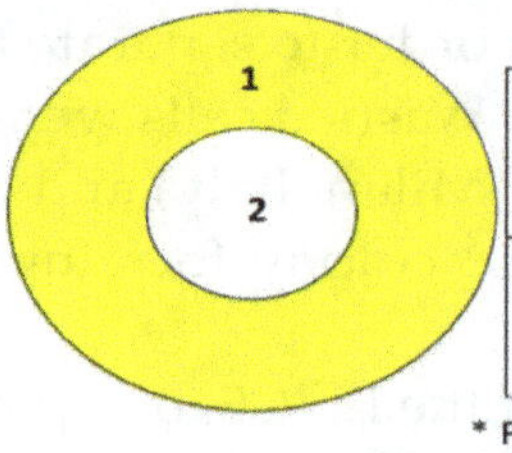

Section	Weight (mg)	GS theoretically in section (mg)*	GS experimentally in section (mg)
1	19.1 ± 1.9	1.32	1.42 ± 0.4
2	38.4 ± 4.5	2.65	2.77 ± 0.9
Total	57.6 ± 3.2	3.97	4.19 ± 0.6

* For evaluation of GS theoretical amount (mg) was used average weight of whole matrix (58 mg ± 2.9) and GS carried (4 ± 0.9)

Figure 5. GS quantification in matrices portions.

4.3. Morphologic Characterization

Data obtained by SEM analysis (Figure 5) showed that fibers morphologies were unchanged after GS addition in polymeric solution. The fibers were in a 700–800 nm range dimension with a smooth surface. No evidence of GS crystals, either on nanofibers surface (Figure 6A,B) or in the electrospun matrices (Figure 6C,D), was highlighted by SEM analysis. Electrospun matrix thickness, as measured by SEM analysis on six replications, resulted to be significantly greater for core portion, 41.81 ± 0.21 μm, with respect to external portion that was 28.61 ± 1.02 μm. The result was due to the electrospinning process on a plane collector and without any restriction, which led to the accumulation of fibers, starting from the collector central part and enlarging the radius as long as conductivity changed as a function of fiber deposition on the collector. As 30 min was fixed as the electrospinning time, this caused the fabrication of matrices with different thickness, decreasing from core to edges. Fibers entanglement, size, and shape did not change in the two different portions analyzed, while fiber density was greater in the electrospun matrices' central portions.

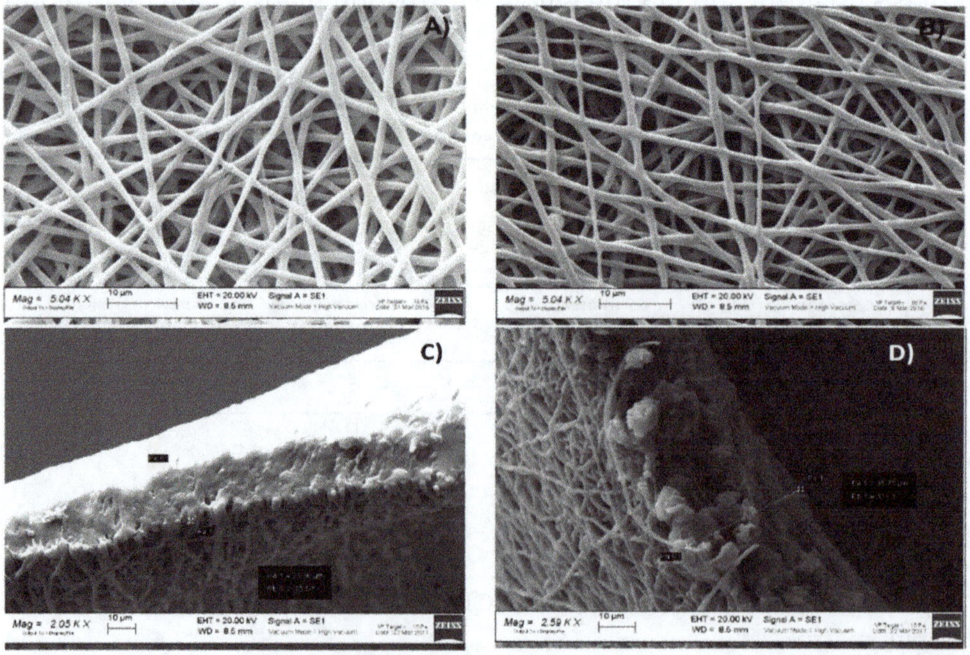

Figure 6. Scanning Electron Microscopy (SEM) images of (**A**) PLA-PCL electrospun matrices (magnification 5.04 KX); (**B**) PLA-PCL/GS electrospun matrices (magnification 5.04 KX); (**C**) orthogonal section of electrospun matrices portion 1 (external edge) (magnification 2.05 KX); and (**D**) orthogonal section of electrospun matrix portion 2 (core) (magnification 2.59 KX).

4.4. GS In Vitro Release in Static and Dynamic Conditions

GS in vitro release profiles obtained either in static or dynamic condition tests were collected in Figure 7, showing that electrospun nanofibers significantly slowed down GS release with respect to drug pristine dissolution profile (Figure 7, orange curve).

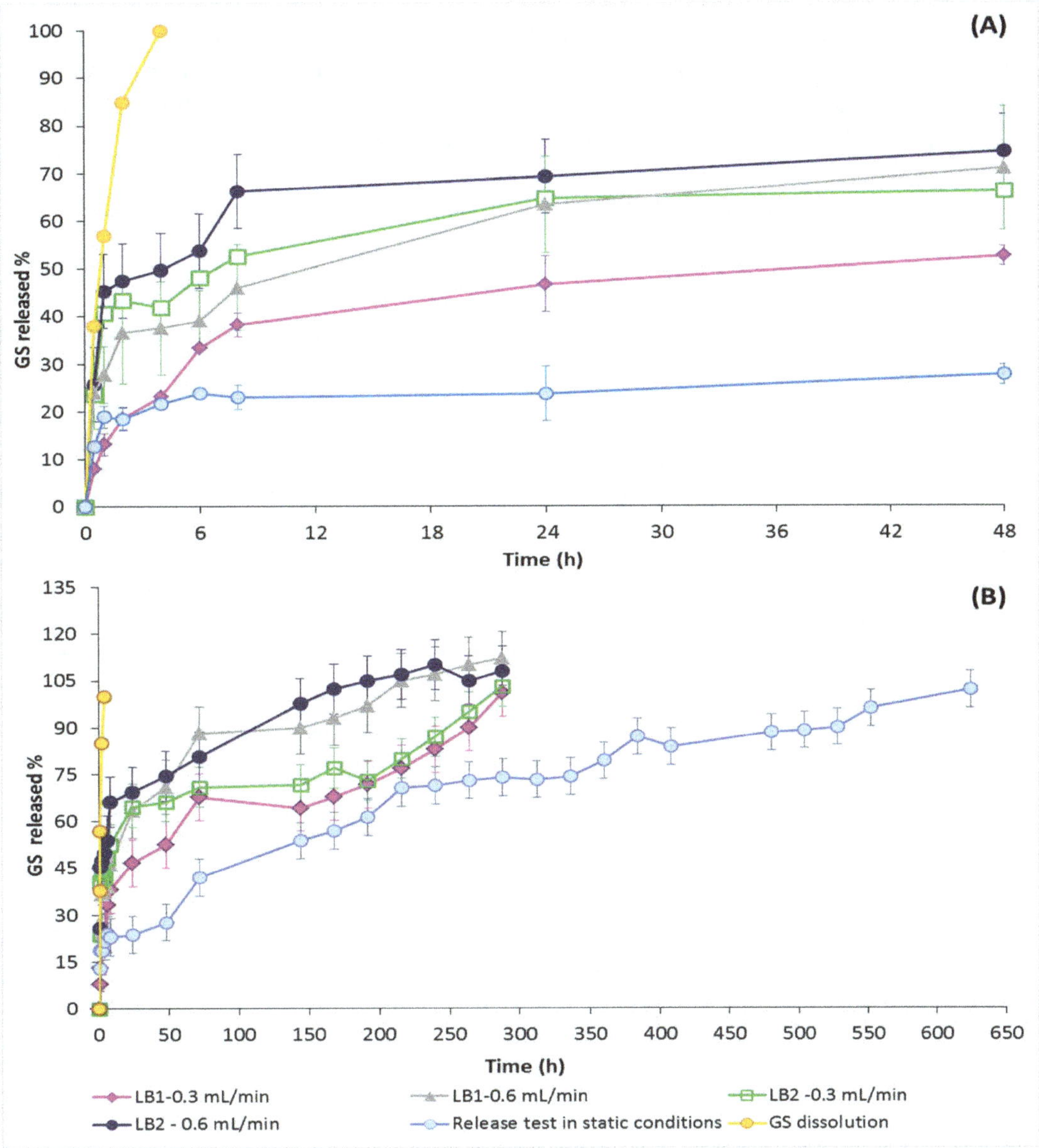

Figure 7. GS in vitro release profiles as tested in static and dynamic conditions: (**A**) GS release in the first 48 h test; and (**B**) in vitro release profiles at GS release completion.

GS release from the electrospun matrices, tested in static conditions, was completed in 624 h (26 days). No differences were highlighted between testing the whole electrospun matrices or a portion of them (data not reported), corroborating that GS was uniformly distributed in the electrospun matrix. Moreover, since GS solubility in water is 100 mg/mL, the in vitro release test on the electrospun matrices was conducted always in sink conditions. For these reasons, the different matrix thicknesses did not play a significant role in GS release. GS release profiles in dynamic conditions using IVTech bioreactors (LB1 and LB2) were reported in Figure 7.

Drug release in dynamic conditions, as expected, was significantly faster with respect to drug release rate in static conditions. In the first 24 h of testing, drug release was faster with LB2 bioreactor, which means that orthogonal flow, independently from flow rate, promoted drug release. However, drug release profiles after the first 24 h showed that the higher flow rate (0.6 mL/min) significantly sped up drug release and the higher flow rates (0.6mL/min) corresponded to significantly faster drug release with both types of flows tested (tangential for orthogonal flow). Moreover, flow direction did not seem to significantly affect the GS release profile when lower the flow rate was applied (0.3 mL/min); however, in this case, complete GS release was achieved in 288 h, both using LB1 and LB2 bioreactors.

Drug burst release (drug released in the first 8 h test) was highlighted in all the in vitro release conditions tested, and it increased by incrementing dissolution medium flow rate and changing from tangential to vertical perfusion flow direction. The results are consistent with GS high water solubility that makes drug release highly sensitive to environmental conditions.

The in vitro release data were elaborated by kinetic release equation models and results are reported in Tables 1 and 2.

Table 1. Kinetic model elaboration of GS release from EL matrices incubated in static conditions in (pH 7.4) at 37 °C.

Models	Intercept	Slope	R^2
Zero-order	0.02	1	0.94
First-order	−1.76	1.2×10^{-2}	0.93
Higuchi	0.01	2.5×10^{-3}	0.97
Korsmeyer-Peppas	−1.88	2.3×10^{-1}	0.77

Table 2. Kinetic model elaboration of GS release from electrospun matrices incubated in dynamic conditions in PBS (pH 7.4) at 37 °C.

	TF-LB1 Bioreactor						**VPF – LB2 Bioreactor**					
Flow Rate (mL/min)	**0.3**			**0.6**			**0.3**			**0.6**		
	Intercept	**Slope**	R^2	**Intercept**	**Slope**	R^2	**Intercept**	**Slope**	R^2	**Intercept**	**Slope**	R^2
Zero order	0.01	0.0001	0.77	0.01	0.0003	0.85	0.02	-7×10^{-5}	0.77	0.03	-7×10^{-5}	0.85
First order	−2.03	0.003	0.63	−1.51	0.003	0.78	−1.59	1.4×10^{-3}	0.82	−1.59	-1.3×10^{-3}	0.84
Higuchi	0.007	0.0015	0.90	0.023	0.004	0.93	0.03	-1.1×10^{-3}	0.98	0.03	-1.1×10^{-3}	0.98
Korsmeyer-Peppas	−2.15	0.25	0.87	−1.56	0.17	0.83	−1.55	-8.86×10^{-2}	0.82	−15,505	-9×10^{-2}	0.96

Electrospun matrices showed drug release was regulated from the Higuchi kinetic model, both in dynamic and static conditions. The Korsmeyer-Peppas slope exponent (n) was between 0.1 and 0.25, which confirms that the pseudo-Fickian diffusional mechanism controlled the GS release from electrospun nanofibers in all the conditions analyzed.

4.5. In Vitro Degradation Test: Mass Loss Analysis

The mass loss results in the 28 days, corresponding to in vitro release test, are reported in Figure 8. They show that matrices' mass loss reached 12% after 28 days incubation in simulated physiologic conditions. The results were consistent with data discussed by the authors in a previously published work [27] on PLA-PCL placebo electrospun matrices, showing GS-loaded PLA-PCL electrospun matrices are stable in the 28 days incubation in the simulated physiologic conditions tested.

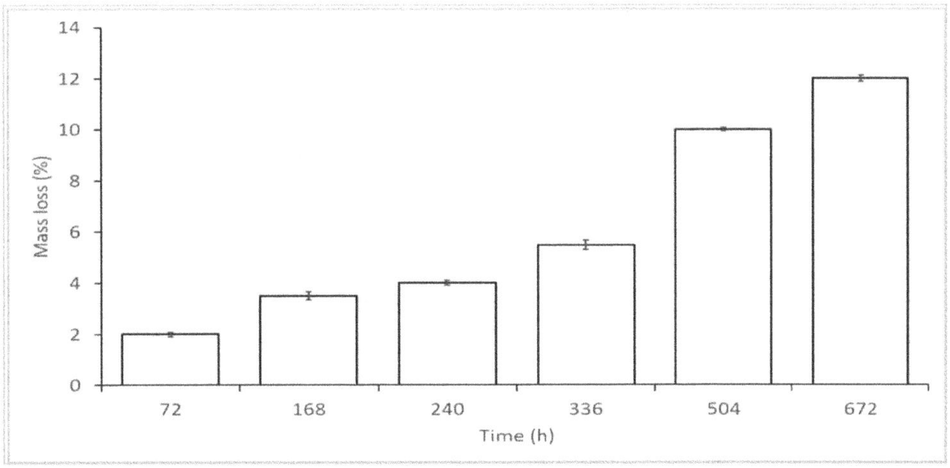

Figure 8. GS-loaded electrospun matrices' mass loss percentage in simulated physiologic conditions (PBS, pH 7.4).

4.6. Antibacterial Activity Measurements

The results of antibacterial activity measurements are reported in Table 3, they show the antimicrobial activity obtained against both *S. aureus* and *E. coli*. In particular, the values of ME were sufficiently high to reach a full antimicrobial effect at the concentrations investigated, comparable to the action of a disinfectant (ME ≥ 4) [32,33].

Table 3. Antibacterial activity of EL-GS evaluated against *S. aureus* and *E. coli*.

Sample Code	Contact Time (h)	Microbicide Effect (ME) vs. *S. aureus*	Microbicide Effet (ME) vs. *E. coli*
EL-GS *	1.0	3.79	5.86
EL-GS	6.0	7.21	8.04
EL-GS	24	10.15	10.37
EL-GS	48	10.48	10.69
EL	1.0	1.0	1.0
EL **	6.0	1.0	1.0
EL	24	0	0
EL	48	0	0

* EL-GS: Electrospun matrices loaded with GS; ** EL: placebo electrospun matrices.

CEN EN 13697 reports ME should be tested after 15 min of contact for disinfectant antibacterial activity determination. Here an antibiotic drug embedded in a polymer matrix was tested; therefore, in a different situation, slightly different time parameters were set (1 h) in order to consider GS release rate from the electrospun matrices.

The antimicrobial effect, being significant after 1 h of contact, increased with time consistently with GS release from the electrospun matrices. Placebo polymeric electrospun matrices show null antimicrobial effect against both microbial strains tested. Considering that in 48 h the EL-GS released about 27.7% GS in the same conditions (see Figure 7B, GS release in static conditions), it can be hypothesized that the antibacterial activity could prolong with time.

5. Discussion

In this work GS was solubilized in DMF, and the mixture solvent system (MC:DMF 70:30) aided the physical stabilization of GS in the polymer solution during the electrospinning process. GS concentration in the final solvent mixture, hence the amount of GS loaded into the electrospun matrices, was strictly dependent on GS solubility in the solvents used. In this experimental condition, uniform distribution of GS inside the electrospun mats was obtained, permitting an accurate dosage of GS, and no crystals were observed by SEM analysis of the electrospun matrices.

GS-loaded electrospun matrices were recently investigated by Coimbra and coll [24], demonstrating the interest in GS local delivery by polymer electrospun matrices. The authors loaded GS into electrospun matrices, starting from a suspension or an emulsion; in all cases, they highlighted similar drug release profiles with great burst release.

The results of the present experimental work highlighted that GS release rate from the electrospun matrices was slowed down with respect to in vitro dissolution of GS powder. Attention was focused on the different in vitro release tests performed, in static conditions and dynamic conditions, and results highlighted that medium flow rate significantly affects drug release rate. This could be explained by a higher differential between drug concentration at the stationary state surrounding the matrices surface and bulk drug concentration, when in vitro release test was carried out in dynamic conditions. The hypothesis was confirmed by high evidence of the phenomenon at the beginning of in vitro release test. Moreover, GS release followed a Higuchi kinetic model, typical of diffusion through porous thin films. The result is consistent with the low values of polymer mass loss obtained, demonstrating that degradation of the PLA-PCL electrospun matrix was not involved in GS release electrospun matrices.

6. Conclusions

The results indicate that there is a good and suitable chance for the future use of electrospun nanofibers as carriers for antibiotics. The electrospun matrices could be applied on severe burns, in order to prevent infections after its implantation into gingival cavities for local infection treatment, or after tooth explant. The advantage is the ability to reach high antibiotic concentrations at the site of action, in the meantime avoiding high system concentrations, thus reducing the drug side effects. Moreover, the prolonged effect of antibiotic at the site of action can reduce administration frequency and improve patient compliance. As far as GS is concerned, further studies should be conducted to ascertain how to reduce GS burst release from the electrospun matrices, meanwhile rendering drug release more independent from environmental conditions.

Author Contributions: S.P. carried out the experiment with support from E.C. Both I.G. and T.M. contributed to the implementation of the research, G.B. performed the SEM experiments, P.G. performed antibacterial activity evaluation. Both B.C. and R.D. wrote and contributed to the final version of the manuscript, B.C. supervised the project.

Acknowledgments: The authors wish to thank PTS (Parco Tecnico Scientifico) of the University of Pavia for providing electrospinning apparatus (Polymerix S.r.l., Via Taramelli 24, Pavia, Italy).

References

1. Sankaran, S.; Deshmukh, K.; Ahamed, M.B.; Pasha, S.K.K. Electrospun Polymeric Nanofibers: Fundamental Aspects of Electrospinning Processes, Optimization of Electrospinning Parameters, Properties, and Applications. In *Polymer Nanocomposites in Biomedical Engineering*; Sadasivuni, K.K., Ponnamma, D., Rajan, M., Ahmed, B., Maadeed, M.A.S.A., Eds.; Springer International Publishing: Cham, Switzerland, 2019; pp. 375–409.
2. Hu, X.; Liu, S.; Zhou, G.; Huang, Y.; Xie, Z.; Jing, X. Electrospinning of polymeric nanofibers for drug delivery applications. *J. Control. Release* **2014**, *185*, 12–21. [CrossRef] [PubMed]
3. Chen, S.; Li, R.; Li, X.; Xie, J. Electrospinning: An enabling nanotechnology platform for drug delivery and regenerative medicine. *Adv. Drug Deliv. Rev.* **2018**, *132*, 188–213. [CrossRef]
4. Kazsoki, A.; Szabó, P.; Domján, A.; Balázs, A.; Bozó, T.; Kellermayer, M.; Farkas, A.; Balogh-Weiser, D.; Pinke, B.; Darcsi, A.; et al. Microstructural Distinction of Electrospun Nanofibrous Drug Delivery Systems Formulated with Different Excipients. *Mol. Pharm.* **2018**, *15*, 4214–4225. [CrossRef] [PubMed]

5. Radacsi, N.; Giapis, K.P.; Ovari, G.; Szabo-Revesz, P.; Ambrus, R. Electrospun nanofiber-based niflumic acid capsules with superior physicochemical properties. *J. Pharm. Biomed. Anal.* **2019**, *166*, 371–378. [CrossRef] [PubMed]
6. Modica de Mohac, L.; Keating, A.V.; De Fátima Pina, M.; Raimi-Abraham, B.T. Engineering of Nanofibrous Amorphous and Crystalline Solid Dispersions for Oral Drug Delivery. *Pharmaceutics* **2018**, *11*, 7. [CrossRef] [PubMed]
7. Padmakumar, S.; Paul-Prasanth, B.; Pavithran, K.; Vijaykumar, D.K.; Rajanbabu, A.; Sivanarayanan, T.B.; Kadakia, E.; Amiji, M.M.; Nair, S.V.; Menon, D. Long-term drug delivery using implantable electrospun woven polymeric nanotextiles. *Nanomed. Nanotechnol. Biol. Med.* **2019**, *15*, 274–284. [CrossRef]
8. Simões, M.C.R.; Cragg, S.M.; Barbu, E.; de Sousa, F.B. The potential of electrospun poly(methyl methacrylate)/polycaprolactone core–sheath fibers for drug delivery applications. *J. Mater. Sci.* **2019**, *54*, 5712–5725. [CrossRef]
9. Rychter, M.; Milanowski, B.; Grzeskowiak, B.F.; Jarek, M.; Kempinski, M.; Coy, E.L.; Borysiak, S.; Baranowska-Korczyc, A.; Lulek, J. Cilostazol-loaded electrospun three-dimensional systems for potential cardiovascular application: Effect of fibers hydrophilization on drug release, and cytocompatibility. *J. Colloid Interface Sci.* **2019**, *536*, 310–327. [CrossRef]
10. Topuz, F.; Uyar, T. Electrospinning of Cyclodextrin Functional Nanofibers for Drug Delivery Applications. *Pharmaceutics* **2019**, *11*, 6. [CrossRef]
11. Khadka, D.B.; Haynie, D.T. Protein- and peptide-based electrospun nanofibers in medical biomaterials. *Nanomed. Nanotechnol. Biol. Med.* **2012**, *8*, 1242–1262. [CrossRef] [PubMed]
12. Wang, B.; Wang, Y.; Yin, T.; Yu, Q. Applications of electrospinning technique in drug delivery. *Chem. Eng. Commun.* **2010**, *197*, 1315–1338. [CrossRef]
13. Persano, L.; Camposeo, A.; Tekmen, C.; Pisignano, D. Industrial Upscaling of Electrospinning and Applications of Polymer Nanofibers: A Review. *Macromol. Mater. Eng.* **2013**, *298*, 504–520. [CrossRef]
14. Liu, S.; Zhou, G.; Liu, D.; Xie, Z.; Huang, Y.; Wang, X.; Wu, W.; Jing, X. Inhibition of orthotopic secondary hepatic carcinoma in mice by doxorubicin-loaded electrospun polylactide nanofibers. *J. Mater. Chem. B* **2013**, *1*, 101–109. [CrossRef]
15. Angkawinitwong, U.; Awwad, S.; Khaw, P.T.; Brocchini, S.; Williams, G.R. Electrospun formulations of bevacizumab for sustained release in the eye. *Acta Biomater.* **2017**, *64*, 126–136. [CrossRef] [PubMed]
16. Goh, Y.-F.; Shakir, I.; Hussain, R. Electrospun fibers for tissue engineering, drug delivery, and wound dressing. *J. Mater. Sci.* **2013**, *48*, 3027–3054. [CrossRef]
17. Abrigo, M.; McArthur, S.L.; Kingshott, P. Electrospun Nanofibers as Dressings for Chronic Wound Care: Advances, Challenges, and Future Prospects. *Macromol. Biosci.* **2014**, *14*, 772–792. [CrossRef] [PubMed]
18. Iqbal, S.; Rashid, M.H.; Arbab, A.S.; Khan, M. Encapsulation of Anticancer Drugs (5-Fluorouracil and Paclitaxel) into Polycaprolactone (PCL) Nanofibers and In Vitro Testing for Sustained and Targeted Therapy. *J. Biomed. Nanotechnol.* **2017**, *13*, 355–366. [CrossRef]
19. Buschle-Diller, G.; Cooper, J.; Xie, Z.; Wu, Y.; Waldrup, J.; Ren, X. Release of antibiotics from electrospun bicomponent fibers. *Cellulose* **2007**, *14*, 553–562. [CrossRef]
20. Al-Enizi, A.M.; Zagho, M.M.; Elzatahry, A.A. Polymer-Based Electrospun Nanofibers for Biomedical Applications. *Nanomaterials* **2018**, *8*, 259. [CrossRef] [PubMed]
21. Wang, X.; Yuan, Y.; Huang, X.; Yue, T. Controlled release of protein from core–shell nanofibers prepared by emulsion electrospinning based on green chemical. *J. Appl. Polym. Sci.* **2015**, 132. [CrossRef]
22. Luu, Y.K.; Kim, K.; Hsiao, B.S.; Chu, B.; Hadjiargyrou, M. Development of a nanostructured DNA delivery scaffold via electrospinning of PLGA and PLA-PEG block copolymers. *J. Control. Release* **2003**, *89*, 341–353. [CrossRef]
23. Ramalingam, R.; Dhand, C.; Leung, C.M.; Ong, S.T.; Annamalai, S.K.; Kamruddin, M.; Verma, N.K.; Ramakrishna, S.; Lakshminarayanan, R.; Arunachalam, K.D. Antimicrobial properties and biocompatibility of electrospun poly-ε-caprolactone fibrous mats containing Gymnema sylvestre leaf extract. *Mater. Sci. Eng. C* **2019**, *98*, 503–514. [CrossRef]
24. Coimbra, P.; Freitas, J.P.; Gonçalves, T.; Gil, M.H.; Figueiredo, M. Preparation of gentamicin sulfate eluting fiber mats by emulsion and by suspension electrospinning. *Mater. Sci. Eng. C* **2019**, *94*, 86–93. [CrossRef]

25. Lian, M.; Sun, B.; Qiao, Z.; Zhao, K.; Zhou, X.; Zhang, Q.; Zou, D.; He, C.; Zhang, X. Bi-layered electrospun nanofibrous membrane with osteogenic and antibacterial properties for guided bone regeneration. *Coll. Surf. B Biointerfaces* **2019**, *176*, 219–229. [CrossRef]
26. Dash, S.; Murthy, P.N.; Nath, L.; Chowdhury, P. Kinetic modeling on drug release from controlled drug delivery systems. *Acta Pol. Pharm.* **2010**, *67*, 217–223.
27. Pisani, S.; Dorati, R.; Conti, B.; Modena, T.; Bruni, G.; Genta, I. Design of copolymer PLA-PCL electrospun matrix for biomedical applications. *React. Funct. Polym.* **2018**, *124*, 77–89. [CrossRef]
28. Dorati, R.; DeTrizio, A.; Genta, I.; Grisoli, P.; Merelli, A.; Tomasi, C.; Conti, B. An experimental design approach to the preparation of pegylated polylactide-co-glicolide gentamicin loaded microparticles for local antibiotic delivery. *Mater. Sci. Eng. C* **2016**, *58*, 909–917. [CrossRef]
29. Dorati, R.; DeTrizio, A.; Spalla, M.; Migliavacca, R.; Pagani, L.; Pisani, S.; Chiesa, E.; Conti, B.; Modena, T.; Genta, I. Gentamicin Sulfate PEG-PLGA/PLGA-H Nanoparticles: Screening Design and Antimicrobial Effect Evaluation toward Clinic Bacterial Isolates. *Nanomaterials* **2018**, *8*, 37. [CrossRef] [PubMed]
30. Peppas, N.A.; Narasimhan, B. Mathematical models in drug delivery: How modeling has shaped the way we design new drug delivery systems. *J. Control. Release* **2014**, *190*, 75–81. [CrossRef] [PubMed]
31. Panotopoulos, G.P.; Haidar, Z.S. Mathematical Modeling for Pharmaco-Kinetic and -Dynamic Predictions from Controlled Drug Release NanoSystems: A Comparative Parametric Study. *Scientifica* **2019**, *2019*, 5. [CrossRef]
32. Yoo, J.H. Review of Disinfection and Sterilization—Back to the Basics. *Infect. Chemother.* **2018**, *50*, 101–109. [CrossRef] [PubMed]
33. EN 13697. *Chemical Disinfectants and Antiseptics—Quantitative Non-Porous Surface Test for the Evaluation of Bactericidal and/or Fungicidal Activity of Chemical Disinfectants Used in Food, Industrial, Domestic and Institutional Areas—Test Method and Requirements (Phase 2, Step 2)*; CEN (CEN European Committee for Standardization): Brussels, Belgium, 2015; pp. 3–34.

8

Monitoring of Antimicrobial Drug Chloramphenicol Release from Electrospun Nano- and Microfiber Mats Using UV Imaging and Bacterial Bioreporters

Liis Preem [1], Frederik Bock [2], Mariliis Hinnu [3], Marta Putrinš [3], Kadi Sagor [3], Tanel Tenson [3], Andres Meos [1], Jesper Østergaard [2,4,*] and Karin Kogermann [1,*]

[1] Institute of Pharmacy, Faculty of Medicine, University of Tartu, Nooruse 1, 50411 Tartu, Estonia; liis.preem@ut.ee (L.P.); andres.meos@ut.ee (A.M.)
[2] Department of Pharmacy, University of Copenhagen, Universitetsparken 2, DK-2100 Copenhagen Ø, Denmark; frederik.bock@sund.ku.dk
[3] Institute of Technology, Faculty of Natural Sciences, University of Tartu, Nooruse 1, 50411 Tartu, Estonia; mariliis.hinnu@ut.ee (M.H.); marta.putrins@ut.ee (M.P.); kadisagor@gmail.com (K.S.); tanel.tenson@ut.ee (T.T.)
[4] LEO Foundation Center for Cutaneous Drug Delivery, Department of Pharmacy, University of Copenhagen, Universitetsparken 2, DK-2100 Copenhagen Ø, Denmark
* Correspondence: jesper.ostergaard@sund.ku.dk (J.Ø.); karin.kogermann@ut.ee (K.K.);

Abstract: New strategies are continuously sought for the treatment of skin and wound infections due to increased problems with non-healing wounds. Electrospun nanofiber mats with antibacterial agents as drug delivery systems provide opportunities for the eradication of bacterial infections as well as wound healing. Antibacterial activities of such mats are directly linked with their drug release behavior. Traditional pharmacopoeial drug release testing settings are not always suitable for analyzing the release behavior of fiber mats intended for the local drug delivery. We tested and compared different drug release model systems for the previously characterized electrospun chloramphenicol (CAM)-loaded nanofiber (polycaprolactone (PCL)) and microfiber (PCL in combination with polyethylene oxide) mats with different drug release profiles. Drug release into buffer solution and hydrogel was investigated and drug concentration was determined using either high-performance liquid chromatography, ultraviolet-visible spectrophotometry, or ultraviolet (UV) imaging. The CAM release and its antibacterial effects in disc diffusion assay were assessed by bacterial bioreporters. All tested model systems enabled to study the drug release from electrospun mats. It was found that the release into buffer solution showed larger differences in the drug release rate between differently designed mats compared to the hydrogel release tests. The UV imaging method provided an insight into the interactions with an agarose hydrogel mimicking wound tissue, thus giving us information about early drug release from the mat. Bacterial bioreporters showed clear correlations between the drug release into gel and antibacterial activity of the electrospun CAM-loaded mats.

Keywords: antibacterial activity; bacterial bioreporters; drug release; electrospinning; microfibers; nanofibers; UV imaging

1. Introduction

Electrospinning is a highly versatile and robust technique that allows production of fibers with diameters from several nanometers to tens of micrometers [1]. Drug-loaded electrospun nanofiber mats have been studied intensively and show potential as drug delivery systems (DDSs) [2] and tissue engineering scaffolds [3,4] due to several advantages, such as huge specific surface area, porosity and the possibility to modify the drug release kinetics [5–7]. Compared to other delivery systems, nano- and microfiber mats enable control and tuning of the drug release kinetics [8] and, hence, design the mats with desired properties [9,10]. For example, for local antibiotic delivery, the desired drug release needs to follow two steps: initial fast release followed by the slow zero-order kinetics over a longer period of time [11]. Novel strategies for attaining sustained release have been proposed, for example via the formation of core-shell structures [12,13], beads [14], or modification of nanofiber mat thickness [15]. The drug release process is affected by several factors, such as the physicochemical properties of the drug and carrier polymer, the structural characteristics of the material system, release environment, and the possible interactions between these factors [16]. It is known that drug release from electrospun fiber mats may vary depending on the material properties and the structure of the mats [9,15,17,18].

Despite the substantial body of literature on electrospun fiber mats and their characterization, there is no standard method for the analysis of drug release from fiber mats. Traditional pharmacopoeial drug dissolution tests have been found useful for the analysis of nanofibers incorporated into capsules or pressed into a tablet [19,20]. However, when electrospun nanofiber mats are intended for the local delivery of drug, e.g., wound therapy, the amount of available liquid is low. Thus, mimicking the actual biorelevant conditions *in vitro* may be challenging using standardized dissolution testing conditions. Researchers have used methods where the amount of dissolution medium is much reduced and size of the sample is close to the actual size of the nanofiber mat used *in vivo* [18,21–23]. Samples are typically collected at predetermined time intervals and analyzed by ultraviolet-visible (UV-VIS) spectrophotometry or high performance liquid chromatography (HPLC).

The biorelevant conditions applied for the drug release studies depend on the exact problem and site of application, and may vary. Hydrogels have been widely used as DDSs for topical applications; however, hydrogels may also provide for a simplistic wound model onto which drug may be released followed by drug diffusion into the hydrogel matrix. Diffusion is one of the major transport mechanisms in the wound [16,24], although swelling and erosion may also play a role depending on the formulation. For some electrospun nanofibers, the release rate has also been explained by desorption of the embedded drug from nanopores in the fibers or from the outer surface of the fibers in contact with the water bath [25]. In addition to the actual testing, simulations have been performed and models proposed that enable prediction of the drug release behavior of the electrospun fiber mats [16,26]. These models enable the design of mats with certain structures in order to achieve a desired drug release kinetics [12].

Recently, a fully automated fiber-optics based dissolution testing systems for *in situ* monitoring of drug release from electrospun fiber mats was proposed [27]. The direct ultraviolet (UV) measurement of dissolved drug within dissolution medium provided the dissolution profile in real-time. UV imaging technology has emerged in pharmaceutical analysis [28]. It has found use for the characterization of different pharmaceutical dosage forms, including monitoring drug release from capsules [29], patches [30], and hydrogels [31,32]. Spatially resolved absorbance values are measured facilitating monitoring of concentrations and concentration gradients by UV imaging, and thereby providing the potential for new insights to the drug dissolution and release processes through real-time monitoring of swelling, precipitation, diffusion, and partitioning phenomena [31,33,34]. Drug release from electrospun fiber mats into hydrogel system has not been investigated before and was of interest within the present study.

In addition to using physical methods in drug release studies, genetically engineered whole-cell bioreporters enable to obtain valuable information during drug release studies. A few of the main advantages of using bioreporters are that they provide physiologically relevant data by measuring only biologically available fraction of the chemical. A typical bioreporter consists of a biological recognition element (i.e., sensor), a transducer, and a reporter protein. Test chemical binds to the sensor element, a transducer initiates the production of the reporter protein, and a signal is produced [35,36]. In parallel to the drug release information, such methods give direct information about the bioactivity of the developed antimicrobial DDSs.

The aim of the current study was to test and compare different drug release model systems for the characterization of electrospun nano- and microfiber antibacterial drug-loaded mats. We studied two different polymeric compositions—polycaprolactone (PCL) alone or in combination with polyethylene oxide (PEO)—with the model antibacterial drug chloramphenicol (CAM). Interestingly, we have previously shown that although these fiber mats with different carrier polymers have different drug release behavior according to the dissolution test results, their antibacterial activity was rather similar in a disc diffusion assay [22]. Therefore, in order to understand drug release from electrospun polymeric fiber mats better, novel characterization methods were acquired in order to elucidate and rationalize drug release behavior. In the current study, the drug release from electrospun fiber mats into buffer solution and agar hydrogel was investigated using HPLC, UV-VIS spectrophotometry, and bacterial bioreporters responding to the antibacterial drug CAM. UV imaging was used for the first time to monitor real-time the drug release and diffusion from electrospun fiber mats into agarose hydrogel. Antibacterial activity testing of the CAM containing fiber mats was performed using disc diffusion assay in order to shed light on the correlation between the drug release and antibacterial activity and, hence, the intended use of electrospun mats as local antibacterial DDSs for wound infections.

2. Materials and Methods

2.1. Materials, Bacteria and Release Media

Drugs, polymers, supplies. The antibacterial agent chloramphenicol (CAM) was used as a model active pharmaceutical ingredient. CAM, hydrophobic carrier polymer polycaprolactone (PCL, Mw $\approx$ 80,000), hydrophilic carrier polymer polyethylene oxide (PEO) (Mw $\approx$ 900,000), and all analytical grade reagents were purchased from Sigma-Aldrich Inc. (Darmstadt, Germany). Ampicillin sodium salt and anhydrous D-glucose used for the bacterial bioreporter preparation were obtained from Carl Roth GmbH + Co. (Karsruhe, Germany) and Fisher Scientific (Waltham, MA, USA), respectively. Type I agarose was purchased from Sigma-Aldrich (St. Louis, MO, USA). Agar hydrogel was prepared using Lennox lysogeny broth (LB) agar (Difco Laboratories, Detroit, MI, USA). FavorPrep Plasmid DNA Extraction Mini Kit and FavorPrep(TM) GEL/PCR Purification Mini Kit was purchased from Favorgen Biotech Corp. (Changzhi Township, Pingtung, Taiwan).

Bacteria. Bacteria (*Staphylococcus aureus* DSM No.: 2569) were obtained from Leibniz Institute DSMZ-German Collection of Microorganisms and Cell Cultures. *Escherichia coli* MG1655 strain [37] was used for biosensor construction. Cloning was performed in *E. coli* strain DH5α [38].

Buffers and agarose hydrogel for drug release testing by UV imaging. For the preparation of the phosphate buffer solution used as a dissolution medium, sodium dihydrogen phosphate dihydrate ($NaH_2PO_4 \cdot 2H_2O$, Merck, Darmstadt, Germany) was dissolved in distilled water. The pH of the solution (67 mM phosphate buffer) was adjusted to pH 7.40 using 5M sodium hydroxide solution. The 0.5% (*w*/*V*) agarose hydrogel was prepared by dissolving type I agarose in an appropriate volume of phosphate buffer kept at 98 °C for 45 min in a water bath. The gels were cast in the quartz cells, and allowed to settle for 30 min prior to commencing the release experiments.

Buffers and agar hydrogels for drug release and antibacterial activity testing. Drug release studies were conducted using phosphate buffered saline (1x PBS). Lennox lysogeny broth (LB) agar with a concentration of 1.5% (*w*/*V*) (*S. aureous*) and MOPS minimal medium [39] with 1.5% (*w*/*V*) agar (*E. coli*) were used for drug diffusion and antibacterial activity testing with bacteria.

2.2. Preparation and Characterization Methods

Preparation of electrospinning solutions and fiber mats. Fiber mats were prepared using an ESR200RD robotized electrospinning system (NanoNC, Seoul, Republic of Korea). Fiber mats with different compositions were prepared in order to provide different drug release kinetics. The exact compositions of the solutions used for electrospinning and electrospinning conditions are shown in Table 1.

Table 1. Composition of the electrospun formulations and electrospinning parameters.

Formulations	Materials/Polymer	Materials/Solvent	Distance (cm)	Flow Rate (ml/h)	Applied Voltage (kV)
PCL	PCL 12.5% (*w/V*), CONTROL	Chloroform:methanol (3:1 *V/V*)	14	1.0	9
PCL/CAM	PCL 12.5% (*w/V*) + CAM (4% *w/w*, solid state)	Chloroform:methanol (3:1 *V/V*)	14	1.0	9
PCL/PEO	PCL 10% + PEO 2% (*w/V*), CONTROL	Chloroform:methanol (3:1 *V/V*)	17	2.5	12
PCL/PEO/CAM	PCL 10% (*w/V*) + PEO 2% (*w/V*) + CAM (4% *w/w*, solid state)	Chloroform:methanol (3:1 *V/V*)	17	2.5	12

Key: CAM, chloramphenicol; CONTROL, formulation without CAM; PCL, polycaprolactone; PEO, polyethylene oxide.

A mixture of chloroform:methanol (3:1) (*V/V*) was used as a solvent system for the preparation of PCL and PCL/PEO systems, and a total of 10 mL was electrospun using rotation (20 rpm) and moving stage (speed 25 mm/min, distance 140 mm). For the preparation of the electrospinning solution, the polymers were dissolved in the solvent system under stirring overnight. The desired CAM concentration in the fibers was 4% (dry solid state %) and CAM was added together with the polymer into the solvent system immediately after the preparation. The electrospun fiber mats were collected onto aluminum foil and put into ziploc bags. The samples were kept in a desiccator at 0% relative humidity above silica gel to avoid humidity induced changes in the mats.

Morphology and solid state characterization of electrospun fiber mats. Morphology and diameter of electrospun fiber mats were investigated using scanning electron microscopy (SEM). Samples were mounted on aluminum stubs and magnetron-sputter coated with 3 nm gold layer in argon atmosphere prior to microscopy. Solid state characterization of the electrospun fiber mats and drug-loaded fiber mats was performed as described previously using attenuated total reflection-Fourier transform infrared (ATR-FTIR) spectroscopy (IRPrestige-21 spectrophotometer (Shimadzu Corp., Kyoto, Japan) with Specac Golden Gate Single Reflection ATR crystal (Specac Ltd., Orpington, UK) and verified with X-ray diffraction (XRD) (D8 Advance, Bruker AXS GmbH, Karlsruhe, Germany) [22]. The thickness of the fiber mats was verified using a Precision-Micrometer 533.501 (Scala Messzeuge GmbH, Dettingen, Germany) with the resolution of 0.01 mm. The thickness of the mats was 0.07 ± 0.01 mm for the PCL fiber (0.05 ± 0.01 mm with CAM) and 0.08 ± 0.01 mm for the PCL/PEO fiber (0.08 ± 0.01 mm with CAM) mats.

Drug loading and distribution in fiber mats. High performance liquid chromatography (HPLC) (Shimadzu Prominence HPLC with LC20, PDA detector SPD-M2QA, controlled by LC Solution software (1.21 SP1 Shimadzu); Shimadzu Europa GmbH, Duisburg, Germany) was used to determine the CAM concentration in the electrospun fiber mats and to evaluate its distribution uniformity throughout the fiber mats. Analyses were performed according to the official European Pharmacopoeia method for a related substance CAM sodium succinate. Briefly, CAM-loaded fiber samples were cut into 1 cm^2 pieces, weighed, and dissolved in chloroform and methanol (3:1 *V/V*). The HPLC measurements were performed using an octadecylsilyl column (Phenomenex, Luna C18(2), 250 × 4.6 mm, 5 μm). The flow rate was 1.0 mL/min, and injection volume was 20 μL. The mobile phase consisted of 2% phosphoric acid R, methanol R and water R in the volume ratio 5:40:55. A wavelength of 275 nm was used.

2.3. Drug Release Studies

2.3.1. Drug Release Testing into Buffer Solution and Agar Hydrogel by UV-VIS Spectrophotometry and HPLC

Drug release to buffer solution and agar hydrogel was investigated using UV-VIS spectrophotometry and HPLC, respectively.

Release to phosphate buffer solution: The *in vitro* drug release of CAM from electrospun PCL and PCL/PEO fiber mats was carried out as described previously [22]; however, a more frequent sampling protocol was used. Briefly, 4 cm^2 samples ($N = 3$) cut from the mats were weighed and placed into 20 mL of 1× PBS (pH 7.4) at 37 °C in 50 mL plastic tubes. The tubes were put into a dissolution apparatus vessel (Dissolution system 2100, Distek Inc., North Brunswick, NJ, USA) containing water maintained at 37 °C using rotation (paddle system, 100 rpm). Aliquots of 2 mL were removed and replaced with the same amount of 1× PBS at set time points. The aliquots were analyzed using UV-spectrophotometry (Shimadzu UV-1800, Shimadzu Europa GmbH, Duisburg, Germany) at 278 nm.

Release to agar hydrogel: The amount of drug released into agar plates was investigated by sampling different zones of the agar (illustrated with a figure in Section 3.4). Pieces of fiber mat (PCL/CAM and PCL/PEO/CAM fiber mat discs, with a diameter of 1 cm) were weighed, put onto pre-warmed LB agar plates, kept at 37 °C, and removed at set time points. Zones of the agar were cut out, the agar sample was put into ethanol (96%) and sonicated for 15 min. This extraction process was repeated twice and the obtained ethanol solutions were combined. The vials with ethanol solutions were left under a fume hood without caps, for the ethanol to evaporate. The residues left in the vials were dissolved in 1.5 mL of ethanol (96%) and the amount of CAM analyzed with HPLC. In the present study, the limit of detection for CAM was 1 μg/mL. Triplicate measurements were performed. The extraction efficacy was tested separately confirming that two times extraction resulted in 100% efficacy (Appendix A, Table A1).

2.3.2. UV Imaging for Drug Release Monitoring in Hydrogel

Complementary to the traditional HPLC method, an Actipix D200 Large Area Imager (Paraytec Ltd., York, England) controlled by Actipix D200 acquisition software ver. 3.1.7.4 was used to image the release of CAM from PCL and PCL/PEO fiber mats. These experiments were performed in a heating cabinet from Edmund Bühler TH30 (Bodelshausen, Germany) set to 37 °C. Imaging was performed at four alternating wavelengths: 525 nm, 280 nm, 255 nm, and 214 nm. Images for each wavelength were recorded at a frequency of 0.125 s^{-1} for the release experiments as well as the standard curve. The imaging area (28 × 28 mm^2; pixel size 13.8 μm^2) encompassed three quartz cells (Pion Inc., UK; 62 mm × 4 mm × 7 mm (L × H × W)), allowing three measurements to be performed simultaneously. The fibers were cut to fit the inner dimensions of the quartz cells (7.0 mm in width and 4.0 mm in height). The fibers were positioned perpendicular to the imaging direction in contact with the agarose gel. The fibers were backed by silicone plugs to ensure good contact with the gel and correct alignment. Parafilm was used to seal the quartz cells preventing evaporation of water from the gels. The release of CAM from the fibers was imaged for 3 h at 37 °C. Each imaging experiment allowed measurements of two CAM-containing fibers and one blank fiber (control). The positioning of the fibers in the imaging system (top, middle or bottom row) was randomized.

Standard Curve for quantification by UV imaging. A CAM stock solution (5 mM) in phosphate buffer was used to make the dilutions for the standard curve in 0.5% (*w*/*V*) agarose gel. These were made by mixing 1.5 mL 1% (*w*/*V*) agarose in phosphate buffer with a defined volume of CAM solution and phosphate buffer to obtain 3 mL of the mixture. The 1% (*w*/*V*) agarose solution and the phosphate buffer were both heated in water bath (98 °C) to facilitate mixing leading to a homogeneous mixture. The gels were cast in the quartz cells, and allowed to settle for 30 min prior to the experiments. As reference, a 0.5% (*w*/*V*) agarose gel in phosphate buffer without CAM was used.

2.4. Antibacterial Activity Studies—Drug Release and Effect on Bacterial Growth

2.4.1. Antibacterial Activity Testing

The antibacterial activity of released CAM on agar plates was investigated at different time points mimicking the drug diffusion tests into agarose hydrogel during UV imaging studies. Overnight culture (20 h) of *S. aureus* DSM No.: 2569 was grown from DMSO stock (100 uL to 3 mL of LB). Preparation of all bacterial DMSO stocks used in the present study is described in Appendix B. The culture was diluted to optical density (OD) 0.05 in LB and 100 μL was plated onto pre-warmed LB agar plates (1.5% (*w*/*V*)). PCL/CAM and PCL/PEO/CAM fiber discs, and a positive CAM filter paper control were applied onto each plate. At specific time points, the discs were removed and the LB plates were incubated at 37 °C for 24 h prior to measurement of the inhibition zones.

2.4.2. Bioreporter Plasmid and Strain Preparation

All cloning was performed using CPEC cloning method [40]. Plasmid vector backbone was low-copy pSC101 plasmid. *Timer* reporter gene in plasmid pSC101-Ptet-Timer [41] was replaced with two fluorescent reporter genes *GFPmut2* [42] and *mScarlet-I* [43]. In order to increase the expression of the green fluorescence protein (GFP) during antibiotic stress additional stress-inducible dnaK1 promoter (PdnaK1) originating from *E. coli* MG1655 genomic DNA was added upstream of the tet-promoter (Ptet). In addition, kanamycin resistance gene *kanR* was replaced with ampicillin resistance gene *ampR*. In order to reduce the expression of *ampR* resulting from reverse direction transcription initiation from PdnaK1, additional rrnB T2 terminator was added between *ampR* and PdnaK1.

In order to construct the ribosomal stalling reporter plasmid pSC101-CAM-bioreporter transcription attenuation-based regulatory *trpL2Ala* region together with a terminator and constitutive T5 promoter from plasmid, pRFPCER-TrpL2A [44] was inserted between *GFPmut2* and *mScarlet-I* ribosomal binding site. mRNA from the reporter gene *mScarlet-I*, and therefore, red fluorescence is only produced when ribosomal stalling occurs, e.g., due to CAM presence (Appendix C).

CPEC products were transformed into *E. coli* DH5α and plasmids were purified using FavorPrep Plasmid DNA Extraction Mini Kit. All plasmids were verified by sequencing. Purified bioreporter plasmid pSC101-CAM-bioreporter was transformed into *E. coli* MG1655 chemical competent cells via heat shock. The transformants were selected on ampicillin (100 μg/mL) containing LB-agar plates after overnight incubation. The full nucleotide sequence of the pSC101-CAM-bioreporter plasmid is provided as Supplementary Materials in GeneBank (gb) file format.

2.4.3. Bioreporter Disc Diffusion Assay

For bacterial bioreporter disc diffusion assay agar plates with defined MOPS minimal medium [39] supplemented with 0.4% (*w*/*V*) glucose as the carbon source and 1.5% (*w*/*V*) agar were prepared in sterile conditions by measuring 20 mL of warm agar medium per plate, and plates were dried for 30 min under laminar flow hood.

Bioreporter strain DMSO stock was thawed, diluted 20× into sterile 1× PBS and 75 μL was plated on each minimal plate. A sterile cotton bud dipped into 1× PBS was used to spread the cells evenly. Plates were left to incubate at 37 °C for 10 h. After incubation, the weighted fiber mats (PCL/PEO/CAM and PCL/CAM) were added to each plate. Individual plates were first scanned with the Amersham Typhoon scanner (GE Healthcare Europe GmbH, Freiburg, Germany) (pixel size 100 μm; green fluorescence: 488 nm laser, 525BP20 filter, PMT voltage 352V; red fluorescence: 532 nm laser, 570BP20 filter, PMT voltage 621V) after adding the mats and re-scanned every hour for 6 h. Scan time for each plate was approximately 6 min. The plates were incubated at 37 °C between the scans.

2.5. Data Analysis

Data are given as average ± standard deviation (SD), unless stated otherwise. Data were analyzed and figures plotted using MS Excel 2017 and/or 2016, GraphPad Prism 7 ver. 7.04 or OriginPro 8.5.

Statistical analysis was performed by two-tailed Student's *t*-test assuming unequal variances ($p < 0.05$) where applicable.

The SDI Data analysis software ver. 2.0.60624 (Paraytec Ltd., York, England) was used to analyze the recordings made on the Actipix D200 system. The CAM molar absorption coefficient determined from the standard curve was used to calculate CAM concentrations in the gels. The analysis was performed at 255 nm, because the linear range of the standard curve covered the absorbance values encountered in the release experiments in contrast to 280 nm. A 6.25 mm wide zone starting from the fiber-gel interface protruding into the gel in the CAM transport direction was defined. For each pixel column, the absorbance was averaged, converted to concentration and plotted as a function of distance from the fiber mat to attain concentration-distance profiles. From the concentration-distance profiles, the area under curve (AUC) was calculated to determine the total amount of CAM released from the fibers.

The inhibition zones free of bacterial growth (diameters, mm) were determined using ImageJ software [45] program version 1.52n. Tests were run at least in triplicate. ImageJ software was also used for obtaining numerical values of fluorescent zones from disc diffusion assay images. Green and red fluorescence images were analyzed separately. 0.8 mm wide lines were chosen as regions of interest for analysis. The 1.5 cm long line was drawn starting from the fiber mat and plot profiles of grey values for these regions were recorded.

3. Results and Discussion

3.1. Preparation and Characterization of Electrospun Fiber Mats

In order to test the suitability of the UV imaging technique and different drug release model systems for monitoring drug release from electrospun fiber mats, different mats were electrospun by varying the polymers (hydrophilic PEO vs. hydrophobic PCL) and incorporating the antibacterial drug CAM into the fibers (Table 1). The preparation and morphological and physicochemical characterization of these electrospun antibacterial CAM-loaded fibers has been performed previously [22]. As shown previously, the prepared PCL and PCL/CAM mats consisted of nanofibers within the average size range from 370 to 496 nm (SD ± 339 nm), whereas PCL/PEO and PCL/PEO/CAM mats were in the micrometer size range with an average diameter of 2.9 μm (SD ± 1.1 μm). Solid state transformation from crystalline CAM to amorphous CAM was confirmed with drug-loaded electrospun fiber mats (data not shown). In agreement with previous findings [22], CAM was homogeneously distributed within the electrospun fiber mats (data not shown) and CAM content matched with the theoretical values (Table 2).

Table 2. Average CAM concentrations within the electrospun fiber mats ($N = 3$–7). Formulation compositions and electrospinning parameters are shown in Table 1.

Electrospun Fiber Formulations	Theoretical CAM Content/%	Measured CAM Content/% ± SD
PCL/CAM	4	4.0 ± 0.2
PCL/PEO/CAM	4	3.8 ± 0.3

Key: CAM, chloramphenicol; SD, standard deviation.

3.2. Drug Release into Buffer Measured by UV-VIS Spectrophotometry

Initially, traditional dissolution testing into buffer solution was performed and CAM concentrations were determined using UV-VIS spectrophotometry. The PCL/CAM and PCL/PEO/CAM mats are different in terms of their wettability and swelling properties. PCL/PEO/CAM mats are more hydrophilic and swell when exposed to an aqueous medium [22]. The PCL/CAM mats are more hydrophobic, although the presence of CAM tends to increase the wetting of the mat and provide access for the buffer to enter the fibers. Thus, PCL/CAM fiber mats provided the expected and desired prolonged

CAM release whilst PCL/PEO/CAM mats due to the hydrophilic nature of PEO exhibited a faster drug release in buffer solution (Figure 1).

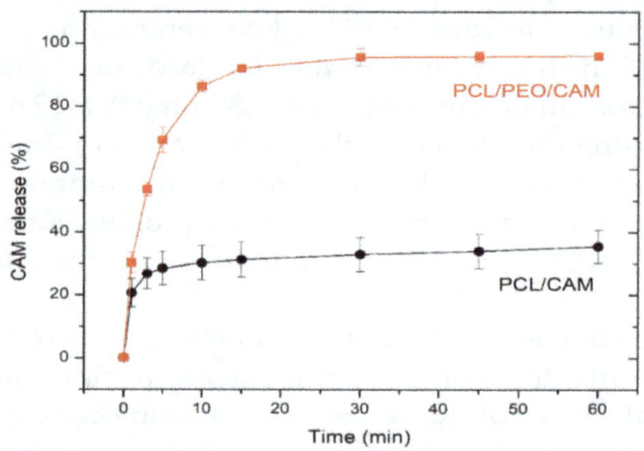

Figure 1. Relative release of CAM from PCL/PEO/CAM (■) and PCL/CAM (●) fiber mats into phosphate buffered saline at pH 7.40 and 37 °C. Data are averages ± SD of at least triplicate samples. Analyses performed using UV-VIS spectrophotometry (reference is made to Table 1 for fiber composition and preparation conditions).

Frequent sampling revealed a significant CAM burst release (up to 15 min of release testing) from both fiber mats. There were only minor differences in triplicate measurements and in the behavior of the fiber mats verifying the reproducibility of the measurements. In a recent study, the free drug (terbinafine hydrochloride) on the surface of fibers was removed after rinsing in distilled water and the amount of released drug quantified in a wound dressing-skin model utilizing filter paper as a matrix [21]. The rinsing procedure most likely removed the drug burst release. In the present study, no pretreatment of the mats was performed and the mats were analyzed directly. It is likely that if burst released amounts were removed the drug release would be even more different between the mats and most of CAM would be removed from PCL/PEO/CAM fibers mats during the pretreatment. For understanding drug release and *in vivo* activity relationships, the mats should not be pretreated; however, such pretreatment might be important if *in vitro* tests are performed to illustrate only the differences between the fiber mats in respect of their prolonged drug release.

3.3. *Antibacterial Activity of Electrospun Fiber Mats*

Despite the different morphologies and behavior (e.g., swelling, drug release into buffer), statistically significant differences in the inhibition zones on agar plate between the PCL/CAM and PCL/PEO/CAM fiber mats were not observed during previous antibacterial activity testing [22]. In the present study, it was of interest to investigate further how the drug is released from the electrospun mat into a gel which more closely resembles the wound matrix (e.g., agar and agarose hydrogels) and how this translates into antibacterial effect. Hydrogels have more similar hydrodynamic conditions to wound tissue as compared to aqueous solutions and thus provide more biorelevant testing option. We developed a modified disc diffusion assay, where the mats were physically removed from the surface of the solid growth medium at specified time points and the antibacterial effect of the released drug on model bacteria *S. aureus* DSM No.: 2569 was determined by measuring the size of the inhibition zones after 24 h. The faster CAM release from PCL/PEO/CAM mats compared to the PCL/CAM mats observed in buffer solution (Figure 1) correlated with larger inhibition zones (Figure 2). The differences were larger at the earlier time points. Control filter paper impregnated with CAM confirmed that the wetting of the sample is the major triggering factor for further drug release and diffusion.

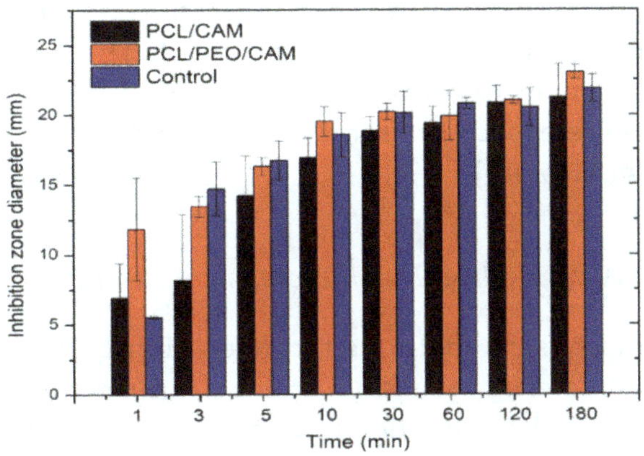

Figure 2. Inhibition zone diameters measured after 24 h on agar plates. X-axis indicates exposure time of discs (PCL/PEO/CAM or PCL/CAM fiber mats) onto the hydrogel. *S. aureus* DSM No.: 2569 was used for the study. Filter paper wetted with CAM solution and dried (same CAM concentration) served as a control. Key: CAM, chloramphenicol; PCL, polycaprolactone; PEO, polyethylene oxide. Data are averages ± SD of at least triplicate samples.

3.4. Drug Release into Agar Hydrogel Measured by HPLC

The extent of CAM release from the mats and diffusion into the agar hydrogel was quantified using HPLC upon extraction of CAM from the agar hydrogel. The agar on the plates was divided into five concentric circular zones (Figure 3A) and the CAM concentration in each zone was determined. The experimental design is detailed in the Materials and Methods and Appendix A (Tables A1 and A2). The amount of drug released from electrospun mats to the agar plates at different time points at 37 °C is summarized in Figure 3.

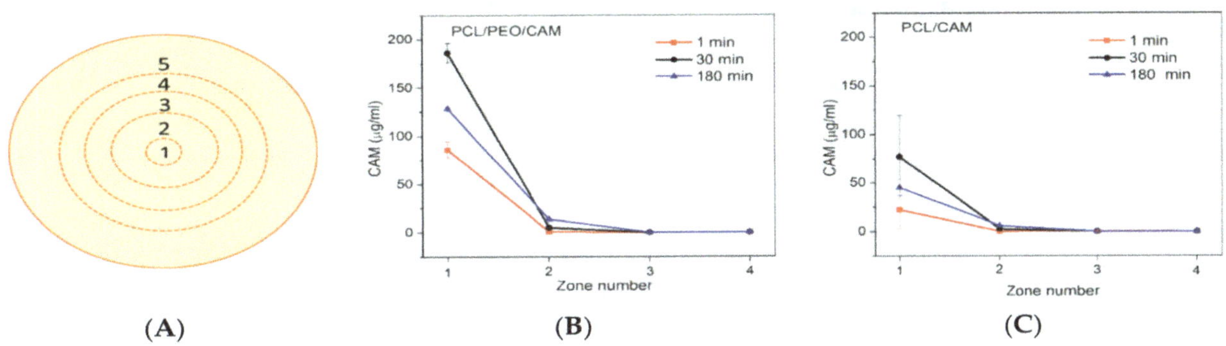

Figure 3. (**A**) Schematic illustrating the division of the agar plate into zones. Zones 1-5 are numbered starting from the inner circle. Zone diameters: 1.0 cm, 3.0 cm, 4.4 cm, 5.8 cm, and 8.6 cm. Concentrations of released CAM (detection limit of 1 μg/mL) from PCL/PEO/CAM (**B**) and PCL/CAM fiber mats (**C**) into 1.5% (*w/V*) agar hydrogel at 37 °C in different time points (1 min, 30 min, 180 min) and into different zones (1–4). Error bars represent standard deviation, $N = 3$. Key: CAM, chloramphenicol; PCL, polycaprolactone; PEO, polyethylene oxide.

The drug diffusion patterns for PCL/CAM and PCL/PEO/CAM fiber mats were qualitatively similar (Figure 3). These findings are consistent with the disc diffusion assay results (see for Figure 2). It is clear that most of the drug is present in the 1 cm diameter section (zone 1) right below the fiber mat at the early time points of the release experiment. As time passed, less drug was recovered in the inner circle (zone 1) and relatively more in zone 2 (larger circle around the mat). CAM release from PCL/PEO/CAM fiber mat was fast followed by slower diffusion further into the agar hydrogel (Figure 3B). Interestingly, after 120 min, the drug was not detectable in the 3rd zone. After 24 h (1440 min), the CAM had reached the outer circle (Appendix A, Table A2). PCL/CAM fiber mats on the other hand showed that less drug was released within the same time period compared to the

PCL/PEO/CAM fiber mat (Figure 3C). The CAM concentration distribution differences are visible in Figure 3, mainly for zone 1 but to some extent also for zone 2. This may explain why it is not always possible to detect differences in the inhibition zones between different fiber mats in a disc diffusion assay although the drug may be released differently from the delivery vehicle and, therefore, lead to different antibacterial efficacy *in vivo* [46].

3.5. Detecting CAM Release into Agar Hydrogel with Bioreporter Strain

In addition to chemical and physical methods for determining the CAM concentrations during the release, it is also possible to use bacterial bioassays. Hence, simultaneously to the antibacterial effects, the drug release can be monitored. We genetically engineered reporter bacteria (*E. coli* MG1655) to produce dose-dependent quantifiable green and red fluorescent signals in the presence of antibacterial drug CAM. The CAM-bioreporter has GFP as a control protein for expression and a red mScarlet-I as a reporter protein. Exact working mechanism of the bacterial bioreporter is provided in Appendix C. In the presence of CAM GFP signal (green) will be reduced due to protein synthesis inhibition, and mScarlet-I signal (red) will increase due to transcription continuation as a result of ribosomal stalling in the transcription attenuation system. Therefore, the CAM release and diffusion can be illustrated in different time points (selected time points 60, 180, and 360 min) using fluorescence data (Figure 4).

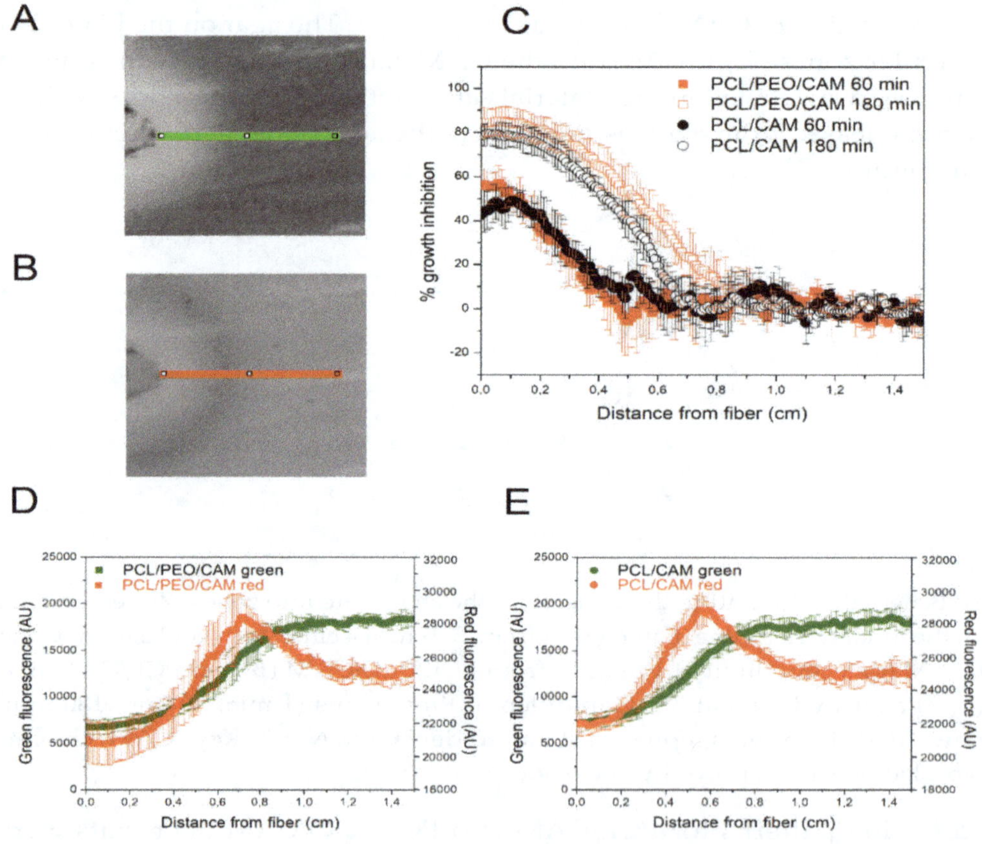

Figure 4. (**A**,**B**). Shows the analyzed region of interest (0.8 mm × 1.5 cm) of bioreporter chloramphenicol (CAM)-containing fiber disc diffusion assay from green fluorescence (**A**) and red fluorescence (**B**) scan images. Green fluorescence images in different time points (60 min and 180 min) allow estimating bacterial growth inhibition due to CAM released from PCL/PEO/CAM and PCL/CAM fiber mats (**C**). Combined green and red fluorescent figures at 6 h reveal the fluorescence levels that can be correlated with the released CAM from PCL/PEO/CAM (**D**) and PCL/CAM fiber mats (**E**). Data are presented as average of three experiments (± SD). Key: CAM, chloramphenicol; PCL, polycaprolactone; PEO, polyethylene oxide.

It is clearly seen that bacterial growth is inhibited close to the fiber mats (inhibition zones surrounding the mats) where CAM concentrations are the highest, which matches with the agar diffusion test results (Figures 2 and 3). Fluorescent bacteria surrounding the inhibition zones reveal the distance from the mat where the CAM levels above the minimum inhibitory concentration (MIC) can still be detected. Compared to the agar hydrogel diffusion tests (Figures 2 and 3), bacterial bioreporter study results on agar hydrogel did not reveal large differences between the PCL/CAM and PCL/PEO/CAM fiber mats with the respect of released drug amounts and its effect on bacteria (Figure 4C). Growth inhibition was very slightly more pronounced in PCL/PEO/CAM fiber mat (fast release) after 60 min of incubation; however, this difference was statistically insignificant and disappears in later time points (180 min). In later time points (6 h) red fluorescence detected from bacteria enabled determining the CAM concentrations even below MIC (in sub-MIC concentrations) (Figure 4D,E). After 6 h of incubation, the peak of the reporter protein signal is located further (approximately 0.75 cm) from the mat in case of PCL/PEO/CAM fiber mat (fast release) (Figure 4D) compared from PCL/CAM fiber mat (slow release; located approximately 0.60 cm) (Figure 4E). This indicates that effective CAM concentration was achieved on larger area (at a further distance from the fiber mat) with PCL/PEO/CAM fiber mat, although the difference between the two fiber mats was minor. Most likely, this is due to the fact that most of the differences between the two different electrospun fiber mats can only be seen in early time points which cannot be distinguished using fluorescent bacteria in these settings.

3.6. Drug Release into Agarose Hydrogel Using UV Imaging

The assessment of CAM release by cutting of zones from agar plates followed by extraction and analysis of the drug is both a destructive and laborious sampling procedure. The fast release of CAM cannot be monitored using bioreporter bacteria that require time for growth and detectable signal production. Therefore, UV imaging was investigated as a potentially less labor intensive and more robust (reproducible/repeatable) approach for monitoring CAM release from the electrospun fiber mats. An additional benefit of the non-intrusive imaging method is the high spatial as well as temporal resolution offered. Due to a lack of transparency of the agar plates used in antibacterial activity tests, a hydrogel matrix based on agarose was applied instead. Moreover, the Actipix D200 Large Area Imager allowed imaging of three samples in parallel enabling comparison. Images visualizing the release and diffusion of CAM at different time points are shown in Figure 5A.

Diffusion into the viscous agarose hydrogel resembles the conditions encountered both during *in vitro* disc diffusion testing (agar hydrogel) as well as *in vivo* where the drug has to be released from the electrospun fiber and diffuse into the wound. The UV imaging results reveal that PCL/CAM fibers provide slower drug release into the gel whereas PCL/PEO/CAM fibers release the drug faster (Figure 5A). The concentration-distance profiles shown in Figure 5B,C correspond to the images in Figure 5A. In addition, the average amount of CAM released was quantified based on the UV images (Figure 6). When comparing the two mats, differences were observed with respect to the total amount of released drug mainly at the early time points (Figure 6).

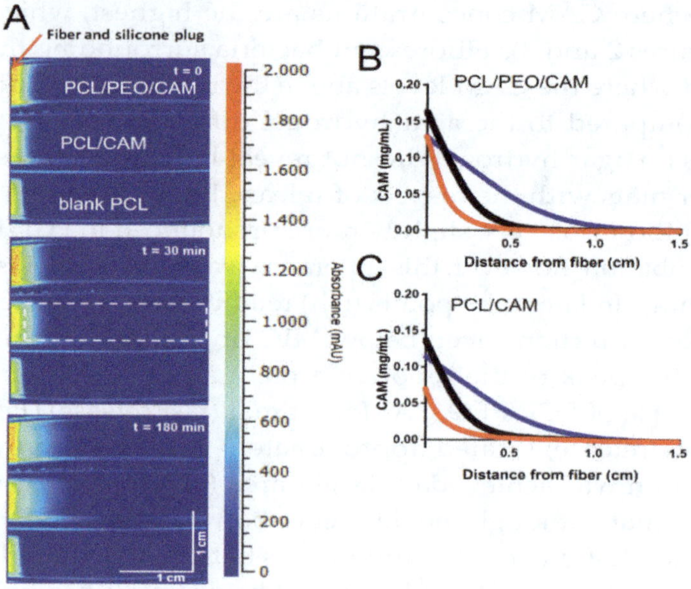

Figure 5. (**A**) Representative images of CAM release from fibers and diffusion into 0.5% (*w*/*V*) agarose hydrogel at 37 °C. Top is PCL/PEO/CAM, middle is PCL/CAM and bottom is PCL/Blank fibers (control). The zone used for the quantification of the CAM absorbance is shown in the middle row at 30 min. Representative concentration-distance profiles for PCL/PEO/CAM (**B**) and PCL/CAM (**C**) fibers diffusing into 0.5% (*w*/*V*) agarose hydrogel at 37 °C. The red, black and blue line is for 0 min (immediately after starting the experiment), 30 min and 180 min, respectively. Key: CAM, chloramphenicol; PCL, polycaprolactone; PEO, polyethylene oxide.

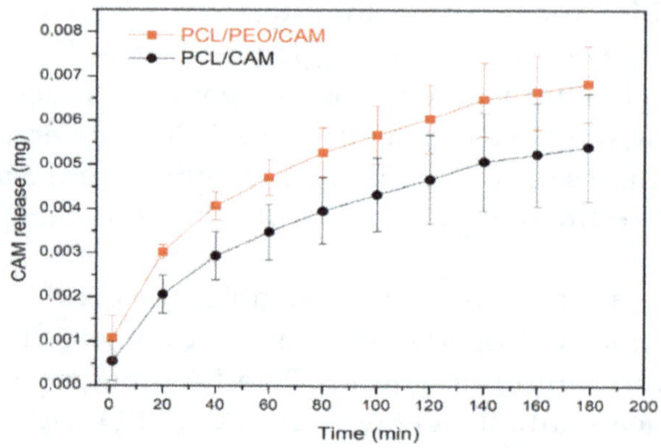

Figure 6. Amount of CAM released from PCL/PEO/CAM (■) and PCL/CAM (●) fiber mats into 0.5% (*w*/*V*) agarose hydrogel at 37 °C based on UV imaging experiment data. Error bars represent one standard deviation, $N = 5$. Key: CAM, chloramphenicol; PCL, polycaprolactone; PEO, polyethylene oxide.

Only slight differences between the PCL/CAM and PCL/PEO/CAM fiber mats with respect to their drug release behavior were detected in average drug release profiles, although these were not statistically significant and can be considered as more of a tendency.

3.7. Comparison between Different Drug Release Model Systems

Irrespective of the *in vitro* release model system (testing approach) employed, the release of CAM was found to be faster from the PCL/PEO fiber mats as compared to the PCL fiber mats (Figure 7). However, the extent to which the release differed tended to vary between the model systems.

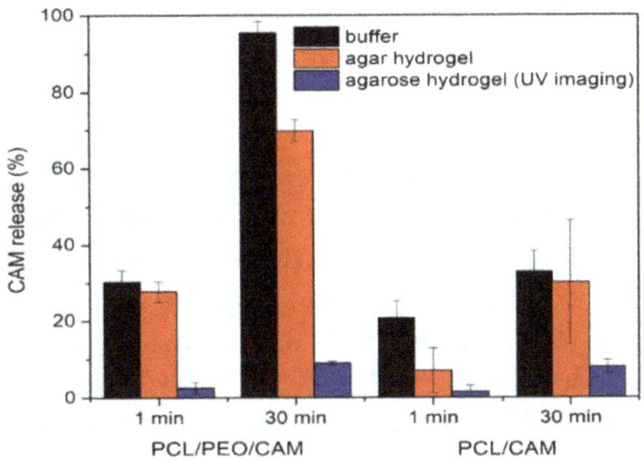

Figure 7. Amount of CAM released from PCL/PEO/CAM and PCL/CAM fiber mats into phosphate buffered saline at pH 7.40 and 37 °C and 1.5% (*w/V*) agar hydrogel at 37 °C and 0.5% (*w/V*) agarose hydrogel at 37 °C. Data are averages ± SD of at least triplicate samples. Analyzes performed using UV-VIS spectrophotometry (CAM concentration in a buffer solution), HPLC (CAM concentration extracted from hydrogel) and UV imaging (CAM concentration within hydrogel) (reference is made to Table 1 for fiber composition and preparation conditions). Key: CAM, chloramphenicol; PCL, polycaprolactone; PEO, polyethylene oxide.

Drug release into buffer revealed that after 30 min the PCL/PEO/CAM fibers had released nearly all CAM into the buffer, whereas only a minor amount (approximately 30%) of drug was released from PCL/CAM fiber mats (Figure 7). When the CAM release into hydrogel was monitored by agar disc diffusion and extraction method, the amount of CAM released from PCL/PEO/CAM fiber mat after 30 min was approximately 70% and the released CAM amount from PCL/CAM mat was similarly approximately 30% (with huge variability between 17–48% for individual PCL/CAM fiber mats). UV imaging, however, showed that the differences with respect to the amount of drug released into the agarose hydrogel between PCL/CAM and PCL/PEO/CAM fiber mats after 30 min were less pronounced as compared to the differences in CAM release into buffer (Figure 7). It was also seen that much less CAM was released and diffused to the region of analysis from both fiber mats (approximately 9% and 8% for PCL/PEO/CAM and PCL/CAM fiber mats, respectively) within the same time period. Most likely, less CAM is released from the fiber mats into the hydrogel according to the UV imaging due to the different geometries of the setup. In the UV imaging setup, diffusion is limited to one direction perpendicular to the mat, whereas diffusion in the agar setup may occur in three dimensions. The latter will favor a relatively larger release of CAM. We believe that the concentration may be more likely to build up at the interface in the UV imaging setup. As might be expected due to the similarity of the release matrices (hydrogel), the UV imaging drug release and diffusion profiles matched more with the drug release into agar hydrogel extraction (Figures 3–5) than release and dissolution into buffer test (Figure 1). The contact and/or of the mats with the hydrogels may be different between the agar and agarose hydrogels. It is not known whether the agar hydrogel may contain components interacting, and thereby facilitating the release of CAM. Similarly to UV imaging, less pronounced differences between the two different electrospun CAM-loaded fiber mats were also observed with bacterial bioreporters (Figure 4C). It is due to the fact that the drug has to diffuse away from the mat before it will be detected (UV imaging and bacterial bioreporters), whereas in the agar hydrogel extraction method, the area under the fiber mat will be included into the total released and detected drug amount.

The differences with respect to CAM release from the mats observed using the *in vitro* release testing model systems are related to the different properties of the release media (volume, agitation, and viscosity), its capability to penetrate into the fiber mat, the sample size of fiber mats, effect of shaking, and geometry of the setup. It is believed that drug diffusion and wetting of the samples were the rate-limiting steps for the drug release from fiber mat into agar and agarose hydrogels. The release into buffer solution, however, was more affected by the hydrodynamics of the buffer measurements. For the different fiber mats agitation led to increased erosion and/or disintegration of the PCL/PEO/CAM fiber mats as compared to the PCL/CAM fiber mats.

In terms of repeatability the model systems and analytical methods were all comparable. It can be seen that larger variations in drug release between replicates were detected for PCL/CAM fiber mats compared to PCL/PEO/CAM fiber mats. This was seen with both drug release model systems (buffer vs. hydrogel) as well as different techniques (UV-VIS spectrophotometry, HPLC, UV imaging, and bacterial bioreporters). This might be explained by the different wettability of the PCL/CAM fiber mats compared to PCL/PEO/CAM fiber mats as discussed previously for PCL and PCL-drug loaded fiber mats [15]. The hydrophilicity of the PCL/PEO/CAM fiber mats makes them wet more homogeneously, whereas for PCL/CAM fiber mats the sample-to-sample variations in wettability may also cause variability in the drug release behavior.

Compared to agar diffusion assay (extraction of CAM from hydrogel), the UV imaging was easier to conduct. Although for both these methods the size of sample, the release environment (hydrogel) and static conditions resembled the *in vitro* antibacterial activity testing conditions. Bacterial bioreporter study enabled to monitor the CAM release into agar hydrogel during diffusion in later time points where even sub-MIC concentration of CAM was determined based on the green and red fluorescence intensity. The method has the advantage of revealing the released antibacterial drug effect directly on bacteria.

For polymer fiber mats as wound matrices it is favorable to have the burst effect. The extent of the burst release is often associated with device geometry, surface characteristics of host material, heterogeneous distribution of drug within the polymer matrix, intrinsic dissolution rate of drug, and heterogeneity of matrices [16]. From the drug release experiments we see that the burst release is smaller with the hydrogels for hydrophilic PCL/PEO/CAM and hydrophobic PCL/CAM fiber mats compared to the buffer solution (Figure 7). Larger differences in the burst release between the samples were observed with hydrophobic PCL/CAM fiber mats (Figure 7). For the drug release to occur from the PCL fiber mat, the medium needs to penetrate into the electrospun fiber mat to cause the diffusion of the drug to the exterior. Initially, the diffusion is affected by the electrospun mat composition and the fiber characteristics, as for PCL/PEO/CAM fiber mats the release was also affected by swelling and dissolution of PEO. As a second step, the diffusion further into the wound and reaction with the surrounding tissue and environment is important [47]. It is clear that the buffer release method shows higher burst release as compared to the *in vitro* antibacterial activity testing. Sadri et al. have measured tetracycline release in a dialysis bag mimicking the human skin-like conditions and shown that the burst release effect is reduced most likely due to the diffusion through the bag, which modified the release [48]. The gels *in vitro* and the wound tissue *in vivo* can be envisioned to provide a diffusion barrier or matrix minimizing burst release effects. Local transport mechanisms determine the volume in which the drug is distributed; thus, understanding these mechanisms is essential for optimizing the effectiveness of local delivery [47]. The *in vitro* methods that enable to most closely mimic the *in vivo* conditions are likely to enable accurate predictions of the drug release and transport in the wound environment. Moreover, it is important to understand the effect on bacteria. Therefore, the response of the bacteria to the active antibiotic concentration has to be measured directly. Here, we have shown that genetically engineered bioreporter systems can be used for this purpose.

4. Summary and Conclusions

All tested drug release model systems enabled to study the drug release from electrospun fiber mats. UV imaging provided faster, non-intrusive real-time information on chloramphenicol (CAM) release and diffusion with higher spatial and temporal resolution as compared to the release methods relying on release from fiber mats directly into buffer solution as well as to the agar plates followed by destructive sampling. The data were similar in terms of sensitivity in detecting differences between the electrospun fiber mat compositions in comparison to the more laborious drug release testing setups. Furthermore, the UV imaging and release into hydrogel method appeared to mimic the *in vitro* antibacterial activity testing conditions to a large degree, while release into buffer solution overestimated the burst release effects.

Advanced antibacterial disc diffusion assays enabled to distinguish small differences in the antibacterial activity of the differently designed electrospun fiber mats, these slight differences were also visualized using UV imaging as well as modified drug release and diffusion into hydrogel model systems. These results suggest that diffusional resistance to drug release observed in the hydrogel based systems may emulate the *in vivo* conditions of the wound matrix.

Author Contributions: Conceptualization, M.P., T.T., J.Ø., and K.K.; methodology, L.P., F.B., M.H., K.S., M.P., T.T., A.M., J.Ø., and K.K.; validation, L.P., F.B., M.H., M.P., A.M., J.Ø., and K.K.; formal analysis, L.P., F.B., M.H., and K.S.; investigation, L.P., F.B., M.H., K.S., M.P., T.T., A.M., J.Ø., and K.K.; resources, T.T., J.Ø., and K.K.; data curation, M.P., J.Ø., and K.K.; writing—original draft preparation, J.Ø. and K.K.; writing—review and editing, L.P., F.B., M.H., M.P., T.T., A.M., J.Ø., and K.K.; visualization, L.P., F.B., M.H., M.P., J.Ø., and K.K.; supervision, M.P., T.T., J.Ø., and K.K.; project administration, K.K.; funding acquisition, T.T., J.Ø., and K.K.

Acknowledgments: K.K. would like to thank the Estonian National Commission for UNESCO and the Estonian Academy of Sciences and the L'ORÉAL–UNESCO international L'ORÉAL Baltic program "For Women In Science" for the fellowship in 2018. MSc Georg-Marten Lanno and MSc Aleksandr Simaško (University of Tartu) and M.I. Andersen (University of Copenhagen) are thanked for the laboratory work. MSc J. Aruväli and Prof K. Kirsimäe are acknowledged for their help in conducting the SEM measurements.

Appendix A. Drug Release Into Agar Hydrogel

Table A1. Confirmation of extraction efficacy.

mg/Samples	% Extracted		
0.119	66.6%	E1	1x extraction
0.122	68.2%	E2	
0.119	66.6%	E3	
	67.1%		
0.186	**103.9%**	E1	2x extraction
0.191	106.8%	E2	
0.177	98.9%	E3	
	103.2%		

Two times extraction used in the present study provides approximately 100% efficacy.

Table A2. Percentage of total amount of drug CAM recovered from all sections on the agar plate. The release of CAM into agar hydrogel was monitored from PCL/PEO/CAM fiber mats.

Zone	5 min	10 min	15 min	30 min	60 min	120 min	1440 min
1	86.8	80.6	78.1	88.5	66.6	62.6	11.8
2	13.2	19.4	21.9	11.5	33.4	37.4	54.6
3	0.0	0.0	0.0	0.0	0.0	0.0	26.9
4	0.0	0.0	0.0	0.0	0.0	0.0	6.3
5	0.0	0.0	0.0	0.0	0.0	0.0	0.4

Appendix B

DMSO stocks preparation. Overnight culture was diluted 100 times into fresh LB medium (100 µL on bacteria in 10 mL medium) and grown aerobically at 37 °C to an OD of 0.8–1 (OD600), cultures were chilled on ice and dimethylsulfoxide (DMSO) was added to a final concentration of 8%. 120 µL of suspension was added to PCR tubes and frozen in liquid nitrogen. The tubes were stored at −80 °C and used within 6 months.

Appendix C

Bacterial bioreporters. Bacterial bioreporters are genetically engineered cells, which will produce a measurable signal in response to some chemical or physical environmental change [36]. In the present study, bacteria were developed to report the presence of antibacterial drug CAM by producing fluorescent proteins. Schematics explaining the working principle of bacterial bioreporters are provided in Figure A1.

Our developed CAM-bioreporter has GFP as a control protein for expression and a red mScarlet-I as a reporter protein. When there is no CAM present, only GFP (green) signal is produced by bacteria (Figure A2).

Bacteria exhibit fast translation and green protein production. In the presence of CAM GFP signal (green) will be reduced due to protein synthesis inhibition, and reporter protein mScarlet-I signal (red) will increase due to transcription continuation as a result of ribosomal stalling in the transcription attenuation system.

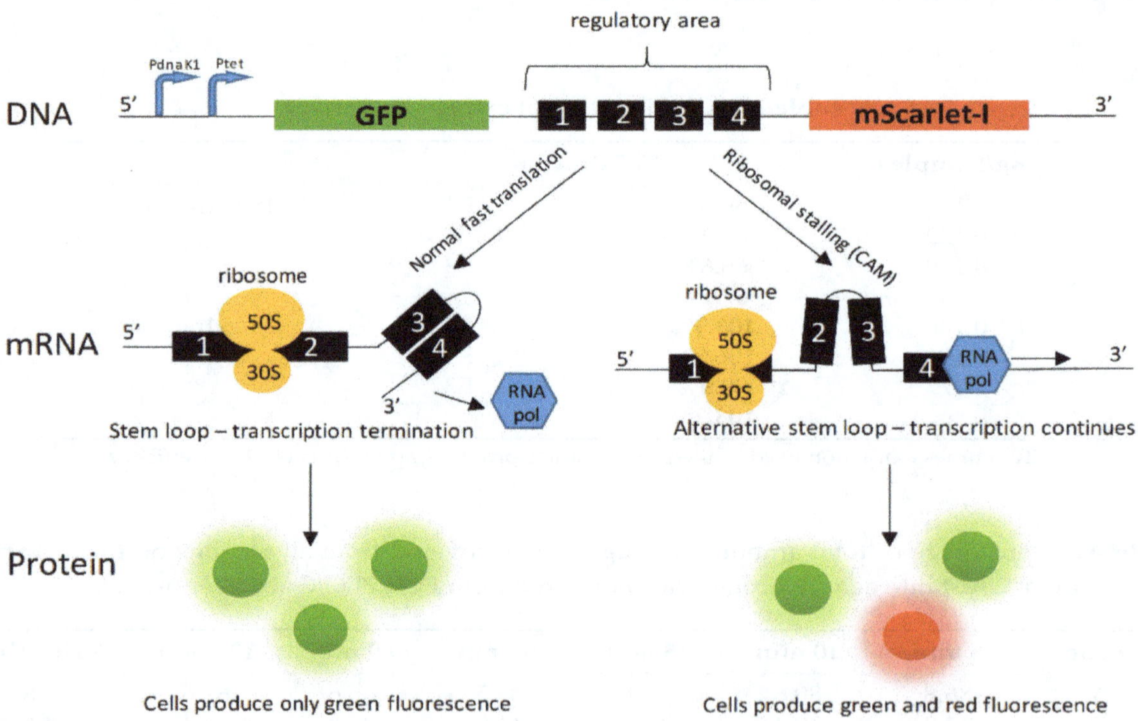

Figure A1. Schematics about bacterial bioreporter system working principle. Key: CAM—chloramphenicol; GFP—green fluorescent protein; mRNA—messenger RNA; 30S/50S—ribosomal subunits; RNA pol—RNA polymerase; PdnaK1 and Ptet—transcription promoters.

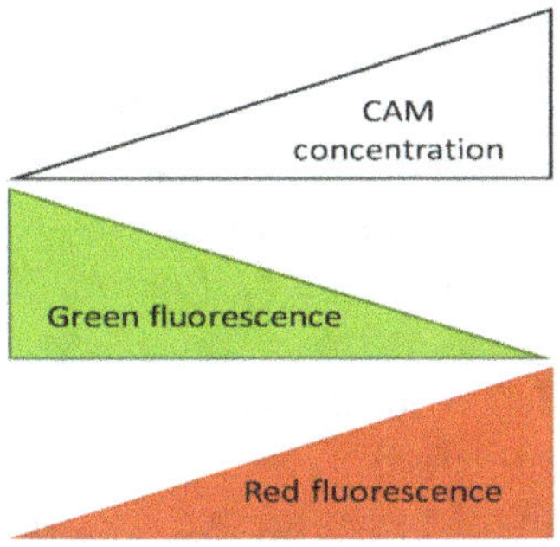

Figure A2. Simplified schematics about bacterial bioreporter system working principle. Key: CAM—chloramphenicol.

References

1. Weng, L.; Xie, J. Smart electrospun nanofibers for controlled drug release: Recent advances and new perspectives. *Curr. Pharm. Des.* **2015**, *21*, 1944–1959. [CrossRef] [PubMed]
2. Torres-Martinez, E.J.; Cornejo Bravo, J.M.; Serrano Medina, A.; Pérez González, G.L.; Villarreal Gómez, L.J. A summary of electrospun nanofibers as drug delivery system: Drugs loaded and biopolymers used as matrices. *Curr. Drug Deliv.* **2018**, *15*, 1360–1374. [CrossRef] [PubMed]
3. Sill, T.J.; von Recum, H.A. Electrospinning: Applications in drug delivery and tissue engineering. *Biomaterials* **2008**, *29*, 1989–2006. [CrossRef] [PubMed]
4. Ye, K.; Kuang, H.; You, Z.; Morsi, Y.; Mo, X. Electrospun nanofibers for tissue engineering with drug loading and release. *Pharmaceutics* **2019**, *11*, 182. [CrossRef] [PubMed]
5. Liu, Y.; He, J.-H. Bubble electrospinning for mass production of nanofibers. *Int. J. Nonlinear Sci. Numer. Simul.* **2007**, *8*, 393–396. [CrossRef]
6. Sultanova, Z.; Kaleli, G.; Kabay, G.; Mutlu, M. Controlled release of a hydrophilic drug from coaxially electrospun polycaprolactone nanofibers. *Int. J. Pharm.* **2016**, *505*, 133–138. [CrossRef] [PubMed]
7. Thakkar, S.; Misra, M. Electrospun polymeric nanofibers: New horizons in drug delivery. *Eur. J. Pharm. Sci.* **2017**, *107*, 148–167. [CrossRef]
8. Gao, S.; Tang, G.; Hua, D.; Xiong, R.; Han, J.; Jiang, S.; Zhang, Q.; Huang, C. Stimuli-responsive bio-based polymeric systems and their applications. *J. Mater. Chem. B* **2019**, *7*, 709–729. [CrossRef]
9. Chou, S.F.; Carson, D.; Woodrow, K.A. Current strategies for sustaining drug release from electrospun nanofibers. *J. Control. Release* **2015**, *220*, 584–591. [CrossRef]
10. Singh, A.; Rath, G.; Singh, R.; Goyal, A.K. Nanofibers: An effective tool for controlled and sustained drug delivery. *Curr. Drug Deliv.* **2018**, *15*, 155–166. [CrossRef]
11. Blanchemain, N.; Laurent, T.; Chai, F.; Neut, C.; Haulon, S.; Krump-konvalinkova, V.; Morcellet, M.; Martel, B.; Kirkpatrick, C.J.; Hildebrand, H.F. Polyester vascular prostheses coated with a cyclodextrin polymer and activated with antibiotics: Cytotoxicity and microbiological evaluation. *Acta Biomater.* **2008**, *4*, 1725–1733. [CrossRef]
12. Liu, X.; Shao, W.; Luo, M.; Bian, J.; Yu, D.-G. Electrospun blank nanocoating for improved sustained release profiles from medicated gliadin nanofibers. *Nanomaterials* **2018**, *8*, 184.
13. Chew, S.Y.; Wen, J.; Yim, E.K.; Leong, K.W. Sustained release of proteins from electrospun biodegradable fibers. *Biomacromolecules* **2005**, *6*, 2017–2024. [CrossRef] [PubMed]
14. Gaharwar, A.K.; Mihaila, S.M.; Kulkarni, A.A.; Patel, A.; Di Luca, A.; Reis, R.L.; Gomes, M.E.; Van Blitterswijk, C.; Moroni, L.; Khademhosseini, A. Amphiphilic beads as depots for sustained drug release integrated into fibrillar scaffolds. *J. Control. Release* **2014**, *187*, 66–73. [CrossRef] [PubMed]
15. Zupančič, Š.; Preem, L.; Kristl, J.; Putrinš, M.; Tenson, T.; Kocbek, P.; Kogermann, K. Impact of PCL nanofiber mat structural properties on hydrophilic drug release and antibacterial activity on periodontal pathogens. *Eur. J. Pharm. Sci.* **2018**, *122*, 347–358. [CrossRef]
16. Fu, Y.; Kao, W.J. Drug release kinetics and transport mechanisms of non-degradable and degradable polymeric delivery systems. *Expert Opin. Drug Deliv.* **2010**, *7*, 429–444. [CrossRef] [PubMed]
17. Natu, M.V.; de Sousa, H.C.; Gil, M.H. Effects of drug solubility, state and loading on controlled release in bicomponent electrospun fibers. *Int. J. Pharm.* **2010**, *397*, 50–58. [CrossRef] [PubMed]

18. Chou, S.-F.; Woodrow, K.A. Relationships between mechanical properties and drug release from electrospun fibers of PCL and PLGA blends. *J. Mech. Behav. Biomed. Mater.* **2017**, *65*, 724–733. [CrossRef] [PubMed]
19. Brettmann, B.K.; Cheng, K.; Myerson, A.S.; Trout, B.L. Electrospun formulations containing crystalline active pharmaceutical ingredients. *Pharm. Res.* **2013**, *30*, 238–246. [CrossRef]
20. Radacsi, N.; Giapis, K.P.; Ovari, G.; Szabó-Révész, P.; Ambrus, R. Electrospun nanofiber-based niflumic acid capsules with superior physicochemical properties. *J. Pharm. Biomed. Anal.* **2019**, *166*, 371–378. [CrossRef]
21. Paskiabi, F.A.; Bonakdar, S.; Shokrgozar, M.A.; Imani, M.; Jahanshiri, Z.; Shams-Ghahfarokhi, M.; Razzaghi-Abyaneh, M. Terbinafine-loaded wound dressing for chronic superficial fungal infections. *Mater. Sci. Eng. C* **2017**, *73*, 130–136. [CrossRef] [PubMed]
22. Preem, L.; Mahmoudzadeh, M.; Putrinš, M.; Meos, A.; Laidmäe, I.; Romann, T.; Aruväli, J.; Härmas, R.; Koivuniemi, A.; Bunker, A.; et al. Interactions between chloramphenicol, carrier polymers, and bacteria–implications for designing electrospun drug delivery systems countering wound infection. *Mol. Pharm.* **2017**, *14*, 4417–4430. [CrossRef] [PubMed]
23. Hu, J.; Prabhakaran, M.P.; Tian, L.; Ding, X.; Ramakrishna, S. Drug-loaded emulsion electrospun nanofibers: Characterization, drug release and *in vitro* biocompatibility. *RSC Adv.* **2015**, *5*, 100256–100267. [CrossRef]
24. Fu, Y.; Kao, W.J. Drug release kinetics and transport mechanisms from semi-interpenetrating networks of gelatin and poly (ethylene glycol) diacrylate. *Pharm. Res.* **2009**, *26*, 2115–2124. [CrossRef] [PubMed]
25. Srikar, R.; Yarin, A.L.; Megaridis, C.M.; Bazilevsky, A.V.; Kelley, E. Desorption-limited mechanism of release from polymer nanofibers. *Langmuir* **2008**, *24*, 965–974. [CrossRef] [PubMed]
26. Nakielski, P.; Kowalczyk, T.; Zembrzycki, K.; Kowalewski, T.A. Experimental and numerical evaluation of drug release from nanofiber mats to brain tissue. *J. Biomed. Mater. Res. Part B Appl. Biomater.* **2015**, *103*, 282–291. [CrossRef] [PubMed]
27. Seif, S.; Graef, F.; Gordon, S.F.; Windbergs, M. Monitoring drug release from electrospun fibers using an in situ fiber-optic system Diss. *Technol.* **2016**, *23*, 6–12.
28. Østergaard, J. UV imaging in pharmaceutical analysis. *J. Pharm. Biomed. Anal.* **2018**, *147*, 140–148. [CrossRef]
29. Asare-Addo, K.; Walton, K.; Ward, A.; Totea, A.-M.; Taheri, S.; Alshafiee, M.; Mawla, N.; Bondi, A.; Evans, W.; Adebisi, A.; et al. Direct imaging of the dissolution of salt forms of a carboxylic acid drug. *Int. J. Pharm.* **2018**, *551*, 290–299. [CrossRef]
30. Østergaard, J.; Meng-Lund, E.; Larsen, S.W.; Larsen, C.; Petersson, K.; Lenke, J.; Jensen, H. Real-time UV imaging of nicotine release from transdermal patch. *Pharm. Res.* **2010**, *27*, 2614–2623. [CrossRef]
31. Ye, F.; Yaghmur, A.; Jensen, H.; Larsen, S.W.; Larsen, C.; Østergaard, J. Real-time UV imaging of drug diffusion and release from Pluronic F127 hydrogels. *Eur. J. Pharm. Sci.* **2011**, *43*, 236–243. [CrossRef] [PubMed]
32. Ye, F.; Larsen, S.W.; Yaghmur, A.; Jensen, H.; Larsen, C.; Østergaard, J. Real-time UV imaging of piroxicam diffusion and distribution from oil solutions into gels mimicking the subcutaneous matrix. *Eur. J. Pharm. Sci.* **2012**, *46*, 72–78. [CrossRef] [PubMed]
33. Østergaard, J.; Lenke, J.; Jensen, S.S.; Sun, Y.; Ye, F. UV imaging for *in vitro* dissolution and release studies: Initial experiences. *Diss. Technol.* **2014**, *21*, 27–38. [CrossRef]
34. Ye, F.; Larsen, S.W.; Yaghmur, A.; Jensen, H.; Larsen, C.; Ostergaard, J. Drug release into hydrogel-based subcutaneous surrogates studied by UV imaging. *J. Pharm. Biomed. Anal.* **2012**, *71*, 27–34. [CrossRef] [PubMed]
35. Daunert, S.; Barrett, G.; Feliciano, J.S.; Shetty, R.S.; Shrestha, S.; Smith-Spencer, W. Genetically engineered whole-cell sensing systems: Coupling biological recognition with reporter genes. *Chem. Rev.* **2000**, *100*, 2705–2738. [CrossRef] [PubMed]
36. Van der Meer, J.R.; Belkin, S. Where microbiology meets microengineering: Design and applications of reporter bacteria. *Nat. Rev. Microbiol.* **2010**, *8*, 511–522. [CrossRef]
37. Blattner, F.R.; Plunkett, G.; Bloch, C.A.; Perna, N.T.; Burland, V.; Riley, M.; Collado-Vides, J.; Glasner, J.D.; Rode, C.K.; Mayhew, G.F.; et al. The complete genome sequence of *Escherichia coli* K-12. *Science* **1997**, *277*, 1453–1462. [CrossRef]
38. Sambrook, J.; Russell, D. *Molecular Cloning: A Laboratory Manual*, 3rd ed.; Cold Spring Harbor Laboratory Press: New York, NY, USA, 2012.
39. Neidhardt, F.C.; Bloch, P.L.; Smith, D.F. Culture medium for enterobacteria. *J. Bacteriol.* **1974**, *119*, 736–747.
40. Quan, J.; Tian, J. Circular polymerase extension cloning for high-throughput cloning of complex and combinatorial DNA libraries. *Nat. Protoc.* **2011**, *6*, 242–251. [CrossRef]

41. Murina, V.; Kasari, M.; Takada, H.; Hinnu, M.; Saha, C.K.; Grimshaw, J.W.; Seki, T.; Reith, M.; Putrinš, M.; Tenson, T.; et al. ABCF ATPases involved in protein synthesis, ribosome assembly and antibiotic resistance: Structural and functional diversification across the tree of life. *J. Mol. Biol.* **2019**, *431*, 3568–3590. [CrossRef]
42. Cormack, B.P.; Valdivia, R.H.; Falkow, S. FACS-optimized mutants of the green fluorescent protein (GFP). *Gene* **1996**, *173*, 33–38. [CrossRef]
43. Bindels, D.S.; Haarbosch, L.; van Weeren, L.; Postma, M.; Wiese, K.E.; Mastop, M.; Aumonier, S.; Gotthard, G.; Royant, A.; Hink, M.A.; et al. mScarlet: A bright monomeric red fluorescent protein for cellular imaging. *Nat. Methods* **2016**, *14*, 53–56. [CrossRef] [PubMed]
44. Osterman, I.A.; Prokhorova, I.V.; Sysoev, V.O.; Boykova, Y.V.; Efremenkova, O.V.; Svetlov, M.S.; Kolb, V.A.; Bogdanov, A.A.; Sergiev, P.V.; Dontsova, O.A. Attenuation-based dual-fluorescent-protein reporter for screening translation inhibitors. *Antimicrob. Agents Chemother.* **2012**, *56*, 1774–1783. [CrossRef] [PubMed]
45. Schneider, C.A.; Rasband, W.S.; Eliceiri, K.W. NIH image to ImageJ: 25 years of image analysis. *Nat. Methods* **2012**, *9*, 671–675. [CrossRef] [PubMed]
46. Mekkawy, A.I.; El-Mokhtar, M.A.; Nafady, N.A.; Yousef, N.; Hamad, M.A.; El-Shanawany, S.M.; Ibrahim, E.H.; Elsabahy, M. *In vitro* and *in vivo* evaluation of biologically synthesized silver nanoparticles for topical applications: Effect of surface coating and loading into hydrogels. *Int. J. Nanomed.* **2017**, *12*, 759–777. [CrossRef] [PubMed]
47. Weiser, J.R.; Saltzman, W.M. Controlled release for local delivery of drugs: Barriers and models. *J. Control. Release* **2014**, *190*, 664–673. [CrossRef] [PubMed]
48. Sadri, M.; Mohammadi, A.; Hosseini, H. Drug release rate and kinetic investigation of composite polymeric nanofibers. *Nanomed. Res. J.* **2016**, *1*, 112–121.

9

Aptamers as Delivery Agents of siRNA and Chimeric Formulations for the Treatment of Cancer

Ana Paula Dinis Ano Bom [1], Patrícia Cristina da Costa Neves [1], Carlos Eduardo Bonacossa de Almeida [2], Dilson Silva [1] and Sotiris Missailidis [1,*]

1 Instituto de Tecnologia em Imunobiológicos (Bio-Manguinhos), Fundação Oswaldo Cruz. Av. Brasil, 4365-Manguinhos, Rio de Janeiro/RJ CEP 21040-900, Brazil; adinis@bio.fiocruz.br (A.P.D.A.B.); Pcristina@bio.fiocruz.br (P.C.d.C.N.); dilson.silva@bio.fiocruz.br (D.S.)

2 Laboratório de Radiobiologia, Divisão de Física Médica, Instituto de Radioproteção e Dosimetria, Comissão Nacional de Energia Nuclear. Av. Salvador Allende S/N., Rio de Janeiro/RJ CEP 22783-127, Brazil; ce.bonacossa@gmail.com

* Correspondence: sotiris.missailidis@bio.fiocruz.br

Abstract: Both aptamers and siRNA technologies have now reached maturity, and both have been validated with a product in the market. However, although pegaptanib reached the market some time ago, there has been a slow process for new aptamers to follow. Today, some 40 aptamers are in the market, but many in combination with siRNAs, in the form of specific delivery agents. This combination offers the potential to explore the high affinity and specificity of aptamers, the silencing power of siRNA, and, at times, the cytotoxicity of chemotherapy molecules in powerful combinations that promise to delivery new and potent therapies. In this review, we report new developments in the field, following up from our previous work, more specifically on the use of aptamers as delivery agents of siRNA in nanoparticle formulations, alone or in combination with chemotherapy, for the treatment of cancer.

Keywords: siRNA; aptamers; cancer; nanoparticles

---

1. Introduction

Small interfering RNA siRNA suppress expression of genes by targeting the mRNA expression. Targeted delivery of siRNA to specific cells is highly desirable for safe and efficient RNAi-based therapeutics [1]. However, the half-life of nucleic acids in the bloodstream is short due to the degradation by endo or exonucleases and rapid clearance [2]. One strategy to solve this challenge is developing siRNA delivery systems. Nanoparticles can be defined as particles less than 100 nm in diameter, these systems can be composed by different materials and are employed according to their purpose [3,4]. For this area, the most widely used systems are polymeric particles, nanoemulsions, nanocrystals, solid lipid nanoparticles, and liposomes [5]. The organic particles used for drug delivery application are micelles, liposomes, polymers, dendrimers, and nanogels. They have versatile surface building blocks for efficient endocytosis and loading [6]. There are numerous advantages to using nanoparticles: (I) Increased bioavailability, (II) dose proportionality, (III) decreased toxicity, (IV) smaller dosage form, (V) stability of drugs dosage forms, and (VI) increased active agent surface area resulting in a faster dissolution [7]. Ideally, nanoparticles should be stable in circulation to protect and deliver their therapeutic load (drug) into recipient tissue; have good penetration and retention in the target tissue so that drug release occurs within the therapeutic window; and ultimately be organically excreted to avoid long term accumulation toxicity [8]. Approaches to drug targeting and delivery may be facilitated by the enhanced permeability and retention (EPR) effect. This effect occurs due to the large endothelial tissue fenestrations which are characteristic of the rapid growth of tumor blood vessels. Therefore, the nanoparticles passively diffuse through the microenvironment targeting the tumor tissues [8].

Although nanocarrier technology has improved, its lack of target specificity limits its widespread use, to overcome this issue and address the lack of specificity is the generation of functionalized nanoparticles, i.e., second generation nanoparticles [8]. Nanoparticle surface functionalization occurs through the fixation of a ligand that interacts with specific tissue-specific receptors, to optimize the administration of the target, selectively transporting it to the binding site [9]. One of the advantages of taking drugs directly to specific tissues is the ability to use relatively more toxic and efficient drugs with less risk of collateral damage to other body tissues. In the case of cancer, drugs could be targeted at tumors, avoiding the systemic side effects of traditional therapies. The functionalization includes surface conjugation of chemicals or bio molecules, like folic acid, biotin molecules, peptides, antibodies, aptamers, short, single stranded RNA or DNA oligonucleotides, proteins, and oligosaccharides, to enhance the properties and hit the target with high precision [10]. In order to provide targetability, aptamers have been widely used due to (I) their capacity of binding to target proteins with a high affinity and specificity, (II) having already been shown to have antibody-like characteristics, and (III) the fact that they are relatively smaller and less immunogenic. All of these useful properties make aptamers attractive in therapeutic and diagnostic fields [11].

2. Aptamer in the Delivery of Therapeutic Nanoparticles Containing siRNA, shRNA, and miRNA

The origin of siRNA nanoparticles targeted delivery through aptamers dates to 1998. Guo et al. treated T cells with an RNA nanoparticle consisting of a dimer of the packaging RNA (pRNA) derived from the DNA-packaging motor of bacteriophage phi29 loaded with a siRNA for survivin mRNA and conjugated with a CD4 specific aptamer [12]. Hu et al. used the same platform to create a nanoparticle containing an siRNA for ICAM 1 conjugated with aptamer FB4 directed against the mouse transferrin receptor. The in vitro results showed a decreased of ICAM-1 expression and blocked the adhesion of monocytes [13].

From this date, many types of platforms and supports were developed so that siRNA could be targeted through aptamers. To target cells using aptamers, Afonin et al. designed multifunctional siRNA nanoparticles aiming at the silence of multiple HIV-1 genes [14]. To show the feasibility of siRNA delivery using nanorings, Li et al. developed a nanorings construct functionalized with J18 RNA aptamers specific for the human epidermal growth factor receptor (EGFR) [15]. The nanoring design can achieve cell-targeting properties, but the internalization and functional effects of siRNAs bound to aptamer-nanorings were not studied [16]. Zhao et al. developed a nanoparticle to treat anaplastic large cell lymphoma (ALCL). The nanocarrier incorporated both anaplastic lymphoma kinase (ALK) siRNA and a CD30 aptamer onto nano-polyethyleneimine-citrate leading to growth arrest and apoptosis in vitro [17]. Powell et al. tested the possibility of conjugating an aptamer A6 which can bind to human epidermal growth factor receptor 2 (HER-2) receptors on breast cancer cells to P-gp siRNA siRNA-containing nanoparticles. The knockdown of P-gp was increased significantly, decreasing a resistance to chemotherapeutics in the cells [18]. To overcome multi-drug resistance (MDR), an MD- specific aptamer-conjugated grapefruit-derived nanovectors (GNVs) was used for co-delivery of siRNA and doxorubicin (DOX), resulting in a potent anti-tumor activity [19].

Stable nucleic acid lipid particles (SNALPs) also used to deliver siRNA through aptamers. In this study, the authors coupled the transferrin receptor aptamer in SNALP loaded with siRNA. The aptamer-targeting enhanced siRNA uptake and target gene knockdown in cells [20]. Another aptamer–liposome–siRNA delivery system was developed by Alshaer et al. In this model, siRNA complexed with protamine and aptamer anti-CD44, a cell surface biomarker overexpressed in many tumors, was used as targeting delivery for the first time [21]. They confirmed the silencing disease-related genes in tumors [18].

To target prostate cancer cells, Kim et al. used shRNAs against the gene BCL-xL and the PSMA (prostate-specific membrane antigens) aptamer (A10–3) conjugated to a polyethyleneimine (PEI)-PEG construction. In order to amplify the therapeutic response and use different drugs in synergy, the authors also included DOX in aptamer-functionalized nanoparticle, and this approach led to the death of the cancer cells, demonstrating the effectiveness of the combination therapy [22]. Likewise, the PSMA aptamer was used to target delivery of miRNA (miR-15a and miR-16–1) identified as tumor suppressor genes in prostate cancer. The nanoparticle based on polyamidoamine and PEG allowed selective killing of prostate cancer cells [23]. Xu et al. used a multifunctional envelope-type nanoparticle platform constituted of two polymers that co-incorporate siRNA. For the nanoparticle functionalization was used *S,S*-2-(3-(5-amino-1-carboxypentyl)ureido)pentanedioic acid (ACUPA) ligand that can specifically bind to PSMA. This study reached an efficient gene silencing in prostate cancer tumor cells in vivo [24].

Lv et al. used Polyamidoamine (PAMAM) dendrimers functionalized with EGFR aptamers to co-deliver shRNA to survivin and erlotinib. Survivin shRNA is used to activate apoptosis while erlotinib is a tyrosine kinase inhibitor. This therapeutic approach in association with Chloroquine acted synergistically to reverse erlotinib resistance in EGFR mutation-positive of non-small-cell-lung cancer (NSCLC) [25].

Another strategy is use of siRNA-aptamer chimera to compose the nanoparticle, and the siRNA-aptamer chimera has emerged as a promising approach for efficient delivery of siRNA to specific cell types, owing to its low immunogenicity, ease of chemical synthesis and modification, and the outstanding targeting specificity of the aptamer [26]. However, in some cases, endosome escape has been reported. To avoid this problem, it has been used siRNA-aptamer chimeras in nanocarriers. Bagalkot and Gao developed a new technology for linking siRNA-aptamer chimeras to carrier nanoparticles [27]. In this new technology, the siRNA block should become the anchor point for interaction with cationic nanoparticles for reduced enzymatic degradation and nonspecific interaction with cells and tissues, whereas the aptamer block should stay on the outside with minimized interaction with the nanoparticle surface. This approach opened new opportunities in targeted delivery based on siRNA-aptamer chimeras.

In recent study, to evaluate cell viability and genes expression in metastatic breast cancer cells, Jafari et al. designed chitosan nanoparticles for co-delivery of Docetaxel and insulin-like growth factor receptor 1 (IGF-1R) siRNA. Docetaxel is a cytotoxic anti-cancer drug approved for the treatment of metastatic breast cancer. IGF-1R signaling is important in tumor growth, development, and its metastasis. The MUC1 aptamer was conjugated to a chitosan based nanocarrier. MUC1-aptamers have been used to targeted drug delivery to several types of cancers, including breast cancer cells [28]. Another study in the cancer field shows an efficiency of EGFR aptamer-conjugated liposome loaded with special AT-rich sequence binding protein 1 (SATB1) siRNA. The genome organizer (SATB1) expression decreased in vitro and in vivo studies with a consequent decrease in choriocarcinoma [29]. A novel targeted delivery platform to mediated gene-silencing in cancer cells was described by Ayatollahi et al.; the 10-bromodecanoic acid (10C) and 10C-PEG was loaded with shRNA plasmid for specific knockdown of BCL-xL protein and was conjugated to AS1411 aptamer for targeting to nucleolin on cancer cells [30]. A synergistic cancer cell death was achieved using a (AS1411) nucleolin aptamer-carbon nanotubes (CNTs) as biological carriers containing BCL-xL-specific shRNA and DOX [31].

Recently, a new types of siRNA delivery by aptamers have been demonstrated. Xu et al. used the three-way-junction (3WJ) RNA to couple epithelial cell adhesion molecule (EpCAM) aptamers aiming to deliver Delta-5-Desaturase (D5D) siRNA. This enzyme acts on dihomo-γ-linolenic acid DGLA, preventing the production of 8-hydroxyloctanoic acid (8-HOA), which is important for inhibiting histone deacetylation in cancer [32]. Li et al. combined pRNA dimers with siRNA and aptamer, and they demonstrated that pRNA, which is a component of a phi29 bacteriophage, can be useful for efficient siRNA delivery. The pRNA-siRNA-aptamer was encapsulated in folate and PEG functionalized chitosan nanoparticles. In that study, the aptamer used was FB4 for a transferrin domain, and the siRNA was c-myc [33]. Wu et al. demonstrated that functionalized cationic nanobubbles decorated with PSMA aptamers are able to carry and deliver FoxM1 siRNA to prostate cancer positive cells and xenographic tumors [34]. One recent study developed a programmable DNA nanostructure that is considered a potential system for drug delivery for non-small cell lung cancer. DNA Prism nanostructure conjugated with MUC-1 aptamers to deliver Rab26 siRNA presented a great cellular uptake efficiency and anti-tumoral activity [35].

In the field of theranostics, this approach can be useful. Theranostics is defined as nanomedicine that can deliver therapeutics to an intended region, diagnose disease, and follow the progression of disease [36]. Recently, interdisciplinary research in this field, which applies theranostics to diagnose and treat cancer, has explosively progressed. Kim et al. 2017 developed a theranostic liposomal system for carrying diagnostic Quantum Dots (QD) and therapeutic siRNA that were coupled to aptamer molecules against EGFR. The theranostic liposomes were evaluated in terms of cancer-targeted siRNA delivery and QD imaging in vitro and in vivo [11]. The anti-EGFR aptamer was used recently as a theranostic delivery system. The authors used two siRNA to provide a combinatorial anti-cancer treatment using BCL-2 siRNA, which interfere with tumor cell proliferation, and siRNA PKC-ι for inhibition of tumor cell migration. Moreover, these vehicles were able to simultaneously delivered QD provided fluorescence signals in internal organs and tumors. This study shows an efficiently delivered targeting of anti-cancer therapeutic siRNAs, as well as fluorescent QDs to tumor tissues, enabling the use of theranostic delivery systems in the treatment and fluorescence imaging of cancers [37].

In this review, we compiled several studies with different types of nanoparticles; despite different types of nanoparticles, aptamer functionalized nanoparticle loading therapeutic siRNA design can generally be done in two ways: (1) incorporated in the nanoparticle itself or (2) conjugated to the nanoparticle surface.

Over the past few years, the investment in therapeutic oligonucleotides (e.g., aptamers, siRNAs, and antisense technology) is constantly increasing. It is projected that clinical testing of aptamer-targeted drugs will materialize over the next 2–5 years However, there are several challenges in the use of aptamers as nanoparticle drivers, including the aptamer structural design, in vivo stability, immunogenicity, cellular uptake, and endosomal escape, that should be considered [16]. There is the possibility of target specificity, RNAi efficacy, and stability of siRNA-aptamers chimeras being affected by chemical modifications. Therefore, it is crucial to find an optimal alternative for each siRNA aptamers chimera to maximize its therapeutic efficacy [38].

In order to increase extracellular stability, incorporation of protective groups, such as thiol-phosphate, 20-fluoro, 20-amino, and 2′-*O*-methyl, in phosphate or sugar of nucleotides improves nuclease resistance of aptamer-siRNA chimeras [39,40]. Another possibility for improving stability is the aptamers PEG conjugation. Furthermore, it has been shown that PEG formulation reduces immune responses in vivo [41]. The thermal stability of siRNA is another parameter to be considered in gene silencing activity when it is conjugated to aptamers [38]. In this context, the computational modeling has been used to guide RNA aptamer truncations, maintaining their functionality, and preventing and minimizing therapy challenges using siRNA.

Several approaches have been developed to facilitate siRNA uptake and nanoparticle entry into endosomes. One possibility is to perform the conjugation of chimeras to short cell penetration cationic peptides (CPPs) that are important for the efficiency in intracellular transport of a variety of macromolecules [42]. Another possibility is the conjugation of the chimeras with peptides from the transactivator of transcription (TAT)region; Diao et al. demonstrated that the survivin siRNA was delivering specifically and efficiently and suppressed tumor growth in prostate cancer in vivo [43]. Inclusion of endosome-disrupting molecules, including PEI and poly (histidine), as well as fusogenic lipids and pH-sensitive lipids in aptamer-siRNA chimeras, have been useful for enhancing siRNA endosomal evasion [24,44,45]. Table 1 summarizes carriers aptamers cited in this section.

Table 1. Aptamers for delivery of siRNA.

siRNA/miRNA/shRNA Target Gene	Carrier Aptamer	Efficacy Tests	Ref.
Survivin	CD4	In vitro knock down antiapoptosis factor survivin	[12]
ICAM 1	FB4 (bind to transferrin receptors)	In vitro results showed a decreased of ICAM-1 expression and blocked the adhesion of monocytes	[13]
Human immunodeficiency virus (HIV)-1	epidermal growth factor receptor (EGFR)	In vitro and in vivo gene silencing	[14]
Anaplastic lymphoma kinase (ALK)	CD30	In vitro results of growth arrest and apoptosis	[17]
P-gp	A6 (bind to human epidermal growth factor receptor 2 (HER-2) receptors)	In vitro results about decreasing of resistance to chemotherapeutics	[18]
P-gp	LA1 (specific to multi-drug resistance (MDR))	In vitro and in vivo anti-tumor activity	[19]
GFP	Transferrin	In vitro enhanced siRNA uptake and target gene knockdown	[20]
Luciferase	CD44	In vitro and in vivo results of targeted gene silencing in CD44-positive breast cancer	[21]
P-gp	HER2	In vitro confirmation of silencing disease-related genes in tumors	[18]
BCL-xL	Prostate-specific membrane antigen (PSMA)	In vitro anti-tumor activity	[22]
Genes in prostate cancer	PSMA	In vitro anticancer effect	[23]
Prohibitin 1	PSMA	In vivo gene silencing in prostate cancer tumor cells	[24]
Survivin	EGFR	In vitro and in vivo antitumor effects	[25]
GFP	PSMA	In vitro GFP silencing/Fluorescence imaging (quantum dots)	[27]
Insulin-like growth factor receptor 1 (IGF-1R)	MUC-1	In vitro augment the targeting of pathways involved in tumorigenesis and metastasis	[28]
Special AT-rich sequence binding protein 1 (SATB1)	EGFR	In vitro and in vivo studies of gene expression decreased	[29]
BCL-xL	Nucleolin	In vitro gene silencing and apoptosis	[30]
BCL-xL	Nucelolin	In vitro gene silencing and tumoricidal efficacy	[31]
D5D	EpCAM	In vitro and in vivo inhibition of D5D expression	[32]
c-myc	Transferrin	In vitro and in vivo anti-tumor activity	[33]
FoxM1	PSMA	In vitro and in vivo anti-tumor activity in prostate cancer cells and xenografts in mice	[34]
Rab26	MUC-1	In vitro anti-tumor activity	[35]
bcl-2	EGFR	In vitro interference of tumor cell proliferation	[11]
bcl-2 and PKC-ι	EGFR	In vivo delivery and therapeutic efficacy	[37]

3. Cancer Immunotherapy Using Aptamers-siRNA

Immunotherapy has emerged as the best clinical alternative for cancer treatment during the last years. It is mostly based in monoclonal antibodies targeting immunological checkpoint pathways, as well as in genetically-engineered cells that directly attack the tumor, like CAR-T cells. Despite the great success of immunotherapy, it works for 20–40% of the patients, depending on tumor type and disease progression stage [46]. So, other classes of molecules and treatments, such as those based in RNA and aptamers, appeared as good alternatives for cancer immunological treatment.

RNA-based immunotherapy is, in concept, more advantageous than those based in recombinant protein expression platforms. It has lower cost, lower immunogenicity, and better penetration in the tumor tissue, which makes it worth developing. In addition, in the last years, a number of pre-clinical and clinical data proved its efficacy, using both aptamer alone and RNAi conjugates.

Antagonistic and agonistic aptamers, acting similar to monoclonal antibodies, were developed to bind to immunomodulating molecules, such as CTLA-4, PD-1, IL-10 R, and LAG-3. The tetrameric antagonistic aptamer selected for CTLA-4, the first one to be developed, was very effective during melanoma murine model studies in vivo [47]. In the same way, multimeric structures of aptamers were shown to have a better performance for agonistic ligands, bringing them together during the activation. It is the case of OX-40 agonistic aptamer, Pratico et al. constructed a multimerized anti OX-40 aptamer using biotinylation and demonstrated a much better biologic effect than the single aptamer, with increased IFN-© production and proliferation, using peripheral blood mononuclear cells as an in vitro model of T cells' activation [48].

Some receptors of the immune system have an interesting characteristic: They get internalized after T cell activation as a feedback mechanism of controlling over-stimulation. Taking advantage of this feature, some aptamers have been developed as delivery systems to siRNA. The first one was 4-1BB aptamer used to deliver siRNA to T cells, aiming to disrupt mTOR pathway and attenuate IL-2R signaling in $CD8^+$ T cells, which, in turn, leads to $CD8^+$ T cells persistence inside the tumor site and its elimination [49]. This same aptamer was used to address siRNA for Smad-4, a protein from TGF-β signaling cascade. TGF-β is a key mediator of immune system suppression during progression. This approach was successful in suppressing the negative effect of TGF-βon infiltrating $CD8^+$ cells elicited by vaccination with tumor antigens [50].

Cluster of Differentiation (CD) aptamers also have been shown as good alternatives for RNAi delivery. CD molecules are used traditionally for identification of subpopulations of immune cells during flow cytometry studies and, as well as 4-1BB, are frequently internalized after cells activation. For example, using CD4 aptamers complexed with short hairpin RNAs (shRNA), it was possible to silence ROR©T pathway, the key for T_H17 cells development, opening a possibility of treatment for a number of conditions, mainly related to autoimmune diseases [51]. In the cancer field, Soldevilla et al. used the previously developed agonistic CD40 aptamer to construct shRNA-aptamer chimeras to inhibit SMG1, a kinase that is essential for nonsense-mediated mRNA decay (NMD) initiation. Mice treated with the CD40 aptamer-shRNA chimera showed higher tumor infiltration of lymphocytes [52,53]. Table 2 summarizes aptamers-siRNAs used for immunotherapy cited in this section.

Table 2. Aptamers and siRNA for immunotherapy.

siRNA Target Gene	Carrier Aptamer	Efficacy Tests	Ref.
IL-2 Rα (CD25)	41-BB	In vitro using CHO cells and murine $CD8^+$ cells and in vivo using C57BL/6 mice adoptively transferred with OT-I cells and breast tumor 4T1 model	[49]
Smad-4	41-BB	In vitro using murine $CD8^+$ cells and in vivo using breast tumor 4T1 model	[50]
RORγT	CD4	In vitro using CD4+ Karpas 299 cells and primary human CD4+ T cells	[51]
SMG-1	CD40 agonist	In vitro using human B-lymphocytes and in vivo using B-cell lymphoma-bearing mice	[52]

4. Tumor-Targeted Aptamers Complexed Directly to siRNAs and Other Agents for Cancer Therapy

Thanks to the unique features of aptamers, such as stability and tumor penetration, its use as tools for delivery of therapeutic agents, including siRNA, has gained great attention from researchers during the last few years.

The idea of a tailored drug for the treatment of a diseased cell avoiding affecting the surrounding healthy cells is not recent, as recalled by Kruspe and Giangrande [54]. It was initially proposed by Paul Ehrlich about one century ago, when he first defined the "magic bullet" and its inherent concept of cell-surface receptor [55]. The route scientists have threaded to reach the current status has grooved a persistent tentative of diverse therapy strategies, some among them based on the conjugation of aptamer with siRNA.

Aptamers, however, due to their anionic characteristics, do not easily transit across the cell lipid bilayer, requiring adequate strategies to overcome the action of those charges, using diverse adjuvants in different structures based on lipids/liposomes, nanoparticles (as seen above), cationic polymers, and peptides.

Aptamer-siRNA conjugates, or AsiCs as they are frequently referred to, comprise an ever-increasing number of structures since 2006 when the delivery of siRNA by an aptamer was described simultaneously by two groups working with prostate membrane antigen (PSMA).

The first aptamer to be conjugated to an siRNA was to treat prostate cancer. The strategy consisted in addressing the tumor trough PSMA, a protein overexpressed in the surface of prostate cancer cells and tumor vascular endothelium, with a PSMA aptamer linked to PLK-1 and BCL-2 siRNAs. The siRNAs were responsible for disrupting the protection against apoptosis of the tumor cells. The tool was successful in eliminating a xenograft prostate cancer in a murine model [56]. After that, many other groups developed similar strategies. Interesting results were obtained for glioblastoma, the most frequent and aggressive primary brain tumor in adults, with a very poor prognosis. Expression and activation of the signal transducer and activator of transcription-3 (STAT3) has been reported as a key regulator of this kind of tumor, so a chimera aptamer antagonistic for PDGFRbr (a receptor overexpressed in glioblastoma, as well as other tumor types) carrying siRNA for STAT 3 was designed. This chimera was able to reduce the anti-apoptotic factors Poly (ADP-ribose) polymerase PARP and BCL-xL, inducing cell death in two glioblastoma lineages in vitro. Moreover, Gint4.T-STAT3 chimera treatment induced significant reduction of tumor growth rate in comparison to control group, as well reduced pro-tumoral factors in a xenograft mouse model of glioblastoma [57]. Similar results were obtained for HER+ breast cancer using a HER-2 sense and antisense bivalent aptamer conjugated to EGFR siRNA. It was able to be delivered to breast cancer cells overexpressing HER-2 and the

EGFR gene was efficiently downregulated in vitro, whilst a xenografted tumor growth was supressed in vivo [58]. Another study from the same group showed the performance of a bivalent HER-2-HER-3 aptamer with an EGFR siRNA between them. It was even better in reducing the expression of all three receptors, in inducing cell cycle arrest and apoptosis in vitro and inhibiting tumor growth with a little of target effect in vivo [59]. Aptamer-siRNA chimeras were also used to overcome multidrug resistance by Jeong et al. They engineered a mucin multiaptamer (E18 units) conjugated to RNAsi for BCL-2, with the intercalation of doxorubicin (DOX) between the double helix of the aptamers. Promising results were obtained using this construct to treat MUC-1 overexpressing MCF-7 breast cancer cells. The complex was efficient in delivering doxorubicin to multi drug resistant MCF-7 cells because of increased endocytosis efficiency due to the cluster effect. BCL-2 RNAsi acted synergistically with DOX, increasing the sensitivity of cells for apoptosis and, in turn, decreasing cell viability [60].

An interesting work has used DOX to inactivate cancer stem cells (CSC) by conjugating this drug to engineered RNA aptamers raised against CSC surface marker epithelial cellular adhesion molecule (EpCAM). A modified DNA-RNA hybrid EpCAM aptamer (10-bp GC at stem region) was loaded with 2,5 molecules of DOX per aptamer and this conjugate was capable to release approximated 89.2% of the intercalated DOX just after endocytosis. The authors proved the release of DOX was dependent on low pH that in turn limited the availability of the drug in systemic circulation and tissue interstitium (physiological pH) to affect sensitive organs. Additionally, the complex Apt-DOX was able to target and deliver DOX to EpCAM positive HT29 colorectal cancer cells in dose and time dependent manner and lead to the accumulation and retention of the drug in the cell nucleus. All these characteristics made this construct very efficient in controlling tumor growth overcoming chemoresistance in both tumorsphere formation assay and immunodeficient mice with LDA xenotransplanted with CSC. The aptamer deliver approach developed by Xiang et al. could in fact improve therapeutic index delivering a sufficient drug dose to the critical subcellular target for enough time to eliminate precisely CSCs [61]. The same group extended the investigation to new approaches to tackle cancer stem cells using EpCAM aptamer. They use the aptamer as a driver to survivin RNAi in colorectal cancer cells, both in vitro as well as in colorectal tumor bearing mice. The combination of the surivin downregulation with the action of 5-fluorouacil cytotoxic chemotherapeutic could increase the lethality of colorectal cancer stem cells, as well as tumor control, in the colorectal cancer xenograph model and, consequently, improvement of animal survival [62].

A proof of concept of an approach using an aptamer-liposomal-DOX to target HER3ECD (epitope to trastuzumab binding epitope antigen) with minimum undesirable toxicity is described by Dou Xi et al. The strategy was to conjugate a single-stranded DNA aptamer against HER3 to liposome to improve targeted delivery with less unspecific action of DOX. The aptamer raised against HER3CD was able to bind to HER3 in MCF-7 $^{HER3+}$, BT 474^{HER3+} but not in 293T $^{HER3-}$ cells. This aptamer originates the apt-Lip-DOX conjugate that in fact increased the sustained drug release and was able to increase the growth inhibition of MCF-7 $^{HER3+}$ and BT 474^{HER3+} cells when compared to liposome-DOX and DOX alone challenge. The Apt-Lip-DOX formulation had many advantages when compared to Lip-DOX treatment. There was a higher uptake and retention by MCF-7 tumors in mice. The survival rate of the animals group treated with the apt-Lip-DOX 60 days after chemotherapy was 40% against 0% of the DOX group attained by 36th day after treatment. It is interesting to notice there was any lethality in the Apt-Lip-DOX treated control group that means a very low toxicity of this construct. Additionally, liver and cardio toxicity in the Apt-Lip-DOX treated group was compared to the control NaCl treated group. Finally, the author have demonstrated that the use of aptamers as a driver to target cells unequivocally reduced the availability of DOX in tissues (reduced biodistribution) other than tumor, reducing significantly the cardio toxicity after chemotherapy when compared to the formulation without aptamer [63].

Prusty et al. (2018) developed a very elegant photo-switchable hybrid-aptameric nanoconstruct that efficiently release DOX at high concentration to HGFR (hepatocyte growth factor receptor–cMet) expressing cells. The HyApNc-DOX nanoconstruct was obtained by the combination of two lipid self-assembly single motifs. The first motif was constituted by a lipid-functionalized aptamer trCLN3 with four lipid-modified dU-phosphoramidite 1 at the 5′end of the aptamer. The so-called trCLN3-L4 retained nanomolar affinity to the cMet receptor in tumor cells despite the modification. The second motif was a lipid functionalized 5′-CG rich hairpin ODN designed to carry DOX by intercalation but with a 2′,6′-dimethylzobenzene (DMAB) photoswitch incorporated in the hairpin nanoscaffold. After UV irradiation, DMAB is responsible for the controlled release of DOX inside cell. A lipid-mediated self-assembly approach to build a multi component supramolecular structure resulted in an improved survival to serum nucleases attack and in a better efficiency in the uptake by the target cell and also a precise subcellular distribution of DOX to the cell nucleus, after endocytosis, when compared to the native aptamer [64].

Another approach using aptamers to deliver DOX was developed to target Glioblastoma multiforme tumor cells. A GMT-3 ssDNA aptamer raised against glioblastoma multiforme A-172 cells demonstrates a high affinity to different glioblastoma cell lines (Kd, ~75 nM). Aptamer GMT-3 charged with DOX (molar ratio 1.2 DOX per aptamer) could selectively bind to and inactivate A-172 glioblastoma cells in comparison to the effect noticed in MCF-7 control cells [65].

A great challenge in the treatment of Glioblastoma using chemotherapeutics is to overcome the blood brain barrier (BBB) and to avoid chemotherapeutic drug deliver to the non-tumor tissues. Luo et al. (2017) developed a nanoconjugate delivery system using AS1411 aptamer as a driver to target nucleolin receptor that is overexpressed in glioblastoma U87 MG cells and neo-vascular endothelial cells in way to deliver chemotherapeutics with more precision. AS 1411-Nucleolin complex undergoes endocytosis inhibiting DNA synthesis inducing apoptosis and also inhibiting angiogenesis, that means it has dual targets. The authors incorporated a more efficient cytotoxic drug to AS1411 synthetizing a poly (L-*c*-glutamyl-glutamine)-paclitaxel nanoconjugate (PGGPTX) to achieve an improvement of aqueous solubility and permanence in plasma. All the results obtained by the group demonstrated that the presence of AS1441 aptamer in the complex AS1411-PGG-PTX improved significantly the U87 MG, as well as neo-vascular endothelial cells uptake and internalization, U87 MG spheroid tumor penetration, and U87 MG cell growth inhibition. The same effect could be demonstrated in vivo with an enhanced accumulation of AS1411-PGG-PTX nanoconjugates in glioblastoma cells, its extended retention time in circulation, and its pronounced penetration in glioblastoma tumors. The authors observed that AS1411-PGG-PTX was able to promote an increase in the survival of the tumor bearing mice and an efficient PCX delivery to glioblastoma tissue with a consequently strong cytotoxic effect [66].

One interesting strategy was used by Balasubramanyam and collaborators in a recently published work, where they designed aptamer-siRNA chimeras with great specificity to cancer expressing EpCAM that can deliver siRNAs against chosen oncogenes. In the case, PLK1, BCL2, and STAT3, three important proteins with high relevance in tumor growth, were selected. They tested various chimeras with positive results in cancer cell lines of breast, lung, head, neck, liver, and retinoblastoma [67].

Li et al. (2017) demonstrated an interesting feature of the aptamers paving the way to the action of neoadjuvant cytotoxic drugs, not necessarily carrying drugs molecules in their own structure. They selected a new ssDNA named HL-1 with high affinity and specificity to Maver-I lymphoma cells (Kd = 70 pmol/L). The aptamer presents a G-quadruplex structure and, once internalized by endocytosis, promoted cell cycle arrest in S-phase in around half of cell population after three days of lymphoma cells treatment. They exploit this effect in a combined treatment of lymphoma cells with a cytotoxic cytarabine. The lethal action of cytarabine is predominant over lymphoma cells in S-phase, and they show that several rounds of aptamer treatment was able to synergistically sensitize these cells to the lethal effect of cytarabine [68].

Pancreatic ductal adenocarcinoma (PDAC) could receive a great benefit from an aptamer target drug deliver approach because it is one with the worst prognosis among all other cancers. The limitation of therapeutic drug treatment dose imposed by the side effects resulted from the non-specificity of the available cancer chemotherapeutics contributes significantly to a poor prognosis. Levy and Kratchmer

(2018) proposed a new treatment approach using the Waz aptamer (anti-transferrin receptor–TfR) and E07 aptamer (anti-epidermal growth factor—EGFR), two receptors overexpressed in PDAC that are internalized by clathrin mediated endocytosis. The product of the conjugation of these aptamers with thiol-reactive membrane-permeable MMAE (MC-VC-PAB-MMAE) bearing a valine-citrulline linker or the membrane-impermeable auristatin derivative MMAF (MC-MMAF) was tested in Panc-1, MIA PaCa-2, and BxPC3 PDAC cell lines, with promising results [69].

Finally, the MUC1 aptamers were also used to deliver chitosan nanoparticles containing both docetaxel and siRNAs for a co-delivery/co-treatment approached. The conjugation of the aptamer to the nanoparticle increased specificity and cellular uptake of the nanoconjugate, whereas a significant impact of the combination therapy was confirmed in terms of cell viability. Furthermore, successful silencing was confirmed. Although this was a preliminary study conducted in vitro, it also demonstrates the potential of this type of approach [70]. Table 3 summarizes all works cited in this section.

Table 3. Aptamers for delivery SiRNA/chemotherapeutics for cancer therapy.

Carrier Aptamers	siRNA or Drug Delivered	Target Cell Lines	Main Effects	Ref.
PDGFRβ (Gint4.T)	STAT-3 siRNA	U87MG and T98G glioblastoma cells	Reduction of anti-apoptotic factors PARP and BCL-xL, inducing cell death in two glioblastoma lineages in vitro. Reduction of tumor growth rate and pro-tumoral factors in a xenograft mouse model of glioblastoma	[57]
HER-2 sense& antisense bivalent	EGFR siRNA	BT474 and SKBR3 breast cancer cells	Downregulation of EGFR in vitro and suppression of xenografted tumor growth in vivo	[58]
bivalent HER-2-HER-3	EGFR siRNA	BT474 and SKBR3 breast cancer cells	Reduction of HER receptors, induction of cell cycle arrest and apoptosis in vitro and inhibition of tumor growth in vivo	[59]
MUC1 multiaptamer	BCL-2 siRNA and Doxorubicin (DOX)	MCF-7 breast cancer cells	More efficiency in delivering doxorubicin. BCL-2 siRNA acted synergistically with DOX increasing the sensitivity of cells for apoptosis	[60]
epithelial cell adhesion molecule (EpCAM)	Doxorubicin (DOX)	EpCAM positive HT29 colorectal cancer cells; SCOV-3 ovarian cancer cell line and T47D breast cancer cell line	Tumor growth control overcoming chemoresistance in both tumorsphere formation assay and in xenotransplanted mice	[61]
EpCAM	Survivin RNAi	EpCAM positive HT29 colorectal cancer cells	The combination of the surivin downregulation with the action of 5-fluorouacil cytotoxic chemotherapeutic could increase the lethality of colorectal cancer stem cells, as well as tumor control, in colorectal cancer xenograph model	[62]
HER-3ECD	Doxorubicin (DOX)	MCF-7 HER3+ and BT 474HER3+ breast cancer cells	Increase in the survival rate in a xenograft mouse model. Reduction of liver and cardio toxicity after chemotherapy when compared to the formulation without aptamer	[63]
cMET	Doxorubicin (DOX)	NCI-H1838 lung cancer cells	Better efficiency in the uptake by the target cell and a precise subcellular distribution of DOX to the cell nucleus, after endocytosis	[64]

Table 3. *Cont.*

Carrier Aptamers	siRNA or Drug Delivered	Target Cell Lines	Main Effects	Ref.
Anti A-172 cells aptamer	Doxorubicin (DOX)	Glioblastoma multiforme tumor cells A-172	Selective binding and inactivation of A-172 glioblastoma cells	[65]
Nucleolin (AS1411)	Paclitaxel (PCX)	Glioblastoma U87 MG cells and neo-vascular endothelial cells	Improvement of cell uptake and internalization, spheroid tumor penetration and cell growth inhibition. Enhanced accumulation of AS1411-PGG-PTX nanoconjugates in glioblastoma cells, retention time in circulation penetration in glioblastoma tumors. Increase survival of the tumor bearing mice and an efficient PCX delivery to glioblastoma tissue with consequently strong cytotoxic effect	[66]
EpCAM	PLK1, BCL2, and STAT3 siRNA	NCC RbC 51 retinoblastoma cells; MCF-7 breast cancer cells; Müller Glial Mio M1 cells; PMI 2650 Head and Neck cancer cells and HepG2 Hepatocellular cells	Cell death induction and tumor reduction on RB xenografts tumor model	[67]
HL-1 (anti Maver-I cells)	Cytarabine	Maver-I lymphoma cells	Aptamer treatment was able to sensitize synergistically lymphoma cells in S-phase to lethal effect of cytarabine	[68]
Waz (anti-transferrin receptor—TfR)	Auristatin modified toxins	Panc-1, MIA PaCa-2, and BxPC3 Pancreas Ductal Adenocarcinoma cells	Aptamer conjugates demonstrated to be toxic to cell lines in different extends	[69]
EGFR	Auristatin modified toxins	Panc-1, MIA PaCa-2 and BxPC3 Pancreas Ductal Adenocarcinoma cells	Aptamer-toxin conjugates demonstrated to be toxic to cell lines in different extends	[69]
MUC1	cMET siRNA and Docetaxel	SKBR3 breast cancer cells	Nanoparticle chitosan increased specificity and cellular uptake of the nanoconjugate and successful silencing was confirmed	[70]

5. Concluding Remarks

Today, there are 42 studies in clinical trials using the term "aptamer", and 64 completed or ongoing studies using the term "siRNA" for treating medical conditions, including: cancer, HIV, and diseases of the immune system (www.clinicaltrial.gov), which indicates that these two therapeutic agents are still on the frontier of knowledge and are tendency in the global market. In a study of market analysis, siRNA and aptamers are the new drugs that biopharmaceutical industries are investing, and the cancer is the most studied disease using this strategy. The global aptamer market was valued at nearly $1.0 billion USD in 2016 and is expected to expand with a CAGR of 20.0% over the period from 2017 to 2025 to attain the value of $5.0 billion USD by the end of 2025. This growth is attributable to technology advances and the introduction of companies at commercial panel. The main players operating in the global aptamer market are AM Biotech (Houston, TX, USA), Aptamer Group (York, UK), Aptamer Sciences Inc. (Gyeongsangbuk-do, Korea), Aptagen LLC (Jacobus, PA, USA), and Base Pair Biotechnologies (Pearland, TX, USA). In regard to siRNA, the therapeutics market is expected to expand significantly until 2025, since the first product approved by FDA is currently available in the market. Major players operating in the global small interfering RNA (siRNA) therapeutics market are GE Dharmacon Lafayette, USA), OPKO Health, Inc. (Miami, FL, USA), Alnylam Pharmaceuticals (Cambridge, MA, USA), Arrowhead Research Corp (Pasadena, CA, USA), Sanofi Genzyme (Cambridge, MA, USA), Genecon Biotechnologies Co., Ltd. (Baesweiler, Germany), Arbutus Biopharma Corp (Burnaby, Canada), Silence Therapeutics AG (London, UK), and Sylentis S.A. (Madrid, Spain) (www.grandviewresearch.com).

Ever since our last revision of the field in 2017 [71], more than 50 new works have been published and revised in this manuscript, which show the potential of this approach. Furthermore, a number of new works have appeared related to nanoparticle formulations of siRNA and other RNA forms, using different types of nanoparticles, and carried successfully by aptamers, whilst some approaches have favored the use of siRNAs in conjunction with chemotherapy agents, with very promising results. A review of some of these technologies in a graphic form is presented in the figure below (Figure 1).

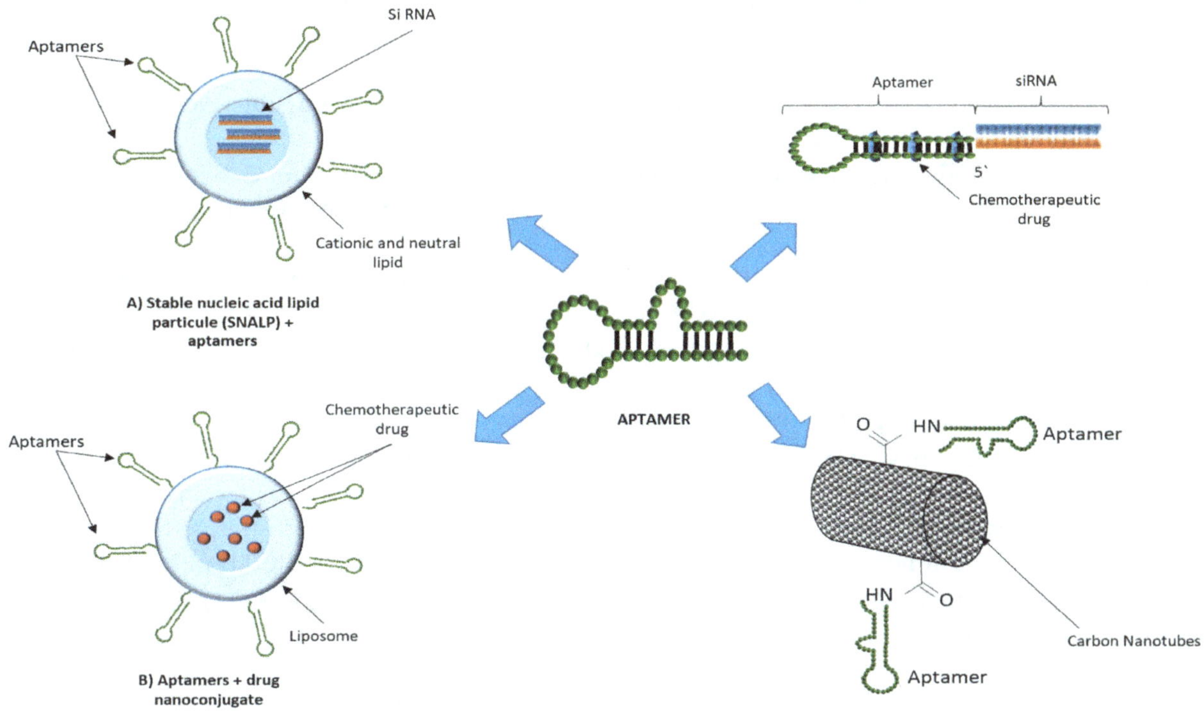

Figure 1. Uses of aptamers in therapeutic delivery.

Harnessing the targeting potential of aptamers, together with the silencing power of siRNAs and a long proved cytotoxic effect of chemotherapeutic agents, and bringing them together into a single therapeutic modality, has shown a great co-operative effect. It offers a therapy delivered directly and specifically to the tumor cell, with important proteins for tumor progression or survival silenced, whilst DNA acting cytotoxic agents act on tumor DNA, causing a specific therapy that has the potential to outmatch other approaches that focus on a single modalities.

Author Contributions: Conceptualization, S.M. and C.E.B.d.A.; writing—original draft preparation: Aptamer in the delivery of siRNA: A.P.D.A.B., Immunotherapy Using Aptamers-siRNA: P.C.d.C.N. and D.S., Aptamers-siRNA Chimeras: C.E.B.d.A., P.C.d.C.N. and D.S.; writing—review and editing, S.M.; supervision, S.M.

References

1. Singh, A.; Trivedi, P.; Jain, N.K. Advances in siRNA delivery in cancer therapy. *Artif. Cells Nanomed. Biotechnol.* **2018**, *46*, 274–283. [CrossRef] [PubMed]
2. Mishra, D.K.; Balekar, N.; Mishra, P.K. Nanoengineered strategies for siRNA delivery: From target assessment to cancer therapeutic efficacy. *Drug Deliv. Transl. Res.* **2017**, *7*, 346–358. [CrossRef] [PubMed]
3. Goldberg, M.S. Improving cancer immunotherapy through nanotechnology. *Nat. Rev. Cancer* **2019**, *19*, 587–602. [CrossRef] [PubMed]
4. Nanjwade, B.K.; Sarkar, A.B.; Srichana, T. Design and Characterization of Nanoparticulate Drug Delivery. In *Characterization and Biology of Nanomaterials for Drug Delivery*; Elsevier: Amsterdam, The Netherlands, 2019.
5. Wang, X.X.; Li, Y.B.; Yao, H.J.; Ju, R.J.; Zhang, Y.; Li, R.J.; Yu, Y.; Zhang, L.; Lu, W.L. The use of mitochondrial targeting resveratrol liposomes modified with a dequalinium polyethylene glycol-distearoylphosphatidyl ethanolamine conjugate to induce apoptosis in resistant lung cancer cells. *Biomaterials* **2011**, *32*, 5673–5687. [CrossRef] [PubMed]
6. Faraji, A.H.; Wipf, P. Nanoparticles in cellular drug delivery. *Bioorg. Med. Chem.* **2009**, *17*, 2950–2962. [CrossRef]
7. Bhushan, B. *Springer Handbook of Nanotechnology*; Bhushan, B., Ed.; Springer: Berlin/Heidelberg, Germany, 2017; ISBN 978-3-662-54355-9.
8. Yao, V.J.; D'Angelo, S.; Butler, K.S.; Theron, C.; Smith, T.L.; Marchiò, S.; Gelovani, J.G.; Sidman, R.L.; Dobroff, A.S.; Brinker, C.J.; et al. Ligand-targeted theranostic nanomedicines against cancer. *J. Control. Release* **2016**, *240*, 267–286. [CrossRef] [PubMed]
9. Guaragna, A.; Chiaviello, A.; Paolella, C.; DAlonzo, D.; Palumbo, G.; Palumbo, G. Synthesis and evaluation of folate-based chlorambucil delivery systems for tumor-targeted chemotherapy. *Bioconjug. Chem.* **2012**, *23*, 84–96. [CrossRef]
10. Eloy, J.O.; Petrilli, R.; Raspantini, G.L.; Lee, R.J. Targeted Liposomes for siRNA Delivery to Cancer. *Curr. Pharm. Des.* **2018**, *24*, 2664–2672. [CrossRef]
11. Kim, M.W.; Jeong, H.Y.; Kang, S.J.; Choi, M.J.; You, Y.M.; Im, C.S.; Lee, T.S.; Song, I.H.; Lee, C.G.; Rhee, K.J.; et al. Cancer-targeted Nucleic Acid Delivery and Quantum Dot Imaging Using EGF Receptor Aptamer-conjugated Lipid Nanoparticles. *Sci. Rep.* **2017**, *7*, 9474. [CrossRef]
12. Guo, P.; Zhang, C.; Chen, C.; Garver, K.; Trottier, M. Inter-RNA interaction of phage θ29 pRNA to form a hexameric complex for viral DNA transportation. *Mol. Cell* **1998**, *2*, 149–155. [CrossRef]
13. Hu, J.; Xiao, F.; Hao, X.; Bai, S.; Hao, J. Inhibition of monocyte adhesion to brain-derived endothelial cells by dual functional RNA chimeras. *Mol. Ther. Nucleic Acids* **2014**, *3*, e209. [CrossRef] [PubMed]
14. Afonin, K.A.; Viard, M.; Koyfman, A.Y.; Martins, A.N.; Kasprzak, W.K.; Panigaj, M.; Desai, R.; Santhanam, A.; Grabow, W.W.; Jaeger, L.; et al. Multifunctional RNA Nanoparticles. *Nano Lett.* **2014**, *14*, 5662–5671. [CrossRef] [PubMed]
15. Li, N.; Ebright, J.N.; Stovall, G.M.; Chen, X.; Nguyen, H.H.; Singh, A.; Syrett, A.; Ellington, A.D. Technical and biological issues relevant to cell typing with aptamers. *J. Proteome Res.* **2009**, *8*, 2438–2448. [CrossRef] [PubMed]
16. Panigaj, M.; Reiser, J. Aptamer guided delivery of nucleic acid-based nanoparticles. *DNA RNA Nanotechnol.* **2016**, *2*, 42–52. [CrossRef]
17. Zhao, N.; Bagaria, H.G.; Wong, M.S.; Zu, Y. A nanocomplex that is both tumor cell-selective and cancer gene-specific for anaplastic large cell lymphoma. *J. Nanobiotechnol.* **2011**, *9*, 2. [CrossRef]
18. Powell, D.; Chandra, S.; Dodson, K.; Shaheen, F.; Wiltz, K.; Ireland, S.; Syed, M.; Dash, S.; Wiese, T.; Mandal, T.; et al. Aptamer-functionalized hybrid nanoparticle for the treatment of breast cancer. *Eur. J. Pharm. Biopharm.* **2017**, *114*, 108–118. [CrossRef]
19. Yan, W.; Tao, M.; Jiang, B.; Yao, M.; Jun, Y.; Dai, W.; Tang, Z.; Gao, Y.; Zhang, L.; Chen, X.; et al. Overcoming Drug Resistance in Colon Cancer by Aptamer-Mediated Targeted Co-Delivery of Drug and siRNA Using Grapefruit-Derived Nanovectors. *Cell. Physiol. Biochem.* **2018**, *50*, 79–91. [CrossRef]
20. Wilner, S.E.; Wengerter, B.; Maier, K.; Borba Magalhães, M.D.L.; Del Amo, D.S.; Pai, S.; Opazo, F.; Rizzoli, S.O.; Yan, A.; Levy, M. An RNA alternative to human transferrin: A new tool for targeting human cells. *Mol. Ther. Nucleic Acids* **2012**, *1*, e21. [CrossRef]

21. Alshaer, W.; Hillaireau, H.; Vergnaud, J.; Mura, S.; Deloménie, C.; Sauvage, F.; Ismail, S.; Fattal, E. Aptamer-guided siRNA-loaded nanomedicines for systemic gene silencing in CD-44 expressing murine triple-negative breast cancer model. *J. Control. Release* **2018**, *271*, 98–106. [CrossRef]
22. Kim, E.; Jung, Y.; Choi, H.; Yang, J.; Suh, J.S.; Huh, Y.M.; Kim, K.; Haam, S. Prostate cancer cell death produced by the co-delivery of Bcl-xL shRNA and doxorubicin using an aptamer-conjugated polyplex. *Biomaterials* **2010**, *31*, 4592–4599. [CrossRef]
23. Wu, X.; Ding, B.; Gao, J.; Wang, H.; Fan, W.; Wang, X.; Zhang, W.; Wang, X.; Ye, L.; Zhang, M.; et al. Second-generation aptamer-conjugated PSMA-targeted delivery system for prostate cancer therapy. *Int. J. Nanomed.* **2011**, *6*, 1747–1756.
24. Xu, X.; Wu, J.; Liu, Y.; Saw, P.E.; Tao, W.; Yu, M.; Zope, H.; Si, M.; Victorious, A.; Rasmussen, J.; et al. Multifunctional Envelope-Type siRNA Delivery Nanoparticle Platform for Prostate Cancer Therapy. *ACS Nano* **2017**, *11*, 2618–2627. [CrossRef]
25. Lv, T.; Li, Z.; Xu, L.; Zhang, Y.; Chen, H.; Gao, Y. Chloroquine in combination with aptamer-modified nanocomplexes for tumor vessel normalization and efficient erlotinib/Survivin shRNA co-delivery to overcome drug resistance in EGFR-mutated non-small cell lung cancer. *Acta Biomater.* **2018**, *76*, 257–274. [CrossRef] [PubMed]
26. Dassie, J.P.; Liu, X.Y.; Thomas, G.S.; Whitaker, R.M.; Thiel, K.W.; Stockdale, K.R.; Meyerholz, D.K.; McCaffrey, A.P.; McNamara, J.O.; Giangrande, P.H. Systemic administration of optimized aptamer-siRNA chimeras promotes regression of PSMA-expressing tumors. *Nat. Biotechnol.* **2009**, *27*, 839–846. [CrossRef]
27. Bagalkot, V.; Gao, X. SiRNA-aptamer chimeras on nanoparticles: Preserving targeting functionality for effective gene silencing. *ACS Nano* **2011**, *5*, 8131–8139. [CrossRef] [PubMed]
28. Jafari, R.; Majidi Zolbanin, N.; Majidi, J.; Atyabi, F.; Yousefi, M.; Jadidi-Niaragh, F.; Aghebati-Maleki, L.; Shanehbandi, D.; Soltani Zangbar, M.-S.; Rafatpanah, H. Anti-Mucin1 Aptamer-Conjugated Chitosan Nanoparticles for Targeted Co-Delivery of Docetaxel and IGF-1R siRNA to SKBR3 Metastatic Breast Cancer Cells. *Iran. Biomed. J.* **2019**, *23*, 21–33. [CrossRef]
29. Dong, J.; Cao, Y.; Shen, H.; Ma, Q.; Mao, S.; Li, S.; Sun, J. EGFR aptamer-conjugated liposome-polycation-DNA complex for targeted delivery of SATB1 small interfering RNA to choriocarcinoma cells. *Biomed. Pharmacother.* **2018**, *107*, 849–859. [CrossRef]
30. Ayatollahi, S.; Salmasi, Z.; Hashemi, M.; Askarian, S.; Oskuee, R.K.; Abnous, K.; Ramezani, M. Aptamer-targeted delivery of Bcl-xL shRNA using alkyl modified PAMAM dendrimers into lung cancer cells. *Int. J. Biochem. Cell Biol.* **2017**, *92*, 210–217. [CrossRef]
31. Taghavi, S.; Nia, A.H.; Abnous, K.; Ramezani, M. Polyethylenimine-functionalized carbon nanotubes tagged with AS1411 aptamer for combination gene and drug delivery into human gastric cancer cells. *Int. J. Pharm.* **2017**, *516*, 301–312. [CrossRef]
32. Xu, Y.; Pang, L.; Wang, H.; Xu, C.; Shah, H.; Guo, P.; Shu, D.; Qian, S.Y. Specific delivery of delta-5-desaturase siRNA via RNA nanoparticles supplemented with dihomo-γ-linolenic acid for colon cancer suppression. *Redox Biol.* **2019**, *21*, 101085. [CrossRef]
33. Li, L.; Hu, X.; Zhang, M.; Ma, S.; Yu, F.; Zhao, S.; Liu, N.; Wang, Z.; Wang, Y.; Guan, H.; et al. Dual Tumor-Targeting Nanocarrier System for siRNA Delivery Based on pRNA and Modified Chitosan. *Mol. Ther. Nucleic Acids* **2017**, *8*, 169–183. [CrossRef] [PubMed]
34. Wu, M.; Zhao, H.; Guo, L.; Wang, Y.; Song, J.; Zhao, X.; Li, C.; Hao, L.; Wang, D.; Tang, J. Ultrasound-mediated nanobubble destruction (UMND) facilitates the delivery of A10-3.2 aptamer targeted and siRNA-loaded cationic nanobubbles for therapy of prostate cancer. *Drug Deliv.* **2018**, *25*, 226–240. [CrossRef] [PubMed]
35. Liu, Q.; Wang, D.; Xu, Z.; Huang, C.; Zhang, C.; He, B.; Mao, C.; Wang, G.; Qian, H. Targeted Delivery of Rab26 siRNA with Precisely Tailored DNA Prism for Lung Cancer Therapy. *ChemBioChem* **2019**, *20*, 1139–1144. [CrossRef] [PubMed]
36. Jeelani, S.; Jagat Reddy, R.C.; Maheswaran, T.; Asokan, G.S.; Dany, A.; Anand, B. Theranostics: A treasured tailor for tomorrow. *J. Pharm. Bioallied Sci.* **2014**, *6* (Suppl. 1), S6. [CrossRef] [PubMed]
37. Kim, M.W.; Jeong, H.Y.; Kang, S.J.; Jeong, I.H.; Choi, M.J.; You, Y.M.; Im, C.S.; Song, I.H.; Lee, T.S.; Lee, J.S.; et al. Anti-EGF receptor aptamer-guided co-delivery of anti-cancer siRNAs and quantum dots for theranostics of triple-negative breast cancer. *Theranostics* **2019**, *9*, 837. [CrossRef] [PubMed]
38. Sivakumar, P.; Kim, S.; Kang, H.C.; Shim, M.S. Targeted siRNA delivery using aptamer-siRNA chimeras and aptamer-conjugated nanoparticles. *Wiley Interdiscip. Rev. Nanomed. Nanobiotechnol.* **2019**, *11*, e1543. [CrossRef]

39. Behlke, M.A. Chemical modification of siRNAs for in vivo use. *Oligonucleotides* **2008**, *18*, 305–320. [CrossRef]
40. Keefe, A.D.; Cload, S.T. SELEX with modified nucleotides. *Curr. Opin. Chem. Biol.* **2008**, *12*, 448–456. [CrossRef]
41. Mohamed, M.; Abu Lila, A.S.; Shimizu, T.; Alaaeldin, E.; Hussein, A.; Sarhan, H.A.; Szebeni, J.; Ishida, T. PEGylated liposomes: Immunological responses. *Sci. Technol. Adv. Mater.* **2019**, *20*, 710–724. [CrossRef]
42. Lächelt, U.; Wagner, E. Nucleic Acid Therapeutics Using Polyplexes: A Journey of 50 Years (and Beyond). *Chem. Rev.* **2015**, *115*, 11043–11078. [CrossRef]
43. Diao, Y.; Liu, J.; Ma, Y.; Su, M.; Zhang, H.; Hao, X. A specific aptamer-cell penetrating peptides complex delivered siRNA efficiently and suppressed prostate tumor growth in vivo. *Cancer Biol. Ther.* **2016**, *17*, 498–506. [CrossRef] [PubMed]
44. Subramanian, N.; Kanwar, J.R.; Athalya, P.K.; Janakiraman, N.; Khetan, V.; Kanwar, R.K.; Eluchuri, S.; Krishnakumar, S. EpCAM aptamer mediated cancer cell specific delivery of EpCAM siRNA using polymeric nanocomplex. *J. Biomed. Sci.* **2015**, *22*, 4. [CrossRef] [PubMed]
45. Tseng, Y.C.; Mozumdar, S.; Huang, L. Lipid-based systemic delivery of siRNA. *Adv. Drug Deliv. Rev.* **2009**, *61*, 721–731. [CrossRef] [PubMed]
46. Sharma, P.; Hu-Lieskovan, S.; Wargo, J.A.; Ribas, A. Primary, Adaptive, and Acquired Resistance to Cancer Immunotherapy. *Cell* **2017**, *168*, 707–723. [CrossRef]
47. Pastor, F.; Berraondo, P.; Etxeberria, I.; Frederick, J.; Sahin, U.; Gilboa, E.; Melero, I. An rna toolbox for cancer immunotherapy. *Nat. Rev. Drug Discov.* **2018**, *17*, 751–767. [CrossRef]
48. Pratico, E.D.; Sullenger, B.A.; Nair, S.K. Identification and characterization of an agonistic aptamer against the T cell costimulatory receptor, OX40. *Nucleic Acid Ther.* **2013**, *23*, 35–43. [CrossRef]
49. Rajagopalan, A.; Berezhnoy, A.; Schrand, B.; Puplampu-Dove, Y.; Gilboa, E. Aptamer-Targeted Attenuation of IL-2 Signaling in $CD8^+$ T Cells Enhances Antitumor Immunity. *Mol. Ther.* **2017**, *25*, 54–61. [CrossRef]
50. Puplampu-Dove, Y.; Gefen, T.; Rajagopalan, A.; Muheramagic, D.; Schrand, B.; Gilboa, E. Potentiating tumor immunity using aptamer-targeted RNAi to render $CD8^+$ T cells resistant to TGFβ inhibition. *Oncoimmunology* **2018**, *7*, e1349588. [CrossRef]
51. Song, P.; Chou, Y.K.; Zhang, X.; Meza-Romero, R.; Yomogida, K.; Benedek, G.; Chu, C.Q. CD4 aptamer-RORγt shRNA chimera inhibits IL-17 synthesis by human CD4 + T cells. *Biochem. Biophys. Res. Commun.* **2014**, *452*, 1040–1045. [CrossRef]
52. Soldevilla, M.M.; Villanueva, H.; Bendandi, M.; Inoges, S.; López-Díaz de Cerio, A.; Pastor, F. 2-fluoro-RNA oligonucleotide CD40 targeted aptamers for the control of B lymphoma and bone-marrow aplasia. *Biomaterials* **2015**, *67*, 274–285. [CrossRef]
53. Nozari, A.; Berezovski, M.V. Aptamers for CD Antigens: From Cell Profiling to Activity Modulation. *Mol. Ther. Nucleic Acids* **2017**, *6*, 29–44. [CrossRef] [PubMed]
54. Kruspe, S.; Giangrande, P.H. Aptamer-siRNA chimeras: Discovery, progress, and future prospects. *Biomedicines* **2017**, *5*, 45. [CrossRef] [PubMed]
55. Strebhardt, K.; Ullrich, A. Paul Ehrlich's magic bullet concept: 100 Years of progress. *Nat. Rev. Cancer* **2008**, *8*, 473–480. [CrossRef] [PubMed]
56. McNamara, J.O.; Andrechek, E.R.; Wang, Y.; Viles, K.D.; Rempel, R.E.; Gilboa, E.; Sullenger, B.A.; Giangrande, P.H. Cell type-specific delivery of siRNAs with aptamer-siRNA chimeras. *Nat. Biotechnol.* **2006**, *24*, 1005–1015. [CrossRef] [PubMed]
57. Esposito, C.L.; Nuzzo, S.; Catuogno, S.; Romano, S.; de Nigris, F.; de Franciscis, V. STAT3 Gene Silencing by Aptamer-siRNA Chimera as Selective Therapeutic for Glioblastoma. *Mol. Ther. Nucleic Acids* **2018**, *10*, 398–411. [CrossRef] [PubMed]
58. Xue, L.; Maihle, N.J.; Yu, X.; Tang, S.C.; Liu, H.Y. Synergistic Targeting HER2 and EGFR with Bivalent Aptamer-siRNA Chimera Efficiently Inhibits HER2-Positive Tumor Growth. *Mol. Pharm.* **2018**, *15*, 4801–4813. [CrossRef]
59. Yu, X.; Ghamande, S.; Liu, H.; Xue, L.; Zhao, S.; Tan, W.; Zhao, L.; Tang, S.C.; Wu, D.; Korkaya, H.; et al. Targeting EGFR/HER2/HER3 with a Three-in-One Aptamer-siRNA Chimera Confers Superior Activity against HER2+ Breast Cancer. *Mol. Ther. Nucleic Acids* **2018**, *10*, 317–330. [CrossRef]
60. Jeong, H.; Lee, S.H.; Hwang, Y.; Yoo, H.; Jung, H.; Kim, S.H.; Mok, H. Multivalent Aptamer–RNA Conjugates for Simple and Efficient Delivery of Doxorubicin/siRNA into Multidrug-Resistant Cells. *Macromol. Biosci.* **2017**, *17*, 1600343. [CrossRef]
61. Xiang, D.; Shigdar, S.; Bean, A.G.; Bruce, M.; Yang, W.; Mathesh, M.; Wang, T.; Yin, W.; Tran, P.H.L.;

Shamaileh, H.A.; et al. Transforming doxorubicin into a cancer stem cell killer via EpCAM aptamer-mediated delivery. *Theranostics* **2017**, *7*, 4071. [CrossRef]
62. Alshamaileh, H.; Wang, T.; Xiang, D.; Yin, W.; Tran, P.H.L.; Barrero, R.A.; Zhang, P.Z.; Li, Y.; Kong, L.; Liu, K.; et al. Aptamer-mediated survivin RNAi enables 5-fluorouracil to eliminate colorectal cancer stem cells. *Sci. Rep.* **2017**, *7*, 5898. [CrossRef]
63. Dou, X.Q.; Wang, H.; Zhang, J.; Wang, F.; Xu, G.L.; Xu, C.C.; Xu, H.H.; Xiang, S.S.; Fu, J.; Song, H.F. Aptamer–drug conjugate: Targeted delivery of doxorubicin in a HER3 aptamer-functionalized liposomal delivery system reduces cardiotoxicity. *Int. J. Nanomed.* **2018**, *13*, 763–776. [CrossRef]
64. Prusty, D.K.; Adam, V.; Zadegan, R.M.; Irsen, S.; Famulok, M. Supramolecular aptamer nano-constructs for receptor-mediated targeting and light-triggered release of chemotherapeutics into cancer cells. *Nat. Commun.* **2018**, *9*, 535. [CrossRef] [PubMed]
65. Bayraç, A.T.; Akça, O.E.; Eyidoğan, F.İ.; Öktem, H.A. Target-specific delivery of doxorubicin to human glioblastoma cell line via ssDNA aptamer. *J. Biosci.* **2018**, *43*, 97–104. [CrossRef] [PubMed]
66. Luo, Z.; Yan, Z.; Jin, K.; Pang, Q.; Jiang, T.; Lu, H.; Liu, X.; Pang, Z.; Yu, L.; Jiang, X. Precise glioblastoma targeting by AS1411 aptamer-functionalized poly (L-γ-glutamylglutamine)–paclitaxel nanoconjugates. *J. Colloid Interface Sci.* **2017**, *490*, 783–796. [CrossRef] [PubMed]
67. Balasubramanyam, J.; Badrinarayanan, L.; Dhaka, B.; Gowda, H.; Pandey, A.; Subramanian, K.; Subadhra, L.B.; Elchuri, S. V EpCAM Aptamer siRNA chimeras: Therapeutic efficacy in epithelial cancer cells. *bioRxiv* **2019**. [CrossRef]
68. Li, H.; Yang, S.; Yu, G.; Shen, L.; Fan, J.; Xu, L.; Zhang, H.; Zhao, N.; Zeng, Z.; Hu, T.; et al. Aptamer internalization via endocytosis inducing s-phase arrest and priming maver-1 lymphoma cells for cytarabine chemotherapy. *Theranostics* **2017**, *7*, 1204–1213. [CrossRef] [PubMed]
69. Kratschmer, C.; Levy, M. Targeted Delivery of Auristatin-Modified Toxins to Pancreatic Cancer Using Aptamers. *Mol. Ther. Nucleic Acids* **2018**, *10*, 227–236. [CrossRef]
70. Zolbanin, N.M.; Jafari, R.; Majidi, J.; Atyabi, F.; Yousefi, M.; Jadidi-Niaragh, F.; Aghebati-Maleki, L.; Shanehbandi, D.; Zangbar, M.S.S.; Nayebi, A.M. Targeted co-delivery of docetaxel and cMET siRNA for treatment of mucin1 overexpressing breast cancer cells. *Adv. Pharm. Bull.* **2018**, *8*, 383–393. [CrossRef]
71. de Almeida, C.E.B.; Alves, L.N.; Rocha, H.F.; Cabral-Neto, J.B.; Missailidis, S. Aptamer delivery of siRNA, radiopharmaceutics and chemotherapy agents in cancer. *Int. J. Pharm.* **2017**, *525*, 334–342. [CrossRef]

Cell Internalization in Fluidic Culture Conditions is Improved When Microparticles are Specifically Targeted to the Human Epidermal Growth Factor Receptor 2 (HER2)

Inmaculada Mora-Espí [1], Elena Ibáñez [1], Jorge Soriano [1], Carme Nogués [1], Thorarinn Gudjonsson [2,3] and Leonardo Barrios [1,*]

1 Unitat de Biologia Cel·lular, Departament de Biologia Cel·lular, Fisiologia i Immunologia, Facultat de Biociències, Universitat Autònoma de Barcelona, Bellaterra, 08193 Barcelona, Spain; xapaxin@gmail.com (I.M.-E.); Elena.ibanez@uab.cat (E.I.); jorge.soriano@uab.cat (J.S.); carme.nogues@uab.cat (C.N.)

2 Biomedical Center, University of Iceland, 101 Reykjavík, Iceland; tgudjons@hi.is

3 Department of Anatomy, Faculty of Medicine, and Department of Laboratory Hematology, University Hospital, 101 Reykjavik, Iceland

* Correspondence: lleonard.barrios@uab.cat

Abstract: Purpose: To determine if the specific targeting of microparticles improves their internalization by cells under fluidic conditions. Methods: Two isogenic breast epithelial cell lines, one overexpressing the Human Epidermal Growth Factor Receptor 2 (HER2) oncogene (D492HER2) and highly tumorigenic and the other expressing HER2 at much lower levels and non-tumorigenic (D492), were cultured in the presence of polystyrene microparticles of 1 μm in diameter, biofunctionalized with either a specific anti-HER2 antibody or a non-specific secondary antibody. Mono- and cocultures of both cell lines in static and fluidic conditions were performed, and the cells with internalized microparticles were scored. Results: Globally, the D492 cell line showed a higher endocytic capacity than the D492HER2 cell line. Microparticles that were functionalized with the anti-HER2 antibody were internalized by a higher percentage of cells than microparticles functionalized with the non-specific secondary antibody. Although internalization was reduced in fluidic culture conditions in comparison with static conditions, the increase in the internalization of microparticles biofunctionalized with the anti-HER2 antibody was higher for the cell line overexpressing HER2. Conclusion: The biofunctionalization of microparticles with a specific targeting molecule remarkably increases their internalization by cells in fluidic culture conditions (simulating the blood stream). This result emphasizes the importance of targeting for future in vivo delivery of drugs and bioactive molecules through microparticles.

Keywords: microfluidics; coculture; HER2; polystyrene μPs; biofunctionalization

---

1. Introduction

Drug targeting has the potential to improve the therapeutic efficacy and mitigate the non-specific effects of many drugs. In the last years, several types of drug delivery vehicles have been developed, including monoclonal antibodies [1], peptides [2], proteins [3], lipoproteins [4], carbohydrates [5], and polymeric nanoparticles [6,7]. Compared with the number of studies in which nanoparticles (NPs) are used [8–12], only a small number of studies involve the use of microparticles (μPs) [13–15]. It has been reported that small sizes and positive charges favor NP intake by cells [14–16], but in some cases, larger particle sizes could be advantageous for preventing non-specific interactions and internalization into normal non-phagocytic cells or for optimal tissue entrapment and transient retention [17]. Moreover, to target cancer cells, NPs and µPs surfaces can be modified to increase the interaction with plasma membrane-specific markers like the transferrin receptor [18], the folate receptor [19], or the human epidermal growth factor receptor 2 (HER2, also known as ERBB2) [20,21]. HER2 is a receptor tyrosine kinase which is overexpressed by some types of cancer cells and is considered a marker of poor clinical outcome in breast and ovarian cancer [22,23]. Some treatments directed to this target have already been approved and are clinically used, such as the anti-HER2 monoclonal antibody trastuzumab, alone or in combination with emtansine (T-DM1) [24], and the HER2 tyrosine kinase activity inhibitor lapatinib.

Traditionally, in vitro studies on drug carriers and drug release have been performed in static monolayer cell cultures. However, studies in microfluidic environments, mimicking the circulatory system, are currently gaining interest [12]. Compared with static cultures, microfluidic studies allow for better predictions about how a drug or a drug carrier running in a circulating flow, will interact with cells [25–27]. On the other hand, because normal and tumoral cells are intermingled in vivo, cocultures of normal and tumoral cells can better simulate tissue conditions than monocultures [28,29].

The overall objective of the present study was to evaluate the efficiency of targeting µPs to cells in physiological-like conditions (fluidic culture conditions). Two isogenic breast epithelial cell lines were used, one normal (D492) and the other overexpressing HER2 (D492HER2). Moreover, polystyrene µPs of 1 µm in diameter were biofunctionalized with a specific targeting protein, an anti-HER2 antibody, or with a non-specific secondary antibody. The specific objectives of the study were to evaluate and compare the cell internalization of these µPs in different culture conditions: monoculture versus coculture conditions, and static versus fluidic culture conditions.

2. Material and Methods

2.1. Biofunctionalization of Polystyrene µPs

Carboxylate polystyrene µPs of 1 µm in diameter (Polybead® Carboxylate Microspheres. Polysciences, Inc., Warrington, PA, USA) were biofunctionalized with two different targeting molecules: (1) mouse anti-c-ERBB2/c-Neu (Ab-5) clone TA-1 (Millipore, Darmstadt, Germany), herein referred to as antiH, and (2) goat anti-mouse IgG2a secondary antibody Alexa Fluor® 647 conjugate (Life Technologies, Carlsbad, CA, USA), herein referred to as secAb. Biofunctionalization was carried out using the PolyLink Protein Coupling Kit for COOH Microspheres (Polysciences) according to the manufacturer's instructions. The size of the µPs before and after biofunctionalization was analyzed by transmission electronic microscopy (TEM) (JEOL, JEM 2011). Biofunctionalization was evaluated under a fluorescence inverted microscope (Olympus IX71, Olympus, Hamburg, Germany) and by the change in the ζ-potential.

Microscopically, biofunctionalization of µPs with secAb (µP-secAb) was evaluated directly on the basis of their far-red fluorescence emission. On the other hand, µPs biofunctionalized with antiH (µP-antiH) were incubated for 5 min with chicken anti-mouse IgG (H+L) secondary antibody Alexa Fluor® 488 conjugate (1:500. Life Technologies) before the evaluation of green fluorescence emission.

Biofunctionalized and non-biofunctionalized µPs were separately resuspended in H14 culture medium [30] and sonicated for 5 min (Fisherbrand FB15047, Fisher Scientific, Germany) to achieve a monodispersed sample. Their ζ-potential was then measured with a Zetasizer Nano ZS (Malvern Instruments, Malvern, UK).

2.2. Cell Lines

Two isogenic breast epithelial cell lines, D492 and D492HER2, were used in the study. D492 is a non-tumorigenic cell line with stem cell properties that expresses low levels of the HER2 oncogene [30,31]. D492HER2 was generated by overexpressing the HER2 oncogene in D492 and is highly tumorigenic [32]. Both cell lines constitutively express green fluorescent protein (GFP).

The cells were cultured in serum-free H14 culture medium [30,31] at 37 °C and 5% CO_2 (standard conditions). As explained below, cell culture was performed as follows: mono- or cocultures in static conditions, and cocultures in fluidic conditions.

2.3. Cell Cultures in Static Conditions

For monoculture experiments, cells were seeded at a density of 60,000 cells/well in 24-well plates (μ-Plate 24-Well ibiTreat: #1.5 polymer coverslip. ibidi, Martinsried, Germany). For coculture experiments, 30,000 cells of each cell line (D492 and D492HER2) were seeded together in each well. In both cases, the cells were maintained for 24 h in standard culture conditions prior to performing any experiments.

To analyze μP internalization, μPs (μP-antiH or μP-secAb) were sonicated for 5 min, diluted (1:100), counted with a hemocytometer, and then added at a proportion of 45 μP/cell to the cell cultures and incubated for further 24 h in standard culture conditions.

2.4. Cell Cultures in Fluidic Conditions

For these experiments, only cocultures were performed. Before seeding, channel slides (μ-Slides I 0.8 mm ibiTreat, ibidi) were coated with bovine collagen type I (Advanced Biomatrix, San Diego, CA, USA) to enhance cell adhesion. Then, 1.5×10^5 cells of each cell line (D492 and D492HER2) were seeded in H14 medium containing 2% penicillin/streptomycin (Biowest, Nuaillé, France) and incubated in standard culture conditions. After 24 h, the slides were connected to a microfluidic system consisting of a perfusion set (Perfusion Set Red ID 1.6 mm, ibidi) filled with fresh H14 medium containing the μPs (μP-secAb or μP-antiH) and a Fluidic Unit connected to an ibidi Pump, controlled by a pump-control software (ibidi). The microfluidic system was kept at 37 °C and 5% CO_2. The cultures were maintained for 24 h under a unidirectional flow rate fixed at 4.32 mL/min with a shear stress of 1.50 dyn/cm^2 and a pressure of 7.9 mbar, as recommended by the manufacturer.

2.5. Evaluation of Microparticles Internalization

After being cultured in either static or fluidic conditions, the cells were washed three times with phosphate buffer saline (PBS) at room temperature (RT), fixed for 15 min with 4% paraformaldehyde (Sigma-Aldrich, St Louis, MO, USA) in PBS, and washed again with PBS (three times). Next, the fixed cells were permeabilized with 0.1% Triton X-100 (Sigma-Aldrich) in PBS for 10 min at RT, washed with PBS (three times), and blocked with 3% bovine serum albumin (BSA) (Sigma-Aldrich) in PBS for 40 min. PBS with 3% BSA was also employed to dilute the antibodies used in this work.

The cells from the monocultures were incubated with Alexa Fluor® 546 Phalloidin (1:40, Life Technologies) to label actin microfilaments and, in the case of samples with μP-antiH, also with goat anti-mouse IgG1 secondary antibody Alexa Fluor® 647 conjugate (1:150. Life Technologies) for 1 h at RT to detect μP-antiH.

To distinguish between D492 and D492HER2 in cocultures, the cells were first incubated with rabbit anti-HER2 monoclonal antibody (1:200, Cell Signaling, Danvers, MA, USA) overnight at 4 °C. Then, the samples were washed three times with PBS and incubated for 2.5 h at RT with Alexa Fluor® 546 Phalloidin to label actin microfilaments to visualize the cell limit and chicken anti-rabbit IgG (H+L) Alexa Fluor® 405 conjugate secondary antibody (1:150, Life Technologies) to label HER2 in the plasma membrane; for cells incubated with μP-antiH, goat anti-mouse IgG1 secondary antibody Alexa Fluor® 647 conjugate was also used.

Finally, the cells were washed three times with PBS and maintained at 4 °C in PBS until evaluation under a confocal laser scanning microscope (CLSM. Olympus, Tokyo, Japan). Orthogonal projections of z-stacks of at least 100 cells for each cell line were evaluated in each replicate. The xyz sequentially acquired images allowed for assessment of whether the particles were inside the cells or attached to their surfaces.

2.6. Statistical Analyses

At least three replicates of each experiment were performed. To compare μP internalization in each experimental condition and for each cell line, ANOVA with post-hoc Tukey HSD test was used; $p < 0.05$ was considered statistically significant.

3. Results

3.1. Microparticles Characterization after Biofunctionalization

Biofunctionalization did not affect the size of μPs, as can be observed in TEM images (Figure 1A). Moreover, biofunctionalization was confirmed in two ways, microscopically and by analyzing the ζ-potential. As expected, under fluorescence microscopy, μP-secAb emitted far-red fluorescence, and μP-antiH emitted green fluorescence after incubation with an Alexa® 488-conjugated secondary antibody (Figure 1B). Biofunctionalization was also confirmed by changes in the μP surface charge. Non-biofunctionalized polystyrene carboxylate μPs (μP-COOH) showed a ζ-potential value of −32.3 mV, whereas μP-secAb and μP-antiH increased their ζ-potential to smaller negative values of −11.23 mV and −11.5 mV, respectively (Figure 1C).

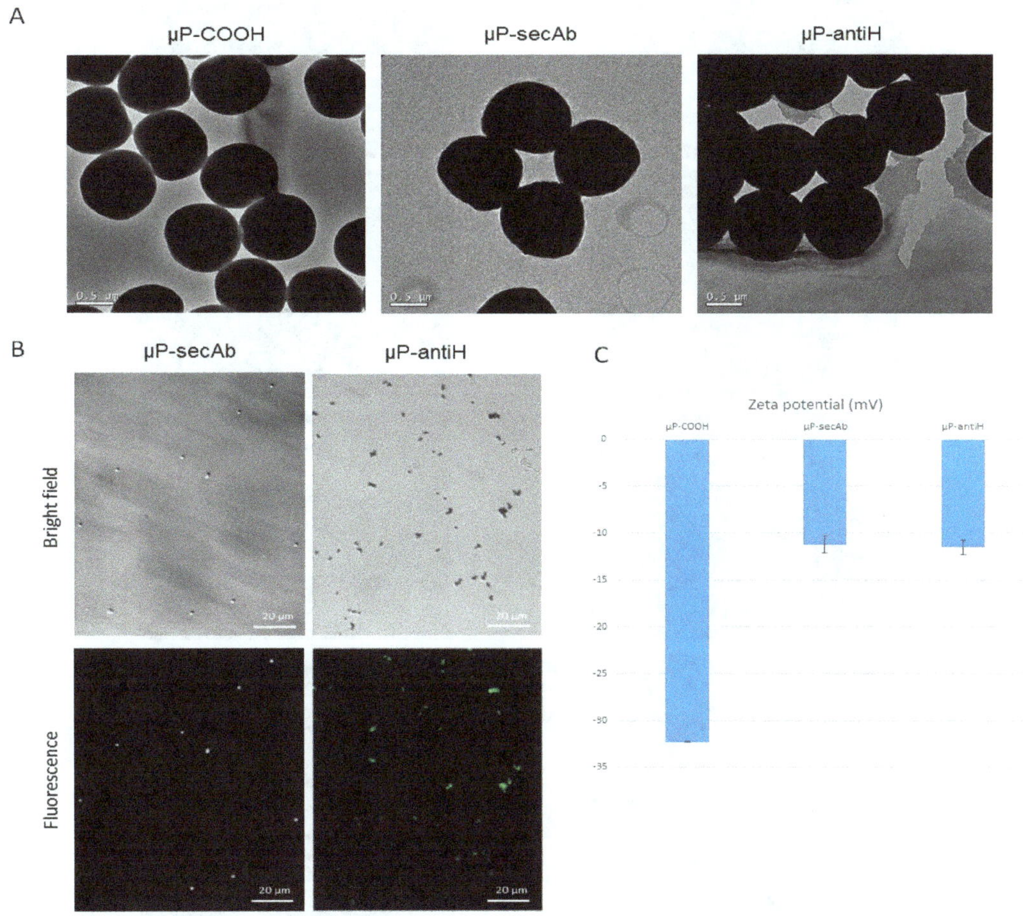

Figure 1. Characterization of microparticles (μP) biofunctionalization. (**A**) Transmission electronic microscopy (TEM) images of microparticles before (COOH) and after biofunctionalization (μP-secAb and μP-antiH). (**B**) Images of microparticles biofunctionalized with a secondary antibody (μP-secAb) or an anti-HER2 antibody (μP-antiH) in bright-field (upper panels) and fluorescence (lower panels) microscopy. (**C**) Zeta potential before (COOH) and after biofunctionalization (μP-secAb and μP-antiH).

3.2. Microparticles Internalization by Cells

The internalization of μPs by cells was evaluated through the orthogonal images captured by a CLSM in both static and fluidic culture conditions (examples in Figures 2 and 3, respectively). Staining of actin filaments was useful to visualize the cell perimeter and, together with the orthogonal projections, allowed us to clearly distinguish between internalized and non-internalized μPs. From these images, the number of cells with at least one internalized μP was scored.

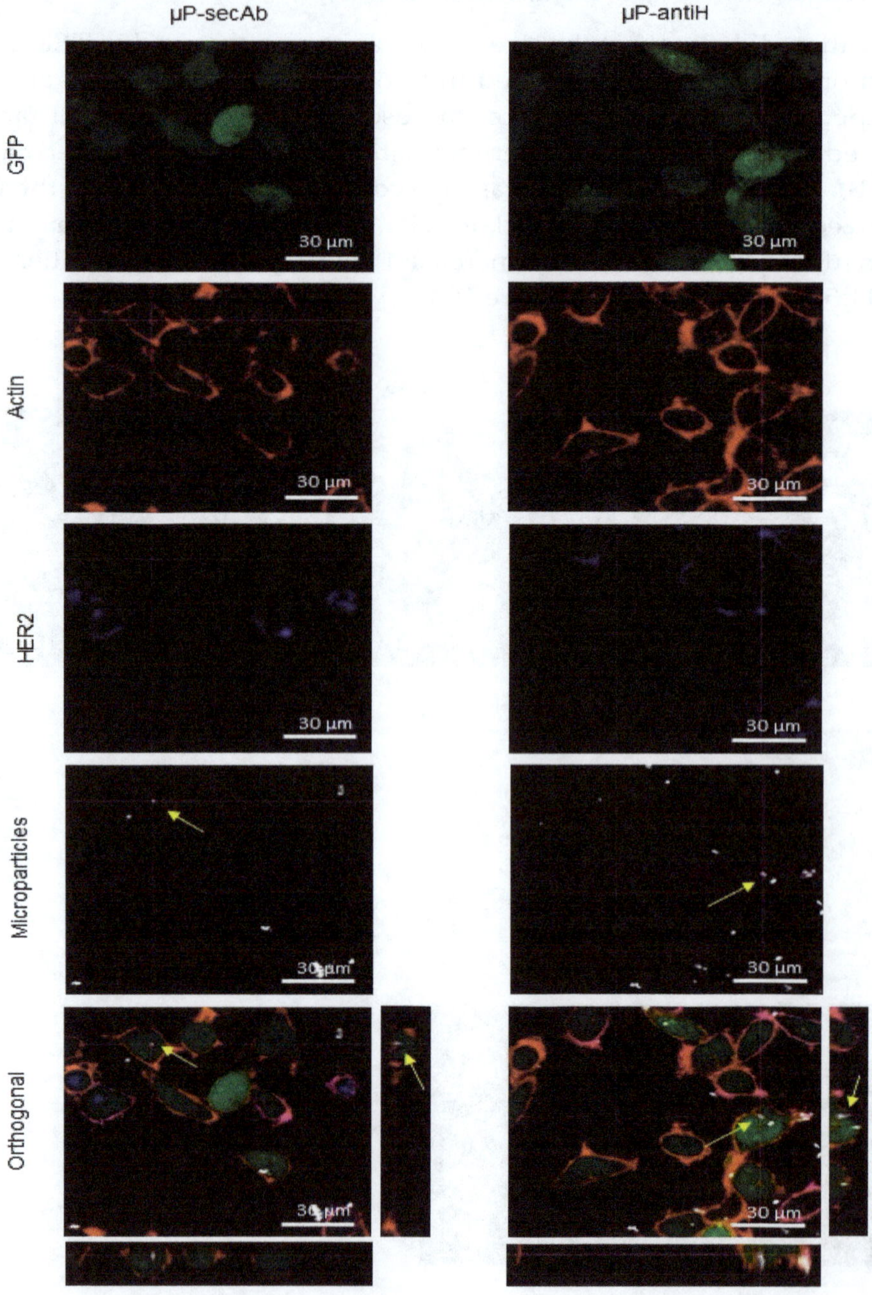

Figure 2. Immunofluorescence analysis by confocal laser scanning microscope (CLSM) of cells cultured in static conditions. Confocal images of D492 and D492HER2 cells cocultured in static conditions and incubated with microparticles biofunctionalized with a non-specific secondary antibody (μP-secAb) or a specific anti-HER2 antibody (μP-antiH). Cells, constitutively expressing green fluorescent protein (GFP, green), were incubated with Alexa Fluor® 546 Phalloidin (red) to label actin microfilaments and Alexa Fluor® 405 conjugate secondary antibody (blue) to label HER2 in the plasma membrane. The arrows point to some examples of μPs located inside the cells.

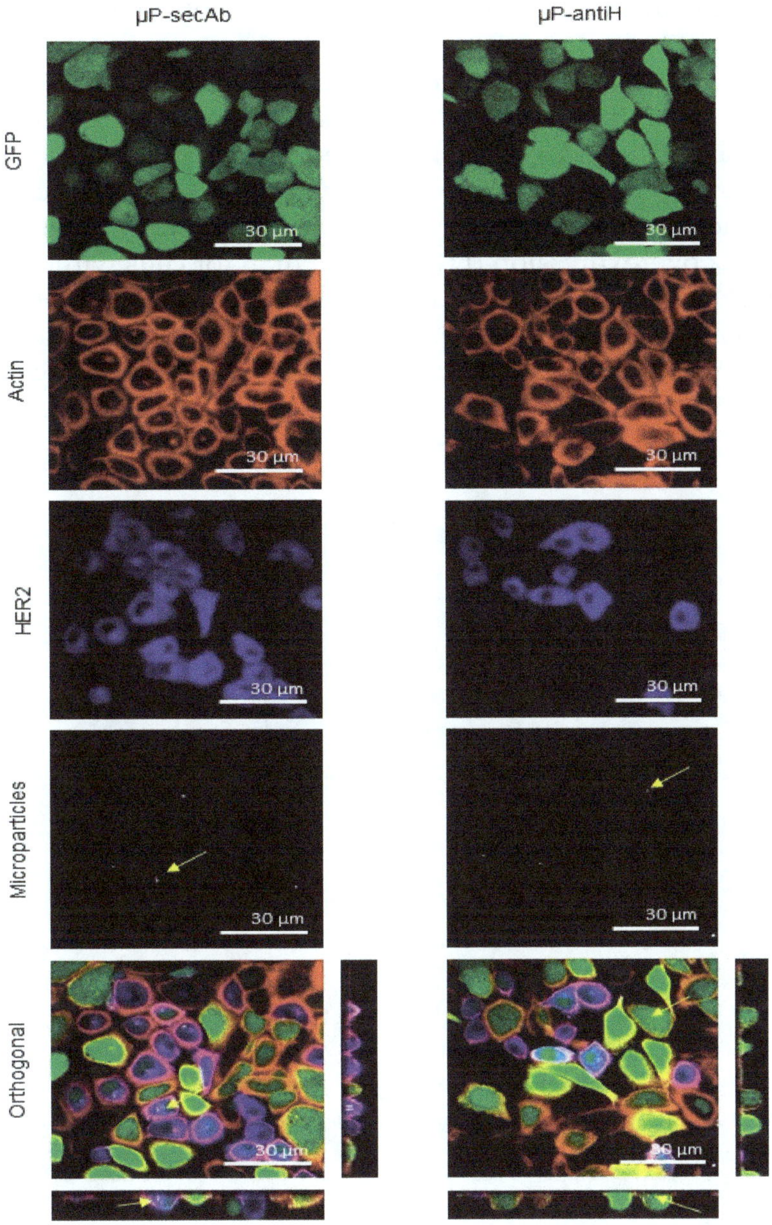

Figure 3. Immunofluorescence analysis by CLSM of cells cultured in fluidic conditions. Confocal images of D492 and D492HER2 cells cocultured in fluidic conditions and incubated with microparticles biofunctionalized with a non-specific secondary antibody (μP-secAb) or a specific anti-HER2 antibody (μP-antiH). The cells, constitutively expressing GFP (green), were incubated with Alexa Fluor® 546 Phalloidin (red) to label actin microfilaments and Alexa Fluor® 405 conjugate secondary antibody (blue) to label HER2 in the plasma membrane. The arrows point to some examples of μPs located inside the cells.

As can be seen in Figure 4, in all conditions, the percentage of D492 cells with internalized microparticles was always higher than that of D492HER2 cells, indicating that D492 cells have an inherent superior capacity to internalize microparticles. Regarding the importance of specific biofunctionalization in μPs recognition and intake by the cells, the internalization related to non-specific binding due to the intrinsic cell endocytic capacity, was represented by the percentage of cells with internalized μPs biofunctionalized with the non-specific antibody (μPs-secAb). In contrast, the internalization related to the specific recognition of μPs by the cells was represented by the increase in the percentage of cells with internalized μPs when these were specifically functionalized (μP-antiH) to recognize a cell membrane receptor (HER2). For both cell lines, the biofunctionalization with a specific targeting antibody (antiH) resulted in higher internalization percentages than the biofunctionalization with a non-specific targeting antibody (secAb). The differences between static monoculture and coculture conditions were not significant. As expected, fluidic culture conditions globally decreased internalization, but again internalization was higher for microparticles which were specifically biofunctionalized (μP-antiH) than for those that were biofunctionalized with a non-specific antibody (μP-secAb). The increase in the percentage of cells with internalized μP-antiH was also higher for cells with HER2 overexpression (D492HER2) than for cells without HER2 overexpression (D492) (Figure 4). Remarkably, the increase in the percentage of cells with internalized μP-antiH with regard to μP-secAb internalization was higher in fluidic conditions than in static conditions, especially in D492HER2 cells (164% versus 77–99% in D492HER2 cells, and 100% versus 22–35% in D492 cells).

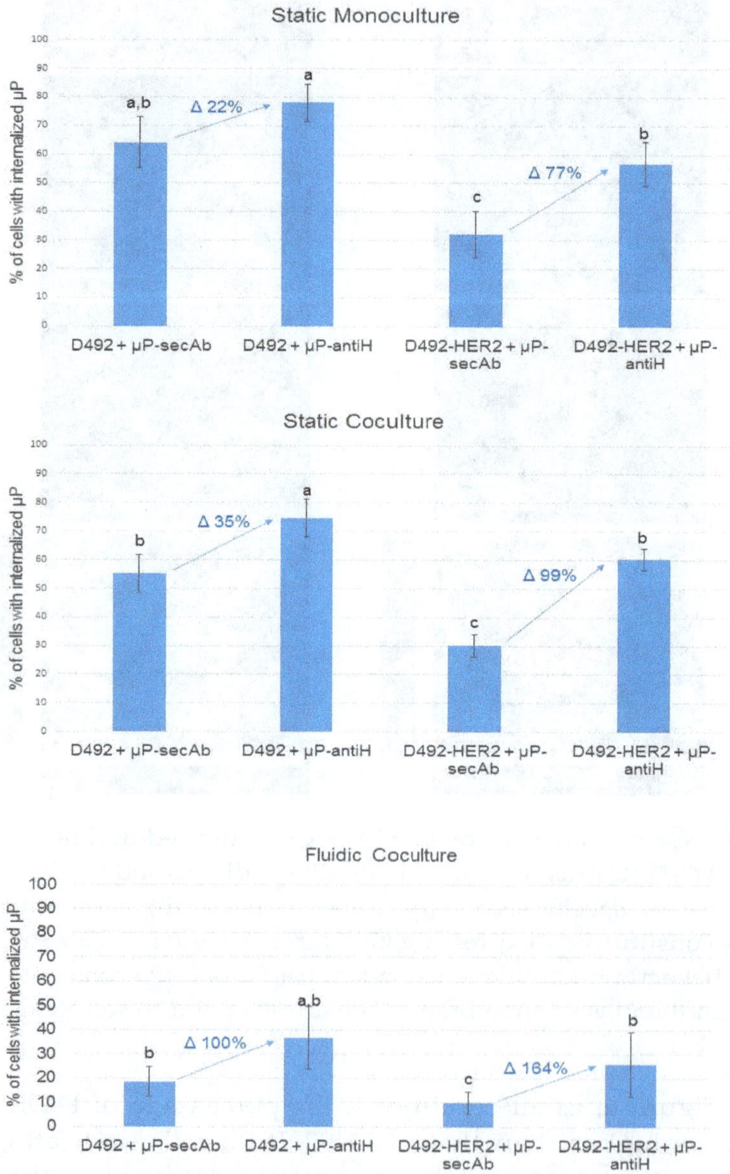

Figure 4. Microparticles internalization by monocultured or cocultured D492 and D492HER2 cells in static and fluidic conditions. Percentages of cells with internalized microparticles biofunctionalized with a non-specific secondary antibody (μP-secAb) or a specific anti-HER2 antibody (μP-antiH). Statistically significant differences are indicated with different letters on top of the bars. An increase of μPs internalization, as a percentage, is indicated in blue together with blue arrows.

4. Discussion

Polystyrene μPs were successfully biofunctionalized with an anti-HER2 antibody or with a secondary antibody, as demonstrated by the detection of fluorescence under a microscope and by changes in their ζ-potential. The reduction in μPs electronegativity could help in their interaction with the plasma membrane, which contains negatively charged saccharides. In fact, it has been described that positively or slightly negatively charged particle surfaces favor cell intake [14,33–35].

The cell lines used in this study are isogenic breast epithelial cell lines. D492 was established by isolating suprabasal cells from a reduction mammoplasty and subsequently immortalizing them using the *E6* and *E7* oncogenes from the human papilloma virus [30,31]. D492 has stem cell properties evaluated by the ability to generate luminal and myoepithelial cells and, in 3D culture, to form branching ductal–alveolar-like structures. D492HER2 was generated by overexpressing the HER2 oncogene in D492 [32]. Interestingly, D492 showed higher percentages of μPs internalization than D492HER2. A possible explanation could be the differences in phenotype between these cells. D492HER2 cells undergo an epithelial to mesenchymal transition (EMT) and express mesenchymal markers, which could reduce their ability to internalize μPs [31,32]. Higher rates of μP internalization have also been described in MCF10A breast epithelial normal cells than in SKBR3 breast epithelial tumoral cells, which also overexpress HER2 [14].

The molecules used to bio-functionalize the μPs also influenced the internalization rates. For both cell lines, the percentage of cells with internalized μP-antiH was higher than that of cells with internalized μP-secAb. This result was expected, since we hypothesized that a specific recognition between the cells and the μPs, such as that afforded by antiH biofunctionalization, could result in an increase in μP internalization. Also as expected, the increase in the percentages of μPs internalization obtained with antiH biofunctionalization was higher for D492HER2 cells, which overexpress HER2, than for D492 cells, which express HER2 at much lower levels [32]. These results clearly indicate that when μPs are biofunctionalized with molecules that specifically interact with plasma membrane receptors, their internalization can be improved, and the level of improvement is related to the number of receptors that are present on the cell surface.

Finally, in relation to the culture conditions, our results indicate that the percentage of cells with internalized μPs clearly decreased in fluidic conditions compared with static conditions. This was probably because the establishment of prior transient contacts between the plasma membrane and the μPs may be more difficult in fluidic conditions or in high shear stress conditions [36,37]. One can hypothesize that in the case of dynamic cultures, specific targeting may be helpful to improve the internalization rates, as it may facilitate the frequency and strength of μPs-cell contacts. Our results agree with this hypothesis because, for both cell lines, the increase of μPs-antiH internalization was higher in fluidic than in static cocultures when compared with μPs-secAb internalization, which opens the door to scale-up studies.

The present results, together with previous research, emphasize the relevance of cell type, specific targeting, and culture conditions such as mono- or cocultures and static or fluidic, to the potential application of NPs and μPs for drug delivery to cancer cells.

5. Conclusions

The present study indicates that, for all culture conditions, μPs biofunctionalized with anti-HER2 antibodies were more efficiently internalized by cells expressing HER2 than μPs biofunctionalized with a non-specific antibody. Moreover, in fluidic culture conditions (simulating the blood stream), the specificity of targeting was still more useful for μP internalization, because the increase in internalization was higher for cells overexpressing HER2. Overall, the results presented emphasize the importance of targeting not only for directing μPs to the appropriate cells but also for achieving reasonable internalization rates, thereby opening the door to the use of microparticles as carriers for drug delivery.

Author Contributions: Conceptualization: E.I., C.N., T.G., and L.B.; Data curation: I.M.-E., J.S., and L.B.; Formal analysis: I.M.-E., J.S., and C.N.; Funding acquisition: C.N.; Investigation: I.M.-E.; Project administration: C.N.; Supervision: L.B.; Validation: E.I., C.N., T.G., and L.B.; Writing—original draft: I.M.-E. and L.B.; Writing—review & editing: I.M.-E., E.I., J.S., C.N., T.G., and L.B.

Acknowledgments: The authors wish to thank the Servei de Microscòpia at the Universitat Autònoma de Barcelona.

References

1. Sato, K.; Nagaya, T.; Choyke, P.L.; Kobayashi, H. Near infrared photoimmunotherapy in the treatment of pleural disseminated NSCLC: Preclinical experience. *Theranostics* **2015**, *5*, 698–709. [CrossRef]
2. You, H.; Yoon, H.E.; Jeong, P.H.; Ko, H.; Yoon, J.H.; Kim, Y.C. Pheophorbide-a conjugates with cancer-targeting moieties for targeted photodynamic cancer therapy. *Bioorg. Med. Chem.* **2015**, *23*, 1453–1462. [CrossRef] [PubMed]
3. Hamblin, M.R.; Newman, E.L. Photosensitizer targeting in photodynamic therapy I. Conjugates of haematoporphyrin with albumin and transferrin. *J. Photochem. Photobiol. B Biol.* **1994**, *26*, 45–56. [CrossRef]
4. Hamblin, M.R.; Newman, E.L. Photosensitizer targeting in photodynamic therapy II. Conjugates of haematoporphyrin with serum lipoproteins. *J. Photochem. Photobiol. B Biol.* **1994**, *26*, 147–157. [CrossRef]
5. Park, S.Y.; Baik, H.J.; Oh, Y.T.; Oh, K.T.; Youn, Y.S.; Lee, E.S. A smart polysaccharide/drug conjugate for photodynamic therapy. *Angew. Chem. Int. Ed.* **2011**, *50*, 1644–1647. [CrossRef] [PubMed]
6. Koopaei, M.N.; Dinarvand, R.; Amini, M.; Rabbani, H.; Emami, S.; Ostad, S.N.; Atyabi, F. Docetaxel immunonanocarriers as targeted delivery systems for HER 2-positive tumor cells: preparation, characterization, and cytotoxicity studies. *Int. J. Nanomed.* **2011**, *6*, 1903–1912.
7. Zheng, Y.; Yu, B.; Weecharangsan, W.; Piao, L.; Darby, M.; Mao, Y.; Koynova, R.; Yang, X.; Li, H.; Xu, S.; et al. Transferrin-conjugated lipid-coated PLGA nanoparticles for targeted delivery of aromatase inhibitor 7alpha-APTADD to breast cancer cells. *Int. J. Pharm.* **2010**, *390*, 234–241. [CrossRef]
8. Calero, M.; Gutiérrez, L.; Salas, G.; Luengo, Y.; Lázaro, A.; Acedo, P.; Morales, M.P.; Miranda, R.; Villanueva, A. Efficient and safe internalization of magnetic iron oxide nanoparticles: Two fundamental requirements for biomedical applications. *Nanomed. Nanotechnol. Biol. Med.* **2014**, *10*, 733–743. [CrossRef]
9. Yang, Q.; Li, L.; Sun, W.; Zhou, Z.; Huang, Y. Dual stimuli-responsive hybrid polymeric nanoparticles self-assembled from POSS-Based starlike copolymer-drug conjugates for efficient intracellular delivery of hydrophobic drugs. *ACS Appl. Mater. Interfaces* **2016**, *8*, 13251–13261. [CrossRef] [PubMed]
10. Liu, X.; Wu, F.; Tian, Y.; Wu, M.; Zhou, Q.; Jiang, S.; Niu, Z. Size Dependent cellular uptake of Rod-like bionanoparticles with different aspect ratios. *Sci. Rep.* **2016**, *6*, 24567. [CrossRef] [PubMed]
11. Chatterjee, D.K.; Fong, L.S.; Zhang, Y. Nanoparticles in photodynamic therapy: An emerging paradigm. *Adv. Drug Deliv. Rev.* **2008**, *60*, 1627–1637. [CrossRef] [PubMed]
12. Chang, J.-Y.; Wang, S.; Allen, J.S.; Lee, S.H.; Chang, S.T.; Choi, Y.-K.; Friedrich, C.; Choi, C.K. A novel miniature dynamic microfluidic cell culture platform using electro-osmosis diode pumping. *Biomicrofluidics* **2014**, *8*, 044116.
13. Patiño, T.; Nogués, C.; Ibáñez, E.; Barrios, L. Enhancing microparticle internalization by nonphagocytic cells through the use of noncovalently conjugated polyethyleneimine. *Int. J. Nanomed.* **2012**, *7*, 5671.
14. Patiño, T.; Soriano, J.; Barrios, L.; Ibáñez, E.; Nogués, C. Surface modification of microparticles causes differential uptake responses in normal and tumoral human breast epithelial cells. *Sci. Rep.* **2015**, *5*, 11371. [CrossRef] [PubMed]
15. Zauner, W.; Farrow, N.A.; Haines, A.M. In vitro uptake of polystyrene microspheres: Effect of particle size, cell line and cell density. *J. Control. Release* **2001**, *71*, 39–51. [CrossRef]
16. Gratton, S.E.A.; Ropp, P.A.; Pohlhaus, P.D.; Luft, J.C.; Madden, V.J.; Napier, M.E.; DeSimone, J.M. The effect of particle design on cellular internalization pathways. *Proc. Natl. Acad. Sci. USA* **2008**, *105*, 11613–11618. [CrossRef]
17. Kutscher, H.L.; Chao, P.; Deshmukh, M.; Sundara Rajan, S.; Singh, Y.; Hu, P.; Joseph, L.B.; Stein, S.; Laskin, D.L.; Sinko, P.J. Enhanced passive pulmonary targeting and retention of PEGylated rigid microparticles in rats. *Int. J. Pharm.* **2010**, *402*, 64–71. [CrossRef]
18. Tros de Ilarduya, C.; Düzgüneş, N. Delivery of therapeutic nucleic acids via transferrin and transferrin receptors: Lipoplexes and other carriers. *Expert Opin. Drug Deliv.* **2013**, *10*, 1583–1591. [CrossRef]

19. Wong, P.T.; Choi, S.K. Mechanisms and implications of dual-acting methotrexate in folate-targeted nanotherapeutic delivery. *Int. J. Mol. Sci.* **2015**, *16*, 1772–1790. [CrossRef]
20. Stuchinskaya, T.; Moreno, M.; Cook, M.J.; Edwards, D.R.; Russell, D. A Targeted photodynamic therapy of breast cancer cells using antibody-phthalocyanine-gold nanoparticle conjugates. *Photochem. Photobiol. Sci.* **2011**, *10*, 822–831. [CrossRef]
21. Awada, G.; Gombos, A.; Aftimos, P.; Awada, A. Emerging drugs targeting human epidermal growth factor receptor 2 (Her2) in the treatment of breast cancer. *Expert Opin. Emerg. Drugs* **2016**, *21*, 91–101. [CrossRef] [PubMed]
22. Slamon, D.; Clark, G.; Wong, S.; Levin, W.; Ullrich, A.; McGuire, W. Human breast cancer: Correlation of relapse and survival with amplification of the HER-2/neu oncogene. *Science* **1987**, *235*, 177–182. [CrossRef] [PubMed]
23. Slamon, D.; Godolphin, W.; Jones, L.; Holt, J.; Wong, S.; Keith, D.; Levin, W.; Stuart, S.; Udove, J.; Ullrich, A.; et al. Studies of the HER-2/neu proto-oncogene in human breast and ovarian cancer. *Science* **1989**, *244*, 707–712. [CrossRef] [PubMed]
24. Lewis Phillips, G.D.; Li, G.; Dugger, D.L.; Crocker, L.M.; Parsons, K.L.; Mai, E.; Blättler, W.A.; Lambert, J.M.; Chari, R.V.J.; Lutz, R.J.; et al. Targeting HER2-positive breast cancer with trastuzumab-DM1, an antibody-cytotoxic drug conjugate. *Cancer Res.* **2008**, *68*, 9280–9290. [CrossRef] [PubMed]
25. Calibasi Kocal, G.; Güven, S.; Foygel, K.; Goldman, A.; Chen, P.; Sengupta, S.; Paulmurugan, R.; Baskin, Y.; Demirci, U. Dynamic Microenvironment induces phenotypic plasticity of esophageal cancer cells under flow. *Sci. Rep.* **2016**, *6*, 38221. [CrossRef] [PubMed]
26. Carvalho, R.M.; Maia, F.R.; Silva-Correia, J.; Costa, B.M.; Reis, R.L.; Oliveira, J.M. A semiautomated microfluidic platform for real-time investigation of nanoparticles' cellular uptake and cancer cells' tracking. *Nanomedicine* **2017**, *12*, 581. [CrossRef] [PubMed]
27. Damiati, S.; Kompella, U.B.; Damiati, S.A.; Kodzius, R. Microfluidic devices for drug delivery systems and drug screening. *Genes* **2018**, *9*, 103. [CrossRef] [PubMed]
28. Tobar, N.; Guerrero, J.; Smith, P.C.; Martínez, J. NOX4-dependent ROS production by stromal mammary cells modulates epithelial MCF-7 cell migration. *Br. J. Cancer* **2010**, *103*, 1040–1047. [CrossRef]
29. Arrigoni, C.; Bersini, S.; Gilardi, M.; Moretti, M. In vitro co-culture models of breast cancer metastatic progression towards bone. *Int. J. Mol. Sci.* **2016**, *17*, 1405. [CrossRef]
30. Gudjonsson, T.; Nielsen, H.L.; Rønnov-jessen, L.; Bissell, M.J.; Petersen, O.W. Isolation, immortalization and characterization of a human breast epithelial cell line with stem cell properties. *Genes Dev.* **2002**, 693–706. [CrossRef]
31. Sigurdsson, V.; Hilmarsdottir, B.; Sigmundsdottir, H.; Fridriksdottir, A.J.R.; Ringnér, M.; Villadsen, R.; Borg, A.; Agnarsson, B.A.; Petersen, O.W.; Magnusson, M.K.; et al. Endothelial induced EMT in breast epithelial cells with stem cell properties. *PLoS ONE* **2011**, *6*, e23833. [CrossRef]
32. Ingthorsson, S.; Andersen, K.; Hilmarsdottir, B.; Maelandsmo, G.M.; Magnusson, M.K.; Gudjonsson, T. HER2 induced EMT and tumorigenicity in breast epithelial progenitor cells is inhibited by coexpression of EGFR. *Oncogene* **2016**, *35*, 4244–4255. [CrossRef]
33. Chithrani, B.D.; Chan, W.C.W. Elucidating the mechanism of cellular uptake and removal of protein-coated gold nanoparticles of different sizes and shapes. *Nano Lett.* **2007**, *7*, 1542–1550. [CrossRef] [PubMed]
34. Dausend, J.; Musyanovych, A.; Dass, M.; Walther, P.; Schrezenmeier, H.; Landfester, K.; Mailänder, V. Uptake mechanism of oppositely charged fluorescent nanoparticles in HeLa Cells. *Macromol. Biosci.* **2008**, *8*, 1135–1143. [CrossRef] [PubMed]
35. Fröhlich, E. The role of surface charge in cellular uptake and cytotoxicity of medical nanoparticles. *Int. J. Nanomed.* **2012**, *7*, 5577. [CrossRef] [PubMed]
36. Farokhzad, O.C.; Khademhosseini, A.; Jon, S.; Hermmann, A.; Cheng, J.; Chin, C.; Kiselyuk, A.; Teply, B.; Eng, G.; Langer, R. Microfluidic System for studying the interaction of nanoparticles and microparticles with cells. *Anal. Chem.* **2005**, *77*, 5453–5459. [CrossRef]
37. Strobl, F.G.; Breyer, D.; Link, P.; Torrano, A.A.; Bräuchle, C.; Schneider, M.F.; Wixforth, A. A surface acoustic wave-driven micropump for particle uptake investigation under physiological conditions in very small volumes. *Beilstein J. Nanothechnol.* **2015**, *6*, 414–419. [CrossRef] [PubMed]

11

Quasi-Dynamic Dissolution of Electrospun Polymeric Nanofibers Loaded with Piroxicam

Urve Paaver [1,*], Jyrki Heinämäki [1], Ivan Kassamakov [2], Tuomo Ylitalo [2], Edward Hæggström [2], Ivo Laidmäe [1] and Karin Kogermann [1]

[1] Institute of Pharmacy, Faculty of Medicine, University of Tartu, Nooruse 1, 50411 Tartu, Estonia; jyrki.heinamaki@ut.ee (J.H.); ivo.laidmae@ut.ee (I.L.); karin.kogermann@ut.ee (K.K.)

[2] Electronics Laboratory, Department of Physics, P.O. Box 64 (Gustaf Hällströmin katu 2a), University of Helsinki, FI-00014 Helsinki, Finland; ivan.kassamakov@helsinki.fi (I.K.); tuomo.ylitalo@helsinki.fi (T.Y.); edward.haeggstrom@helsinki.fi (E.H.)

* Correspondence: urve.paaver@ut.ee

Abstract: We investigated and monitored in situ the wetting and dissolution properties of polymeric nanofibers and determined the solid-state of a drug during dissolution. Piroxicam (PRX) was used as a low-dose and poorly-soluble model drug, and hydroxypropyl methylcellulose (HPMC) and polydextrose (PD) were used as carrier polymers for electrospinning (ES). The initial-stage dissolution of the nanofibers was monitored in situ with three-dimensional white light microscopic interferometry (SWLI) and high-resolution optical microscopy. The physical solid-state characterization of nanofibers was performed with Raman spectroscopy, X-ray powder diffraction (XRPD), and scanning electron microscopy (SEM). We showed that PRX recrystallizes in a microcrystalline form immediately after wetting of nanofibers, which could lead to enhanced dissolution of drug. Initiation of crystal formation was detected by SWLI, indicating: (1) that PRX was partially released from the nanofibers, and (2) that the solid-state form of PRX changed from amorphous to crystalline. The amount, shape, and size of the PRX crystals depended on the carrier polymer used in the nanofibers and dissolution media (pH). In conclusion, the present nanofibers loaded with PRX exhibit a quasi-dynamic dissolution via recrystallization. SWLI enables a rapid, non-contacting, and non-destructive method for in situ monitoring the early-stage dissolution of nanofibers and regional mapping of crystalline changes (re-crystallization) during wetting. Such analysis is crucial because the wetting and dissolution of nanofibers can greatly influence the performance of nanofibrous drug delivery systems in pharmaceutical and biomedical applications.

Keywords: wetting; in situ drug release; nanofibers; electrospinning; poorly water-soluble drug; piroxicam; hydroxypropyl methyl cellulose; polydextrose; scanning white light interferometry

---

1. Introduction

In recent years, advanced polymeric nanofibrous drug delivery systems (DDSs) have been of increasing use in pharmaceutical and biomedical applications. Such systems include oral dispersible thin films, ophthalmic preparations, multifunctional wound dressings, and implanted DDSs [1–3]. These hybrid polymer nanofibers hold great promise with respect to drug therapy and tissue engineering in both human and veterinary medicine. Nanofibers have a unique capability to modify material properties, which could have a paramount effect on drug delivery performance. They possess fiber structure dimensions at the nanoscale and a large outer surface-to-volume ratio, enabling multiple alternatives in drug delivery. The conversion of polymer solutions to nanofibers by solution electrospinning (ES) is affected by material, process, and ambient parameters [3–5]. The geometric and physicochemical properties of nanofibers depend, for example, on the nature of the solution, polymer type, polymer chain conformation, viscosity, elasticity, and electrical conductivity, as well as on solvent polarity and surface tension [4,5]. These structural fiber properties in turn can have a great impact on the dissolution and drug release of fibers [6–11]. To date, however, our understanding on the dissolution (drug release) behavior of polymeric nanofibers and related physicochemical mechanisms is still limited. This is partially due to the fact that the nanofibers are challenging samples for analysis due to their nanoscale size and brittleness.

In the state-of-the art literature there are many examples of how the geometric nanofiber properties (size, size distribution, surface morphology, orientation) and porosity can greatly affect the dissolution (drug release) and therapeutic efficiency of nanofibrous DDSs [6,12–14]. With poorly water-soluble drugs, the limitations in drug release of the nanofibrous DDSs can delay the onset of drug action, cause poor oral bioavailability, and ultimately decrease therapeutic effect. The geometric nanofiber properties can be governed by the adjustment and control of the critical material, process, and environmental parameters in an ES process [5,15,16]. Lately, increasing interest has been focused on developing ES processes which could produce drug-loaded nanofibers of a specific quality and with reproducible drug release. Due to the nanoscale size, controlling the quality and performance of such nanofibers is still challenging. Consequently, the mechanisms of drug release associated with such novel polymeric nanofibrous DDSs remain poorly understood.

Scanning white light microscopic interferometry (SWLI) is a high-depth resolution imaging technique suitable for determining the geometric properties (i.e., fiber shape, diameter, and length), porosity, and surface topography of nanofibrous DDSs [17]. Three-dimensional (3D) SWLI permits rapid, non-contacting and non-destructive imaging of nanofibrous samples, since it requires neither sample preparation nor modification. Recently, we applied SWLI and high-resolution scanning electron microscopy (SEM) equipped with a customized measurement program for 3D surface topography analysis of non-woven nanofibrous mats [17]. In pharmaceutical research, the use of SWLI for investigating and non-contact imaging of the manufacturing processes and final products is still limited. Sandler et al. and Genina et al. used SWLI to image 3D printed multi-layered DDSs [18,19]. Hanhijärvi et al. applied SWLI to investigate the film surface properties of hydroxypropyl methylcellulose (HPMC)-coated tablets [20], while O'Bryan et al. used it to image 3D printed microgels intended for bioprinting applications [21]. Recently, Wickström et al. applied SWLI to characterize the surface texture and surface roughness of antibiotic-loaded fiber-reinforced composite implants [22].

The aim of the present study was to provide insight into the wetting and early-stage dissolution of drug loaded polymeric nanofibers. To gain an understanding of such phenomena, we monitored in situ the wetting and drug release of fibers loaded with a poorly water-soluble drug (piroxicam, PRX), and determined the solid-state of the drug during dissolution. Two hydrophilic polymers were investigated in nanofibers: hydroxypropyl methylcellulose (HPMC) intended for the sustained drug release and polydextrose (PD) intended for the immediate drug release of a poorly water-soluble drug [23,24]. We combined SWLI and high-resolution optical microscopy to image PRX-loaded nanofibers in contact with an aqueous medium, and the physical appearance and solid-state changes of nanofibers were verified with scanning electron microscopy (SEM), Raman spectroscopy, and X-ray diffraction (XRD), respectively. To our knowledge, this is the first time when such imaging and solid-state analyses are applied in a complimentary fashion to investigate the dissolution of polymeric nanofibers.

2. Materials and Methods

2.1. Materials

Commercially available cellulose ether, hydroxypropyl methylcellulose, HPMC (Methocel K100M premium CR, Colorcon Ltd., Dartford, Kent, UK), and polydextrose, PD (STA-LITE L90, 70% aqueous solution of PD, Tate & Lyle Netherlands B.V., Koog Aan De Zaan, KA, Netherlands) (Figure 1) were used as carrier polymers for the ES of nanofibers. The organic solvents were 1,1,1,3,3,3-hexa-fluoro-2-propanol (HFIP) (≥99.0%) (Sigma-Aldrich C.C., St. Louis, MO, USA) and methanol (Lach-Ner, s.r.o., Neratovice,

Czech Republic). Anhydrous piroxicam, (PRX, pure form I, PRXAH I, Letco Medical, Inc., N Livonia, MI, USA) was selected as a model drug for a low-dose poorly water-soluble active substance in nanofibers. In the wetting and dissolution experiments, purified water, hydrochloric acid buffer solution, USP 28 (pH 1.2), and phosphate buffer solution (pH 7.2) were used as dissolution media. The materials for the preparation of buffer solutions were of analytical grade and purchased from Lach-Ner, s.r.o., Neratovice, Czech Republic.

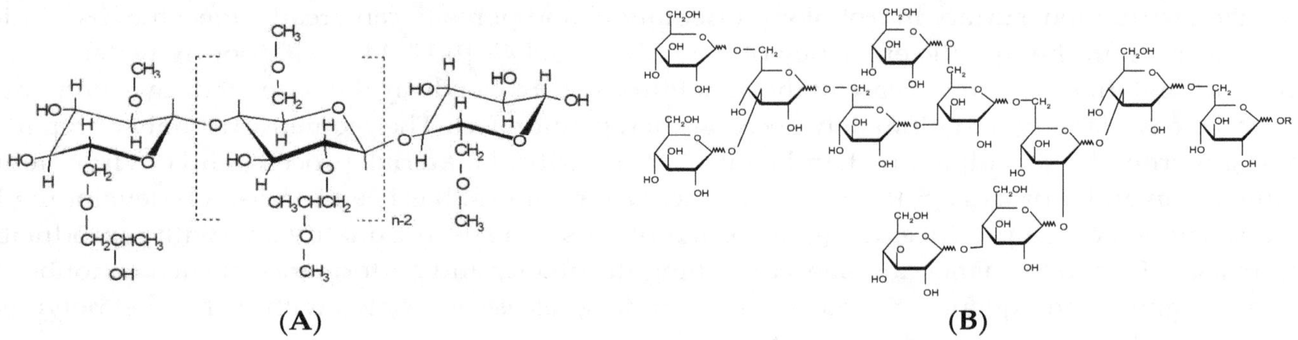

Figure 1. Structural formula of (**A**) hydroxypropyl methylcellulose (HPMC) and (**B**) polydextrose (PD).

2.2. *Preparation of Fiber Mats*

The carrier polymer (HPMC) and model drug (PRX) were first manually dry mixed with a mortar and pestle at three different ratios (1:1, 1:2, and 1:4). Next, the pre-mixtures were dissolved in organic solvent to obtain the 0.8% (w/V) solution of HPMC in HFIP as described in our previous study [16]. With PD, the aqueous solution of PD (70%) alone or the mixture of the aqueous solution of PD (70%) and methanol (5:1) were used for ES. The amount of PRX in the 70% aqueous solution of PD (0.75 mL) used for ES was 20 mg, and 0.75 mL contained 530 mg PD. The drug-loaded nanofibers were fabricated with an in-house ES set-up equipped with a syringe system, automatic syringe pump, spinneret, high-voltage power supply, and a grounded collector plate. The high-voltage power supply system was a Gamma (Gamma High Voltage Research, Model ES3OP-10W/DAM, Ormond Beach, FL, USA). For HPMC solutions, the ES distance and voltage between the spinneret and the collector plate were 8.0 cm and 7 kV, respectively. The pump rate of the automatic syringe pump (KdScientific, Model No: KDS-250-CE, Geneq Inc, Montreal, Quebec, Canada) was 1.0 mL/h. For PD solutions, the ES distance, voltage, and pump rate were 17 cm, 14 kV, and 2.0 mL/h, respectively. The prepared fibers were stored in desiccators (above silica gel, with relative humidity (RH) of 0%) at ambient room temperature (21 ± 2 °C) and in a refrigerator (6 ± 2 °C/RH 0%) prior to use.

2.3. *Physical Appearance and Solid-State Characterization*

The size and surface morphology of fibers were investigated with scanning electron microscopy, SEM (Helios NanoLab 600, FEI Company, Hillsboro, OR, USA). The samples were coated with a 3-nm gold layer in an argon atmosphere using a magnetron sputter prior to SEM imaging. Solid-state characterization of the starting materials and the electrospun fibers were carried out with X-ray diffraction, XRD (D8 Advance, Bruker AXS GmbH, Karlsruhe, Germany), and Raman spectroscopy (B&W Tek Inc., Newark, DE, USA). In XRD, Cu Kα1 radiation (λ= 1.5418 Å, 40 kV, and 40 mA) was used, and data were collected in the range of 5° and 35° 2θ with a step size of 0.2° 2θ. The brittleness of the fibrous mats was detected by visual inspection and manual palpation with tweezers.

2.4. *In Situ Wetting and Dissolution Tests of Fibers*

For in-situ wetting tests, we applied the fiber mats as such and the tablets compressed from these fibers. The initial-stage dissolution of the fiber mats were monitored by a high-resolution optical microscopy (Microscope Leica DMLB equipped with the Leica Germany 5.0× and L50×/0.50 objectives and Canon Power Shot 550 digital camera). A standardized drop (50 μL) of aqueous dissolution media was gently placed in contact with a fiber mat at room temperature (21 ± 2 °C), and the dissolution was monitored by taking micrographs at regular intervals.

Pieces of a fiber mat were manually compressed into small flat-faced tablets (discs) with a miniaturized press (Specac Ltd., Orpington BR5 3FQ, UK) intended for preparing sample discs for infrared (IR) spectroscopy analysis. The compression pressure was 196 MPa (2t/cm^2) and the compression time was 5 s. The tablets (discs) were 12.7 mm in diameter and 0.8–1.0 mm in thickness. For in situ initial-stage dissolution experiments, one micro-pipette drop of purified water (2 μL) was gently placed onto the surface of fibrous tablets at room temperature (21 ± 2 °C). The contact point of the drop onto the tablet surface was kept as constant as possible.

The wetting and early-stage dissolution of fibrous tablets were monitored in situ with an in-house 3D scanning white light microscopic interferometry (SWLI). In SWLI, a light beam passes through an interferometric objective (Nikon, Michelson type, magnification 120×) containing a beam splitter that reflects half the incident beam onto a reference surface and passes the other half onto the test surface (Figure 2). Light reflected from the test and reference surfaces recombines and interferes to form an interferogram. The working principle and structure of SWLI is described elsewhere. For details see Kassamakov et al. [25,26], Hanhijärvi et al. [20], and Paaver et al. [17]. In the present study, we obtained three-dimensional (3D) images featuring 29 nm × 29 nm active pixel size from a 55 × 40 μm^2 area. The time period of 10 min prior to a subsequent drop was required for the complete SWLI analysis of the tablets. Purified water (pH 5.6) and the USP 28 buffer solutions (hydrochloric acid buffer pH 1.2 and phosphate buffer solution pH 7.2) were used as dissolution media. The total number of optical microscopy and SWLI images taken on the course of the in situ dissolution experiments was over 500 (including short video-clips). The number of samples was 3–6 in each analysis.

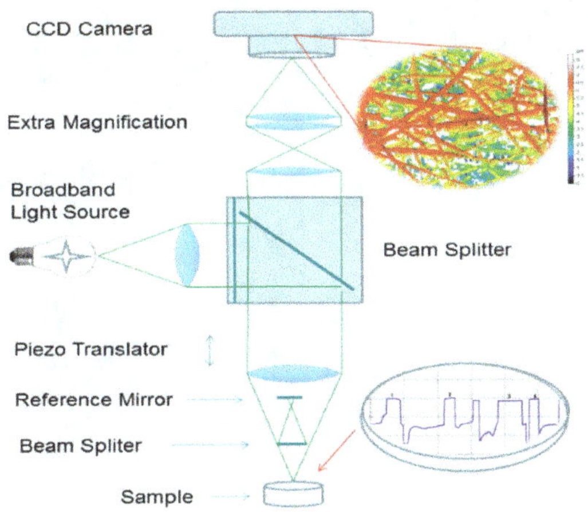

Figure 2. Schematic diagram of scanning white light interferometer (SWLI) and the experimental setup for the in situ wetting and early-stage dissolution of nanofibers.

A high-resolution scanning electron microscope (SEM) (Helios NanoLab 600, FEI Company, Hillsboro, OR, USA) was used as a reference method to the SWLI. A software-based measurement function xT Microscope Control (FEI) was used to measure the horizontal dimensions of the nanofibers. Samples were mounted on aluminum stubs with silver paint and were magnetron-sputter coated with a 3-nm gold layer in an argon atmosphere prior to microscopy. ImageJ (vers. 1.50i) was used for fiber size distribution analysis.

2.5. Dissolution Test

The in vitro dissolution tests of the electrospun nanofiber mats and the pure PRX powder samples were performed using an USP dissolution apparatus I (basket method) in a semi-automated dissolution system (Termostat-Sotax AT7, Sotax AG, Aesch, Switzerland). The concentration of PRX in the dissolution medium was measured at 354 nm by using a UV-VIS spectrophotometer (Ultrospec III, Biochrom Ltd, Cambourne, Cambridge, UK). The dissolution medium was 900 mL of purified water (pH 5.6) and buffer solution (pH 1.2 or pH 7.2) maintained at 37 ± 0.5 °C as described in the USP 28. The basket rotation speed was 50 rpm. The amount of PRX in the powder and nanofiber samples used in the dissolution test was 20 mg. Six parallel tests were performed for each sample.

3. Results and Discussion

3.1. Physical Appearance of Nanofibers

The ES of PRX-loaded fibers with both HPMC and PD polymers resulted in yellowish and white thin fiber mats with a porous internal structure, respectively (Figure 3). HPMC generated fibrous mats with a nanoscale fiber diameter ranging from 100 nm to 400 nm and uniform fiber thickness (Figure 3A,B,E). With PD, we found that due to the hygroscopic nature of PD, the ES of PRX-loaded fibers was possible only in precisely controlled and optimized temperature and humidity conditions (below 30 °C and 40% RH). The PD fiber mat consisted of individual short fibers reaching micron size and a large spread in diameters (Figure 3C,D,F). The diameter of these fibers ranged from 400 nm to 5 µm, and the corresponding fiber mats were brittle (based on palpation with tweezers). A number of spherical beads were observed (SEM) in the electrospun PD fiber mats (Figure 3C). This was due to the high surface tension and low viscosity of the solution. The fiber mats prepared from the mixtures of an aqueous PD solution and methanol, were smaller in diameter, more uniform in radial size, and less brittle (based on visual inspection and palpation with tweezers). The thickness of an entire PD fiber mat ranged from few microns to several tens microns (SWLI).

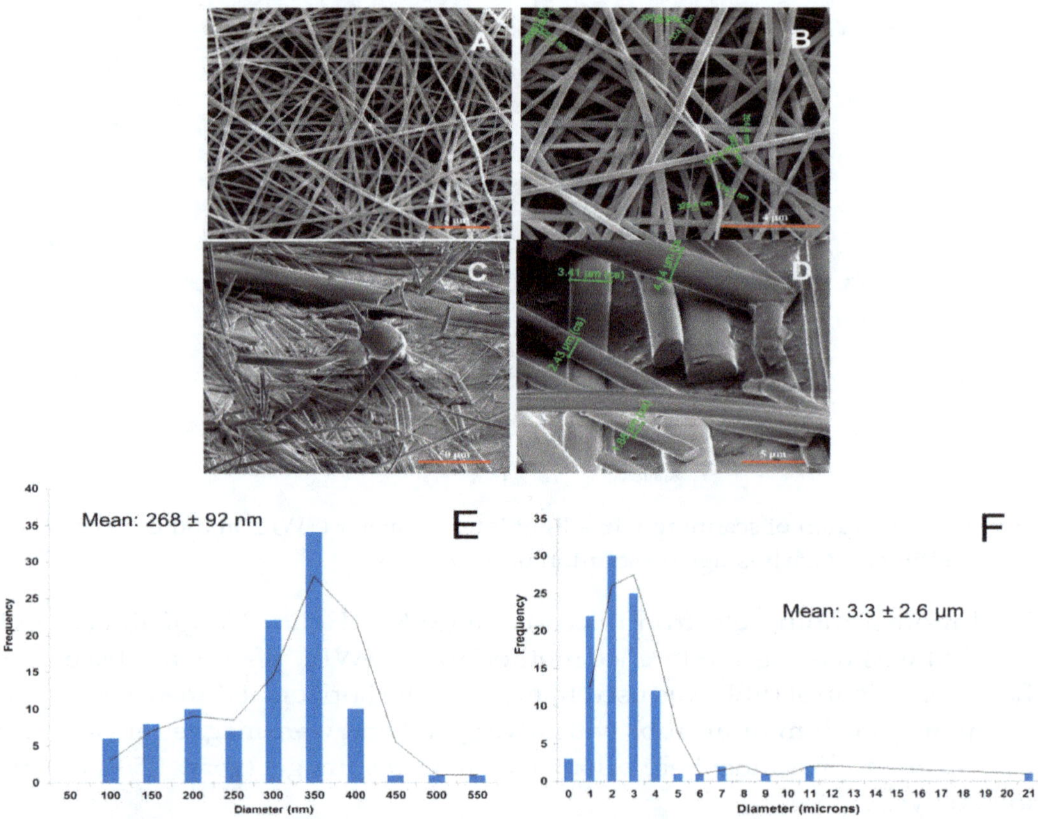

Figure 3. SEM images of piroxicam (PRX)-loaded hydroxypropyl methylcellulose (HPMC) (**A**,**B**) nanofibers and polydextrose (PD) (**C**,**D**) fibers. Magnification of SEM: 5000× (**A**), 10000× (**B**), 600× (**C**), and 5000× (**D**). (**E**) Fiber size distribution of the PRX-loaded HPMC nanofibers; (**F**) Fiber size distribution of the PRX-loaded PD fibers.

3.2. Physical Solid-State Properties of Nanofibers

Recently, we reported that the electrospun HPMC nanofibers loaded with PRX are amorphous, and they remain as an amorphous form during a short storage period [16]. In the present study, we found that the ES of PD fibers loaded with PRX did not generate the corresponding amorphous structure, or the produced PRX amorphous structure was very unstable and immediately recrystallized as also discussed previously [27]. The solid-state properties of the electrospun PD fibers loaded with PRX were investigated immediately after the preparation and after a 1-month short-term storage at 0% RH and low temperature (6 °C). As seen in Figure 4 (I), the XRD patterns of electrospun fiber mats showed an amorphous halo together with the characteristic crystalline reflections of PRX anhydrate form I (PRXAH I) immediately after preparation. The XRD and Raman spectroscopy results (Figure 4 (II)) confirmed that PRX (PRXAH I) had lost some of its crystallinity during ES, but did not stay amorphous. No other crystalline reflections (XRD) or spectral features (Raman) characteristic to the known anhydrous PRX solid-state forms were observed in XRD diffractograms or Raman spectra.

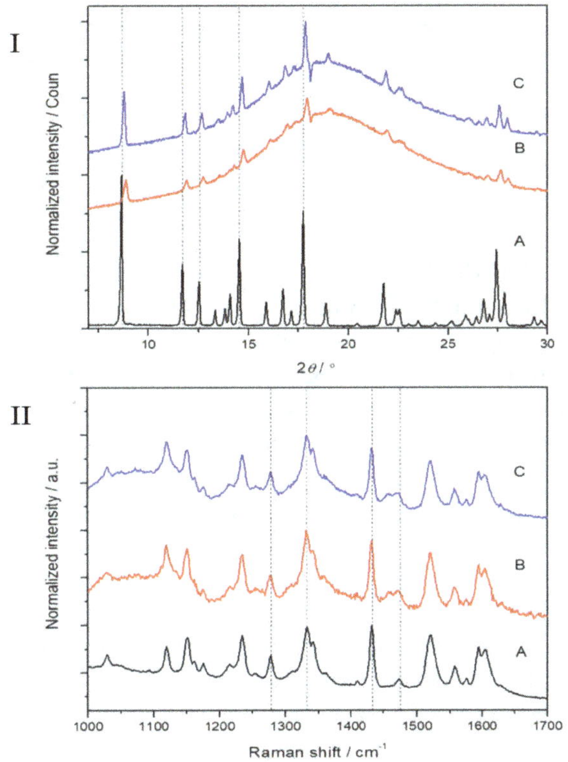

Figure 4. XRD patterns (**I**) and Raman spectra (**II**) of piroxicam (PRX)-loaded polydextrose (PD) fibers. Key: (**A**) PRX anhydrate form I (PRXAH I); (**B**) Fibers immediately after preparation; (**C**) Fibers stored for 30 days at 0% room humidity (RH) and low temperature (6 °C).

3.3. In Situ Wetting and Initial Dissolution of Fibers

Figures 5 and 6 show the high-resolution optical microscopy and SWLI results on the initial stages of the release and dissolution of PRX from the HPMC and PD fiber mats. Since PRX was completely dissolved in the HPMC solution, it is evident that the drug is homogeneously dispersed within nanofibers after ES, and hence the release would be uniform from fiber mats. Figure 5A shows a time-lapse-like snapshot from a high-resolution optical microscope of what happens to the PRX-loaded HPMC nanofiber mats during wetting and initial-stage dissolution. As shown in Figure 5A, the polymeric HPMC-PRX nanofibers dissolved within 1–5 s in the aqueous dissolution media used. According to the literature, PRX exists in an amorphous form in electrospun HPMC nanofibers [16,17,28,29], and the amorphous state of PRX hastened the onset of wetting and premature drug release. In our study, in situ wetting and dissolution monitoring indicated that PRX recrystallizes in a microcrystalline form immediately after wetting and release from the HPMC nanofibers. The PRX microcrystals ranging from 0.2 μm to 12 μm in size were formed after the addition of a standardized drop (50 μL) of purified water, hydrochloric acid (pH 1.2) or phosphate buffer (pH 7.2) solutions onto the HPMC nanofiber mats (Figure 5A,C). The recrystallization of PRX was associated with the formation of larger clusters of microcrystals.

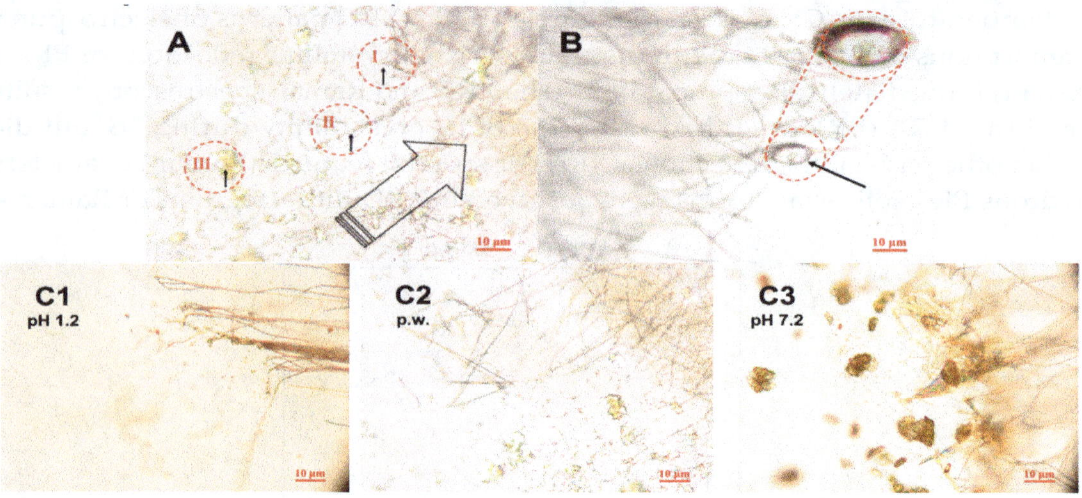

Figure 5. (**A**) Three phases identified in the release and crystallization of piroxicam (PRX) from hydroxylpropyl methylcellulose (HPMC) nanofibers. High-resolution light microscopy image (magnification 50×) validates the results obtained with SWLI (shown in Figure 6): **I**. PRX embedded in the nanofibers. **II**. Crystallization inside or on the nanofibers. **III**. Recrystallization of PRX. The large arrow indicates the propagation direction of the water front. Magnification 50×. (**B**) Representative micrograph on the initial dissolution of PRX–loaded polydextrose (PD) fibers. Visible crystals of PRX evident (highlighted with a black arrow) inside a red circle. Magnification 50×. (**C**) The PRX crystals visible at 30 s after wetting of nanofibers (HPMC:PRX 1:4) by placing a small drop of different dissolution media onto the surface of the fibrous sample: (**C1**) hydrochloric acid buffer solution pH 1.2; (**C2**) purified water, p.w. (pH 5.6); (**C3**) phosphate buffer solution pH 7.2 (22 ± 2 °C). Magnification 50×.

The overall initial-stage dissolution behavior of freely water-soluble PD fibers loaded with PRX was similar, but faster than that observed with the corresponding HPMC nanofibers. As seen in Figure 5B, individual PRX crystals entrapped inside the PD fibers, and the release and dissolution of PRX from the PD fibers progressed via crystal formation. The rapid dissolution of a carrier polymer (PD) fostered the dissolution of PRX. The number and size of the PRX crystals differed from those observed with HPMC nanofibers. With PD, the number of crystals detected was smaller and the size of the crystals slightly larger (ranging from 0.3 μm to 15 μm) than with the HPMC nanofibers. The PRX crystals were located (clustered) inside the PD fibers (Figure 5B), which evidently could advance the dissolution of PRX since PD is a freely water-soluble carrier material. Consequently, this is an interesting approach to use freely water-soluble carrier polymer in electrospun fibers for the improvement of drug dissolution rate. The dissolution behavior of both types of drug-loaded fibers was verified with an established in vitro dissolution test (USP), and the results are shown in the next section (Figures 7–9).

Figure 5C illustrates the status of the HPMC:PRX (1:4) nanofibers at 30 s after wetting the surface of a thin nanofibers sample layer by a small drop (2 μL) of different dissolution media (hydrochloric acid buffer solution at pH 1.2, purified water, or phosphate buffer solution at pH 7.2). The number, shape, and size of the PRX crystals depended on the pH of the dissolution media used. With all dissolution media, the dissolution of nanofibers occurred via immediate crystal formation of PRX (i.e., recrystallization to microcrystals). Rapid changes in the solubility of PRX were also observed with a high-resolution optical microscope. The largest PRX microcrystals and clusters (ranging from few micrometers up to 10 μm) were present with phosphate buffer solution at pH 7.2 (Figure 5C3) and the smallest (0.2–1 μm in size) with hydrochloric acid buffer solution at pH 1.2 (Figure 5C1). It is evident that the recrystallization of PRX associated with the dissolution of HPMC nanofibers is dependent on both the pH and viscosity of dissolution media (in the microenvironment of dissolving nanofibers). Based on our findings, the lower pH of the dissolution media (pH 1.2) induces PRX to recrystallize into small 0.2–1 μm microcrystals in the vicinity of dissolving HPMC nanofibers. In addition, the subsequent formation of microcrystalline clusters occurred slower than that observed with the corresponding nanofibers in the higher pH of dissolution media (pH 7.2). The release of drug from nanofiber mat is shown to be also dependent on the mat thickness [30]. In the present study, the thickness of the HPMC fiber mat was in the range of 2–3 μm (measured by SEM and SWLI).

The SWLI images on the surface of the tablets compressed from the drug-loaded HPMC nanofibers are presented in Figure 6. Figure 6A shows a SWLI image of a tablet surface, where individual fibers are visible: A(I) initial state of tablet (magnification 30×) and A(II) after wetting with 2 μL of water and evaporating for 1 min. In the initial stage, the tablet surface is flat and there is no crystal formation visible. This indicates that PRX is located in nanofibers and most likely is still amorphous. Point A(II) is the first wetting point after adding 2 μL of water and evaporating for 1 min. Figure 6B illustrates the surface of the same tablet after wetting with another 2 μL of water and evaporating for 10 min. Initiation of crystal formation is visible indicating that PRX is partially released from the nanofibers (as seen in Figure 6B). This indicates also that the solid-state form of PRX has changed from amorphous to crystalline form. In contact with water, PRX anhydrate form I transfers to PRX monohydrate before dissolving [27]. It is obvious that PRX monohydrate crystals are visible in SWLI images (Figure 6B,C). Figure 6C shows that the surface of the same tablet after the identical wetting procedure applied to the same spot for a third time. The release of PRX and crystallization occur rapidly, and most likely the crystals of PRX monohydrate are instantly formed in the vicinity of nanofibers. This in turn leads to the retarded quasi-dynamic dissolution of PRX. The present finding is in good agreement with our previous study describing the dissolution behavior of PRX anhydrate and monohydrate forms [31].

In summary, the three phases of the initial-stage dissolution of PRX-loaded HPMC nanofibers were observed with the present compressed tablets and with the corresponding free nanofiber mats studied by SWLI and high-resolution optical microscopy, respectively. These phases are as follows (as shown in Figures 5 and 6): (A) PRX is embedded in the nanofibers (in an amorphous state confirmed by our earlier study [16]), and all nanofibers are intact prior to the water front moving into them; (B) Crystallization of PRX starts inside the nanofibers; (C) Recrystallization of PRX is finalized after drug release from nanofibers.

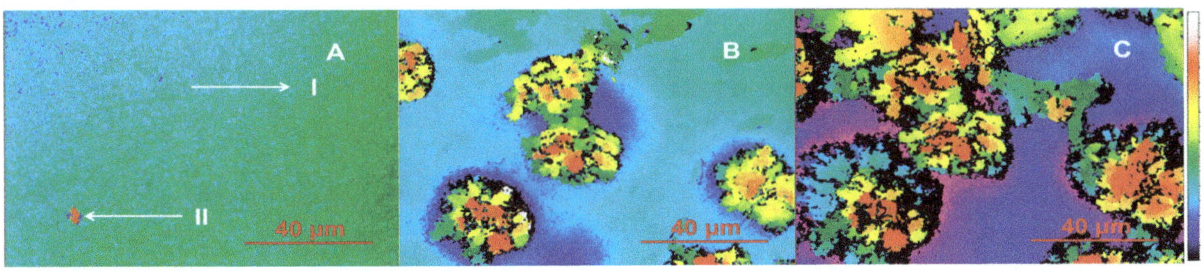

Figure 6. Time-lapse of wetting induced piroxicam (PRX) crystallization on the fixed surface of the tablet consisting of PRX-loaded hydroxypropyl methylcellulose (HPMC) nanofibers. The PRX release is visualized by scanning white light interferometry (SWLI). Key: (**A-I**) Initial state of the tablet; (**A-II**) After wetting with 2 μL of water and evaporating for 1 min; (**B**) After wetting a second time with 2 μL of water and evaporating for 10 min; (**C**) After wetting a third time with 2 μL water and evaporating for 10 min. The scale for height differences is changed according to changes in surface altitude (A—0 to 8 μm; C—0 to 90 μm). The diameter and thickness of tablet (disc) are 12.7 mm and 0.8–1.0 mm, respectively. Magnification 30×.

3.4. Dissolution of Fibers

Figures 7–9 show the early-phase dissolution curves for the PRX anhydrate form I (PRXAH I) in a powder form, the PRX-loaded HPMC nanofibers, and PRX-loaded PD fibers. PRXAH I in a powder form exhibited clearly a longer lag-time in the early-phase dissolution than that observed with the drug-loaded HPMC or PD fiber mats. The early-phase dissolution of PRX anhydrous form I powder was also dependent on the dissolution media used (the amount of PRX dissolved in purified water within the first 15 min was only less than 3%). The present results are also supported by the results on the dissolution behavior of PRX obtained in our previous study [31].

As shown in Figures 7 and 8, the HPMC nanofibers accelerated the immediate dissolution of PRX compared to that obtained with pure PRX anhydrous form I in a powder form. With the drug-loaded HPMC nanofibers, the early-phase dissolution of PRX was fast within the first 3 min followed by a sustained-release phase (Figures 7 and 8). This accelerated dissolution is obviously due to an immediate release of amorphous PRX from the surface of nanofibers and formation of PRX microcrystals in the vicinity of nanofibers (as shown in Figure 5A). The initial drug release from the HPMC nanofibers depended on the dissolution medium, and this finding was in line with the optical microscopy images on the dissolution of HPMC nanofiber mats shown in Figure 5C. The subsequent sustained dissolution phase of PRX observed with the HPMC nanofibers (Figures 7 and 8) is most likely partially due to the gel formation of HPMC as the nanofibers are dissolved, thus forming a hydrophilic gel barrier for the release of drug.

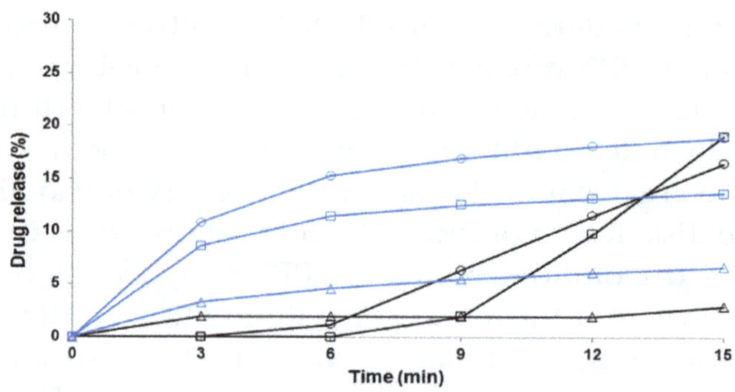

Figure 7. Early-phase dissolution of piroxicam (PRX)-loaded hydroxypropyl methylcellulose (HPMC) nanofibers freely set into the dissolution baskets ($n = 6$). The ratio of a carrier polymer (HPMC) and PRX is 1:1 in the nanofibers. Key: black curve—PRX anhydrate form I (PRXAH I) in a powder form; blue curve—HPMC:PRX nanofibers 1:1; Δ—purified water; ○—pH 7.2; □—pH 1.2. Standard deviation (SD) in each time point is less than 0.5%.

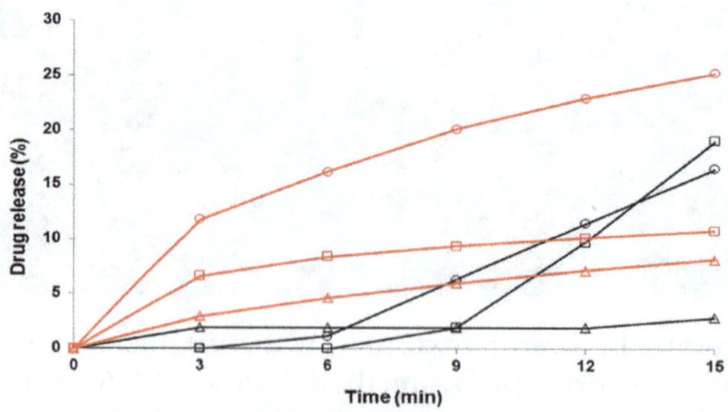

Figure 8. Early-phase dissolution of piroxicam (PRX)-loaded hydroxypropyl methylcellulose (HPMC) nanofibers freely set into the dissolution baskets ($n = 6$). The ratio of a carrier polymer (HPMC) and PRX is 1:4 in the nanofibers. Key: black curve—PRX anhydrate form I (PRXAH I) in a powder form; red curve—HPMC: PRX nanofibers 1:4; Δ—purified water; ○—pH 7.2; □—pH 1.2. Standard deviation (SD) in each time point is less than 0.5%.

With the drug-loaded PD fibers, the initial-stage dissolution of PRX within the first 3 min was somewhat slower than that obtained with the PRX-loaded HPMC nanofibers (Figure 9). This is obviously due to the crystalline state PRX in the PD fibers, thus resulting in a short delay in the onset of dissolution. In spite of a 3-min lag-time, over 70% of PRX was dissolved within 15 min in acidic dissolution medium (pH 1.2) when formulated as PD fibers. The use of methanol as a co-solvent for ES slightly improved the dissolution of PRX from the PD fibers compared to the corresponding fibers electrospun with pure aqueous solution of PD (i.e., without any organic solvent component) (Figure 9).

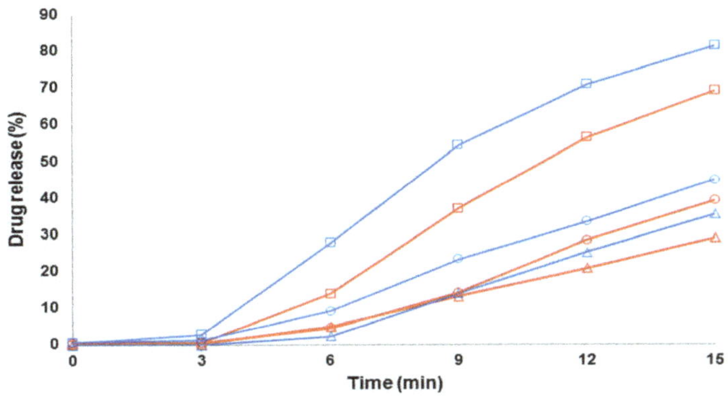

Figure 9. Early-phase dissolution of piroxicam (PRX)-loaded polydextrose (PD) fibers freely set into the dissolution baskets ($n = 6$). Key: red curve—the fibers containing PRX anhydrate form I (PRX AH I) and PD (electrospun from water solution); blue curve—the fibers containing PRXAH I and PD (electrospun from a water-in-methanol 5:1 solution); Δ—purified water; ○—pH 7.2; □—pH 1.2. Standard deviation (SD) in each time point is less than 1.4%.

4. Conclusions

A solution electrospinning (ES) can be used to prepare composite hydroxypropyl methyl cellulose (HPMC) and polydextrose (PD) nanofibers loaded with piroxicam (PRX). The wetting and early-phase dissolution of PRX from these fiber mats are accelerated compared to PRX anhydrate form I in a powder form. With PRX-loaded HPMC nanofiber mats, the dissolution of drug progressed via immediate wetting of the polymeric matrix followed by a lucid recrystallization and dissolution of the drug. A poorly water-soluble PRX recrystallizes in a microcrystalline form after wetting of nanofiber mats, and the further dissolution of PRX is dependent on the pH of the dissolution media. The accelerated dissolution of PRX from freely water-soluble PD nanofibers occurs also via immediate microcrystals formation after wetting. We propose that the present electrospun nanofibers mats loaded with PRX exhibit a quasi-dynamic dissolution behavior. SWLI provides rapid non-contacting and non-destructive in situ monitoring of early-stage dissolution of nanofibers and regional mapping of crystalline changes (re-crystallization) during wetting.

Author Contributions: Conceptualization, U.P., J.H., I.K., T.Y., K.K., and E.H.; methodology, U.P., I.K., T.Y., K.K., and I.L.; investigation, U.P., I.K., and T.Y.; resources, J.H., K.K., and E.H.; writing—original draft preparation, U.P. and J.H.; writing—review and editing, U.P., J.H., I.K., I.L., E.H., and K.K.; visualization, U.P., I.K., and T.Y.; supervision, J.H., I.K., and E.H.; project administration, J.H., E.H., and K.K.; funding acquisition, J.H., E.H., and K.K.

Acknowledgments: J. Aruväli is kindly acknowledged for performing XRPD analyses, J. Kozlova for taking SEM images, and Helder A. Santos for consulting in optical microscopy experiments.

References

1. Rošic, R.; Kocbek, P.; Pelipenko, J.; Kristl, J.; Baumgartner, S. Nanofibers and their biomedical use. *Acta Pharm.* **2013**, *63*, 295–304. [CrossRef] [PubMed]
2. Schiffman, J.D.; Schauer, C.L. A Review: Electrospinning of biopolymer nanofibers and their applications. *Polym. Rev.* **2008**, *48*, 317–352. [CrossRef]
3. Bhardwaj, N.; Kundu, S.C. Electrospinning: A fascinating fiber fabrication technique. *Biotechnol. Adv.* **2010**, *28*, 325–347. [CrossRef] [PubMed]
4. Rošic, R.; Pelipenko, J.; Kocbek, P.; Baumgartner, S.; Bešter-Rogač, M.; Kristl, J. The role of rheology of polymer solutions in predicting nanofiber formation by electrospinning. *Eur. Polym. J.* **2012**, *48*, 1374–1384. [CrossRef]
5. Pelipenko, J.; Kocbek, P.; Kristl, J. Critical attributes of nanofibers: Preparation, drug loading, and tissue regeneration. *Int. J. Pharm.* **2015**, *484*, 57–74. [CrossRef] [PubMed]
6. Sebe, I.; Szabo, P.; Kallai-Szabo, B.; Zelko, R. Incorporating small molecules or biologics into nanofibers for optimized drug release: A review. *Int. J. Pharm.* **2015**, *494*, 516–530. [CrossRef]
7. Torres-Martinez, E.J.; Cornejo Bravo, J.M.; Serrano Medina, A.; Pérez González, G.L.; Villarreal Gómez, L.J. A Summary of Electrospun Nanofibers as Drug Delivery System: Drugs Loaded and Biopolymers Used as Matrices. *Curr. Drug Deliv.* **2018**, *15*, 1360–1374. [CrossRef]
8. Patra, J.K.; Das, G.; Fraceto, L.F.; Campos, E.V.R.; Rodriguez-Torres, M.D.P.; Acosta-Torres, L.S.; Diaz-Torres, L.A.; Grillo, R.; Swamy, M.K.; Sharma, S.; et al. Nano based drug delivery systems: Recent developments and future prospects. *J. Nanobiotechnol.* **2018**, *16*, 71. [CrossRef]
9. Thakkar, S.; Misra, M. Electrospun polymeric nanofibers: New horizons in drug delivery. *Eur. J. Pharm. Sci.* **2017**, *107*, 148–167. [CrossRef]
10. Haider, A.; Haider, S.; Kang, I.K. A comprehensive review summarizing the effect of electrospinning parameters and potential applications of nanofibers in biomedical and biotechnology. *Arab. J. Chem.* **2018**, *11*, 1165–1188. [CrossRef]
11. Lim, C.T. Nanofiber technology: Current status and emerging developments. *Prog. Polym. Sci.* **2017**, *70*, 1–17.
12. Wang, J.; Windbergs, M. Functional electrospun fibers for the treatment of human skin wounds. *Eur. J. Pharm. Biopharm.* **2017**, *119*, 283–299. [CrossRef]
13. Xue, J.; Wu, T.; Dai, Y.; Xia, Y. Electrospinning and Electrospun Nanofibers: Methods, Materials, and Applications. *Chem. Rev.* **2019**, *119*, 5298–5415. [CrossRef]
14. Hu, X.; Liu, S.; Zhou, G.; Huang, Y.; Xie, Z.; Jing, X. Electrospinning of polymeric nanofibers for drug delivery applications. *J. Control. Release* **2014**, *185*, 12–21. [CrossRef]
15. Wang, J.; Hu, X.; Xiang, D. Nanoparticle drug delivery systems: An excellent carrier for tumor peptide vaccines. *Drug Deliv.* **2018**, *25*, 1319–1327. [CrossRef]
16. Paaver, U.; Heinämäki, J.; Laidmäe, I.; Lust, A.; Kozlova, J.; Sillaste, E.; Kirsimäe, K.; Veski, P.; Kogermann, K. Electrospun nanofibers as a potential controlled-release solid dispersion system for poorly water-soluble drugs. *Int. J. Pharm.* **2015**, *479*, 252–260. [CrossRef]
17. Paaver, U.; Heinämäki, J.; Kassamakov, I.; Haeggstrom, E.; Ylitalo, T.; Nolvi, A.; Kozlova, J.; Laidmäe, I.; Kogermann, K.; Veski, P. Nanometer depth resolution in 3D topographic analysis of drug-loaded nanofibrous mats without sample preparation. *Int. J. Pharm.* **2014**, *462*, 29–37. [CrossRef]
18. Sandler, N.; Kassamakov, I.; Ehlers, H.; Genina, N.; Ylitalo, T.; Haeggstrom, E. Rapid interferometric imaging of printed drug laden multilayer structures. *Sci. Rep.* **2014**, *4*, 4020. [CrossRef]
19. Genina, N.; Fors, D.; Vakili, H.; Ihalainen, P.; Pohjala, L.; Ehlers, H.; Kassamakov, I.; Haeggstrom, E.; Vuorela, P.; Peltonen, J.; et al. Tailoring controlled-release oral dosage forms by combining inkjet and flexographic printing techniques. *Eur. J. Pharm. Sci.* **2012**, *47*, 615–623. [CrossRef]
20. Hanhijärvi, K.; Majava, T.; Kassamakov, I.; Heinämäki, J.; Aaltonen, J.; Haapalainen, J.; Haeggström, E.; Yliruusi, J. Scratch resistance of plasticized hydroxypropyl methylcellulose (HPMC) films intended for tablet coatings. *Eur. J. Pharm. Biopharm.* **2010**, *74*, 371–376. [CrossRef]
21. O'Bryan, C.S.; Bhattacharjee, T.; Hart, S.; Kabb, C.P.; Schulze, K.D.; Chilakala, I.; Sumerlin, B.S.; Sawyer, W.G.; Angelini, T.E. Self-assembled micro-organogels for 3D printing silicone structures. *Sci. Adv.* **2017**, *3*, e1602800. [CrossRef]

22. Wickström, H.; Hilgert, E.; Nyman, O.J.; Desai, D.; Şen Karaman, D.; De Beer, T.; Sandler, N.; Rosenholm, M.J. Inkjet Printing of Drug-Loaded Mesoporous Silica Nanoparticles—A Platform for Drug Development. *Molecules* **2017**, *22*, 2020. [CrossRef]
23. Florek, C.A.; Kohn, J.B.; Michniak-Kohn, B.B.; Thakur, R.A. Electrospun Matrices for Delivery of Hydrophilic and Lidophilic Compounds. Available online: https://patentsgooglecom/patent/EP2079416A2/en (accessed on 9 August 2019).
24. Baier, S.; Given, P.; Kanjanapongkul, K.; Weiss, J. Formation of Conjugated Protein by Electrospinning. Available online: https://patentsgooglecom/patent/WO2013151694A1/de (accessed on 9 August 2019).
25. Kassamakov, I.V.; Seppänen, H.O.; Oinonen, M.J.; Hæggström, E.O.; Österberg, J.M.; Aaltonen, J.P.; Saarikko, H.; Radivojevic, Z.P. Scanning white light interferometry in quality control of single-point tape automated bonding. *Microelectron. Eng.* **2007**, *84*, 114–123. [CrossRef]
26. Kassamakov, I.; Hanhijärvi, K.; Abbadi, I.; Aaltonen, J.; Ludvigsen, H.; Haeggström, E. Scanning white-light interferometry with a supercontinuum source. *Opt. Lett.* **2009**, *34*, 1582–1584. [CrossRef]
27. Kogermann, K.; Veski, P.; Rantanen, J.; Naelapää, K. X-ray powder diffractometry in combination with principal component analysis—A tool for monitoring solid state changes. *Eur. J. Pharm. Sci.* **2011**, *43*, 278–289. [CrossRef]
28. Brewster, M.E.; Verreck, G.; Chun, I.; Rosenblatt, J.; Mensch, J.; Van Dijck, A.; Noppe, M.; Ariën, A.; Bruining, M.; Peeters, J. The use of polymer-based electrospun nanofibers containing amorphous drug dispersions for the delivery of poorly water-soluble pharmaceuticals. *Pharmazie* **2004**, *59*, 387–391.
29. Verreck, G.; Chun, I.; Rosenblatt, J.; Peeters, J.; Dijck, A.V.; Mensch, J.; Noppe, M.; Brewster, M.E. Incorporation of drugs in an amorphous state into electrospun nanofibers composed of a water-insoluble, nonbiodegradable polymer. *J. Control. Release* **2003**, *92*, 349–360. [CrossRef]
30. Zupančič, Š.; Preem, L.; Kristl, J.; Putrinš, M.; Tenson, T.; Kocbek, P.; Kogermann, K. Impact of PCL nanofiber mat structural properties on hydrophilic drug release and antibacterial activity on periodontal pathogens. *Eur. J. Pharm. Sci.* **2018**, *122*, 347–358. [CrossRef]
31. Paaver, U.; Lust, A.; Mirza, S.; Rantanen, J.; Veski, P.; Heinamaki, J.; Kogermann, K. Insight into the solubility and dissolution behavior of piroxicam anhydrate and monohydrate forms. *Int. J. Pharm.* **2012**, *431*, 111–119. [CrossRef]

Evaluation of Electrospun Poly(ε-Caprolactone)/Gelatin Nanofiber Mats Containing Clove Essential Oil for Antibacterial Wound Dressing

Irem Unalan [1], Stefan J. Endlein [1], Benedikt Slavik [2], Andrea Buettner [2], Wolfgang H. Goldmann [3], Rainer Detsch [1] and Aldo R. Boccaccini [1,*]

1 Institute of Biomaterials, Department of Materials Science and Engineering, Friedrich-Alexander-University Erlangen-Nuremberg, Cauerstraße 6, 91058 Erlangen, Germany; irem.unalan@fau.de (I.U.); stefan.endlein@fau.de (S.J.E.); Rainer.Detsch@fau.de (R.D.)

2 Chair of Aroma and Smell Research, Department of Chemistry and Pharmacy, Friedrich-Alexander-University Erlangen-Nuremberg, Henkestraße 9, 91054 Erlangen, Germany; benedikt.slavik@fau.de (B.S.); andrea.buettner@fau.de (A.B.)

3 Institute of Biophysics, Department of Physics, Friedrich-Alexander-University Erlangen-Nuremberg, Henkestraße 91, 91052 Erlangen, Germany; wgoldmannh@aol.com

* Correspondence: aldo.boccaccini@ww.uni-erlangen.de

Abstract: The objective of this study was to produce antibacterial poly(ε-caprolactone) (PCL)-gelatin (GEL) electrospun nanofiber mats containing clove essential oil (CLV) using glacial acetic acid (GAA) as a "benign" (non-toxic) solvent. The addition of CLV increased the fiber diameter from 241 ± 96 to 305 ± 82 nm. Aside from this, the wettability of PCL-GEL nanofiber mats was increased by the addition of CLV. Fourier-transform infrared spectroscopy (FTIR) analysis confirmed the presence of CLV, and the actual content of CLV was determined by gas chromatography–mass spectrometry (GC-MS). Our investigations showed that CLV-loaded PCL-GEL nanofiber mats did not have cytotoxic effects on normal human dermal fibroblast (NHDF) cells. On the other hand, the fibers exhibited antibacterial activity against *Staphylococcus aureus* and *Escherichia coli*. Consequently, PCL-GEL/CLV nanofiber mats are potential candidates for antibiotic-free wound healing applications.

Keywords: electrospinning; PCL; gelatin; clove essential oil; antibacterial; biocompatibility

1. Introduction

Microorganisms can quickly enter and instantly grow in open wounds, causing exudate formation, delay in wound healing, and deformation of the skin [1]. Therefore, the most critical issue in the field of wound healing is preventing wound contamination. This drawback could be overcome by using antibacterial wound dressing that protects the area around the wound, providing a suitable moist environment and antibacterial properties [2]. More recently, there has been renewed interest in natural antibacterial agents such as phytotherapeutics for antibiotic-free wound healing applications [3,4]. In particular, essential oils are one of the most promising phytotherapeutics, aiming at the promotion of the wound healing process while minimizing bacterial infections [5–7].

Essential oils (EOs) are natural-based compounds that can provide antibacterial, anti-inflammatory, and antioxidation protection [8]. The antibacterial activity of EOs such as clove, cinnamon, oregano, and lemongrass essential oil depends on the chemical structure of their primary component and concentration [9]. Among these, clove essential oil (CLV) has been medicinally used for centuries for its therapeutic effects [10]. CLV is isolated from the aromatic flower buds of *Eugenia caryophyllata*, which is composed of eugenol (78%), β-caryophyllene (13%), and other compounds such as benzyl alcohol [11]. Its primary components have been widely used due to their medicinal properties such as antioxidant, anti-inflammatory, and antimicrobial activities [12]. Moreover, its antibacterial activity has been demonstrated to be particularly effective against bacterial strains such as *Escherichia coli*, *Staphylococcus aureus*, *Bacillus subtilis*, and *Pseudomonas fluorescens* [13]. On the other hand, the effective dose of CLV has enhanced cell viability [14,15]. According to our knowledge, a few studies related to EOs' influence on in vitro cell migration have been carried out. Aside from this, the application of CLV in wound dressing is limited due to its high volatility and sensitivity to degradation from exposure to oxygen, heat, and light [16]. In order to improve the applicability of CLV, different scaffold preparation methods have been used to develop polymer carriers for CLV, such as casting films [17,18], nanoparticles [19,20] and, more recently, electrospun fiber mats [21].

The electrospinning process is a convenient, versatile, and cost-effective method for fabricating homogeneous and porous macro- or nanofibers [22]. The nanostructure and high surface-area-to-volume ratio of electrospun nanofibers are attractive features to enhance the drug releasing capability for wound healing applications [23]. Poly(ε-caprolactone) (PCL), one of the promising synthetic polymers for wound healing applications, has an excellent processability, good biocompatibility and, compared to natural polymers, high mechanical properties, whereas the biodegradability, cell adhesion, and proliferation responses to PCL are limited [24]. On the other hand, the natural polymer gelatin (GEL) containing molecular components present in the extracellular matrix (ECM) promotes cell adhesion and proliferation properties [25]. Therefore, the combination of PCL and GEL in electrospun fibers should lead to improved mechanical and physical properties coupled with suitable biocompatibility [26]. There are only a limited number of studies reporting the incorporation of natural antimicrobial agents into PCL-GEL electrospun fibers for antibacterial wound dressing applications. For instance, Ramalingam et al. [27] fabricated PCL-GEL hybrid composite mats loaded with *Gymnema sylvestre* for wound dressing applications. Similarly, Fallah et al. [28] developed curcumin (CUR)-loaded electrospun PCL-GEL nanofibers. Their results indicated that the addition of CUR increased the antibacterial activity against both Gram-positive and Gram-negative bacteria [28].

Essential oil incorporated in electrospun fibers for wound dressings are a rather recent technology; therefore, there are no reports on the use of CLV and PCL-GEL for antibacterial wound dressing. In this study, PCL-GEL nanofiber mats containing various concentrations of CLV were fabricated using glacial acetic acid (GAA) as a "benign" (non-toxic) solvent for antibiotic-free wound healing applications. The use of benign solvents in so-called "green" electrospinning has special relevance when using natural products such as EOs [29,30] Here, we investigated the effect of various CLV concentrations (1.5%, 3%, and 6%, *v*/*v*) on morphology, average fiber diameter, contact angle (wettability), cell viability, cell morphology, rate of wound closure, and antibacterial activity. To the best of the authors' knowledge, the cell migration effect of CLV-loaded PCL-GEL nanofiber mats for wound healing applications has not been investigated before.

2. Materials and Methods

2.1. Materials

PCL (Mw = 80 kDa), GEL (~300 g Bloom, Type A), CLV (C8392, CAS number: 8000-34-8), standard eugenol (E51791, 99%), and fetal bovine serum (FBS; F2442) were purchased from Sigma Aldrich (Darmstadt, Germany). Glacial acetic acid (GAA; 87003-241) and dichloromethane (DCM; BDH1113-4LG) were obtained from VWR (Darmstadt, Germany). The microorganism strains of *S. aureus* (ATCC25923) and *E. coli* (ATCC25922) were used. Luria/Miller agar (X969.1) and lysogeny broth medium (Luria/Miller, 6673.1) were supplied by Carl Roth GmbH (Karlsruhe, Germany). Dulbecco's modified Eagle's medium (DMEM, 31885-023), penicillin/streptomycin (PS, 15140-122) and trypsin/EDTA (25200-056) were purchased from Thermo Scientific (Schwerte, Germany). The normal human dermal fibroblast (NHDF) cell line was obtained from Translation Research Center

(TRC) of Friedrich-Alexander-University Erlangen-Nuremberg. All reagents and solvents were of analytical grade.

2.2. Fabrication of PCL-GEL/CLV Nanofiber Mats

For the fabrication of PCL-GEL electrospun nanofiber mats, firstly GEL powder (4.8%, *w*/*v*) was dissolved in the GAA (90%, *v*/*v*) solvent at 45 °C for 4 hours. After the GEL was dissolved, PCL pellets (11.2%, *w*/*v*) were added to the solution and stirred overnight at room temperature. The total polymer concentration of GAA solution was fixed at 16% (*w*/*v*). For the preparation of CLV-incorporated solutions, PCL-GEL solution preparation was followed as explained above. After 30 min of addition of PCL pellets, different ratios of CLV (1.5%, 3%, and 6%, *v*/*v*) were separately added in a dropwise manner to the PCL-GEL solution and stirred overnight at room temperature. Then, each electrospinning solution was carried out under defined and constant ambient conditions (temperature (T): 25 °C and relative humidity (RH): 25%) using a commercially available electrospinning setup (IME's medical electrospinning machines, EC-16 CLI, IME Technologies, Netherlands). The solutions were loaded separately into a 3 mL plastic syringe equipped with a 23G needle and fed at 0.6 mL/h. The aluminum sheet wrapped around the rotating drum collector was placed at a distance of 12 cm from the needle tip to the collector. Electrospinning was conducted by applying a voltage of +19 kV in the needle and −1 kV to the target. Moreover, during the electrospinning process, the gas shield accessory with nitrogen flux was set at 8 mL/min for optimization of the Taylor cone. The samples were then stored at 4 °C in the dark until further analysis.

2.3. Characterization of Nanofiber Mats

The surface morphology of nanofiber mats was analyzed by scanning electron microscopy (SEM, ETH: 2 kV, Everhart-Thornley detector (SE2), AURIGA base 55, Carl Zeiss). The samples were coated with a thin layer of gold (Q150T Turbo-Pumped Sputter Coater/Carbon Coater, Quorum Technologies) before SEM analyses. The average fiber diameter of nanofiber mats was measured from the SEM images using the Image J analysis software (NIH, Bethesda, MD, USA). For calculation of the average fiber diameter and fiber distribution, 50 randomly selected different points were measured.

The contact angle meter (Drop Shape Analyzer, DSA 30, CA Measurement setup, Kruess GmbH, Hamburg, Germany) was used to investigate the wettability of nanofiber mats using a sessile drop method. Briefly, the samples were placed on a glass slide before the test and 8 µl of de-ionized water was dropped on the surface of the nanofiber mats. Four measurements were taken at different locations of the same mats and the average value was obtained.

The functional group of PCL-GEL and CLV-loaded PCL-GEL nanofiber mats PCL-GEL/CLV were analyzed by Fourier-transform infrared spectroscopy (FTIR, IRAffinity-1S, Shimadzu). The spectrum analysis was performed with wavenumbers ranging between 400 and 4000 cm^{-1} and at a spectral resolution of 4 cm^{-1}.

The investigation of the total CLV content in CLV-loaded PCL-GEL nanofiber mats was performed using gas chromatography–mass spectrometry (GC-MS, GC/MSD Systems, GC 7890A, MSD 5975C, Agilent Technologies, Waldbronn, Germany) equipped with a DB-FFAP (Durabond-Free Fatty Acid Phase) capillary column (GC Column, 30 m × 0.25 mm, film thickness 0.25 µm; Agilent Technologies, Santa Clara, CA). Briefly, the calibration curve of eugenol, that is, the main component in the volatile fraction of CLV, was prepared and the eugenol concentration was calculated using the peak area ($y = 77732x + 89964$, $R^2 = 0.9995$). On the other hand, the nanofiber mats (3 mg) were dispersed in DCM (20 mL) for 2 h. Subsequently, the solvent-assisted flavor evaporation technique (SAFE) [31] was used for the isolation of the CLV volatile fraction. The volatile fraction in DCM was dried over sodium sulfate and then filtered. The final volume (100 µL) was obtained using Vigreux and microdistillation at 50 °C [32]. Then, 1 µL of each sample was taken for the GC-MS measurements. The oven temperature was programmed at 40 °C for 2 min and then heated up at 8 °C/min to 240 °C and held for 5 min. Helium was used as carrier gas at a flow rate of 1 mL/min. Mass spectra were recorded in selected ion monitoring (SIM) mode (*m*/*z* ratio 164). Finally, the percentage of encapsulation efficiency was calculated as Equation (1):

$$\text{Encapsulation Efficiency (EE)}(\%) = \frac{M_a}{M_t} \times 100 \quad (1)$$

where M_a and M_t are the actual and theoretical amounts of CLV in nanofiber mats, respectively.

2.4. Antibacterial Assay

The antibacterial activity of CLV-loaded PCL-GEL nanofiber mats was separately tested with *S. aureus* (Gram-positive) and *E. coli* (Gram-negative) bacteria. Initially, the bacterial suspensions were prepared for both bacteria stains in lysogeny broth medium at 37 °C for 24 h. Then, the optical density (OD) (600 nm, Thermo Scientific GENESYS 30, Germany) of the cultivated bacteria was arranged at 0.015. The nanofiber mats (~3 mg) were then cut and were sterilized by UV light irradiation for 30 min. The samples were immersed in lysogeny broth medium, and 20 μL of bacteria suspension was added. Finally, all the samples were incubated at 37 °C for 3, 6, and 24 h and then they were measured at each time interval at 600 nm OD. The relative viability of the bacteria was calculated according to Equation (2):

$$\text{Relative viability } (\%) = \frac{OD_{\text{Sample}}}{OD_{\text{Control}}} \times 100 \quad (2)$$

The lysogeny broth medium and bacterial cell suspension in lysogeny broth medium were used as a blank and control (CNT), respectively. The experiments were performed three times.

2.5. In Vitro Assay

The cell viability, cell morphology, and wound closure rate of NHDF cells were analyzed to gain the first impression of the biological behavior of PCL-GEL, PCL-GEL/CLV1.5, PCL-GEL/CLV3, and PCL-GEL/CLV6 nanofiber mats.

2.5.1. Cell Culture

NHDF cells were cultured in DMEM supplemented with 10% FBS and 1% penicillin/streptomycin in 75 cm^2 cell culture flasks (Nunc, Denmark). Subsequently, NHDF cells were grown to confluency, and then the cells were detached by trypsinization and counted by trypan blue assay using a hemocytometer (Roth, Germany). Counted cells were seeded in 24-well plates at a density of 50.000 cell/well and incubated at 37 °C in a humidified incubator with 5% CO_2 for 24 h. Prior to cell culture experiments, the nanofiber mats were fixed on CellCrown 24 inserts (ScaffdexOy, Tampere, Finland) and sterilized by UV light irradiation for 30 min. After 24 h incubation, the medium of the cell was refreshed, and the samples were immersed in a 24-well plate without touching the cells. Finally, the cells were incubated with samples for a further 48 h.

2.5.2. Cell Viability

The viability of the cells was analyzed by a WST-8 cell counting assay kit (Sigma Aldrich). The basis of this assay is the reduction of yellow-colored tetrazolium salt in WST-8 to form orange formazan crystals by dehydrogenases enzymes secreted by mitochondria of metabolically active cells. The amount of these formazan crystals is directly proportional to the number of living cells. After culturing the cells for 48 h, they were washed with PBS to remove unattached cells and incubated with 5% WST-8 reagent in DMEM for a period of 2h at 37 °C. The absorbance of the dye was measured at 450 nm using a spectrophotometric plate reader (PHOmo, anthos Mikrosysteme GmbH, Germany). The percentage of cell viability was calculated as follows:

$$\text{Cell viability } (\%) = \frac{(\text{Absorbance of control } - \text{ Absorbance of test sample})}{(\text{Absorbance of control } - \text{ Absorbance of blank})} \times 100 \quad (3)$$

All samples were measured in triplicate.

2.5.3. Hematoxylin and Eosin (H&E) Staining

Hematoxylin and eosin (H&E) staining methods were used for analyzing the cell density. Briefly, the cells were washed with PBS and fixed with Fluoro-Fix for 15 min. After that, the cells were stained with Hematoxylin for 20 min and washed with tap water followed by Scott's tap water for 5 min and then further rinsed with de-ionized water. After hematoxylin dying, the cells were stained with 0.4% eosin stain (in a saturated aqueous solution of 60% ethanol and 5% acetic acid) for 5 min. Cells were dehydrated with 95% and 100% ethanol, respectively, and air-dried in a fume hood. Finally, the cell density of the NHDF cells was examined using a light microscope (Primo Vert, Carl Zeiss).

2.5.4. In Vitro Wound Healing Assay (Scratch Test)

In vitro healing assay was performed according to the procedure described in [33]. The experimental set-up for the scratch test is schematically illustrated in Figure 1. Firstly, NHDF cells were seeded at 50,000 cell/well into 24-well plate and were incubated at 37 °C in 5% CO_2 for 24 h. Then, a vertical scratch was created using a 1000 mL sterile pipet tip in the middle of the NHDF monolayer. Subsequently, the nanofiber mats were fixed on CellCrown 24 inserts (ScaffdexOy, Tampere, Finland) and placed in the 24-well plate without touching the surface. Finally, the wound closure rate was monitored at different times (0 h, 4 h, 6 h, and 24 h) and photographed using a light microscope (Primo Vert, Carl Zeiss). The images were analyzed with Image J (NIH, Bethesda, MD, USA). The rate of wound closure was calculated using the following formula:

$$\text{Rate of wound closure (\%)} = \frac{(A_0 - A_t)}{A_0} \times 100 \quad (4)$$

where A_0 is the initial wound area and A_t is the wound area at the designated time.

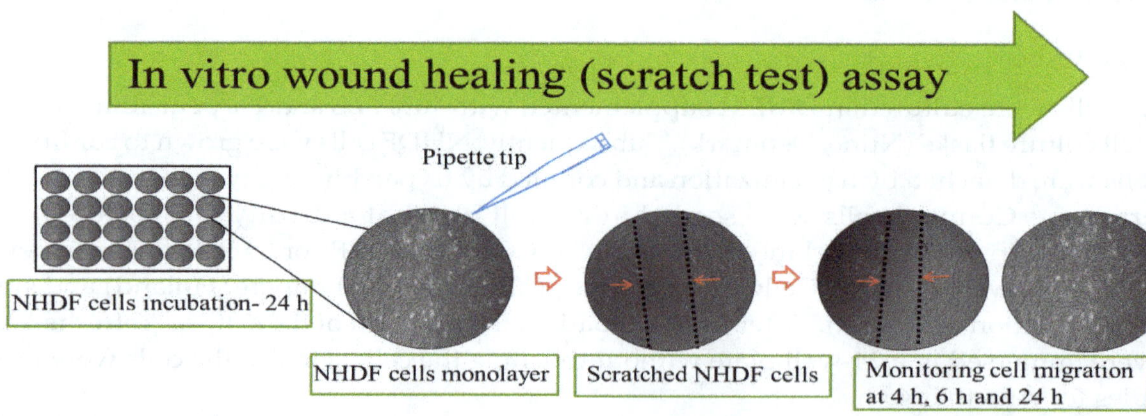

Figure 1. Schematic illustration of in vitro wound healing assay (scratch test) set-up for the study. NHDF: normal human dermal fibroblast.

2.6. Statistical Analysis

Data were analyzed by ANOVA and Bonferroni's test using the Origin (OriginLab, Northampton, MA, USA). The level of significance was determined as $p < 0.05$.

3. Results

3.1. Surface Morphology of PCL-GEL/CLV Nanofiber Mats

The morphology of PCL-GEL, PCL-GEL/CLV1.5, PCL-GEL/CLV3, and PCL-GEL/CLV6 nanofiber mats was investigated. The results revealed that all samples had a smooth, uniform, and bead-less morphology. Figure 2 and Table 1 show the fiber distribution and average fiber diameter, separately. The average fiber diameters were 241 ± 96, 285 ± 67, 300 ± 73, and 305 ± 82 nm for PCL-GEL, PCL-GEL/CLV1.5, PCL-GEL/CLV3, and PCL-GEL/CLV6, respectively. The results indicate that the fiber diameter had increased with the addition CLV compared to PCL-GEL.

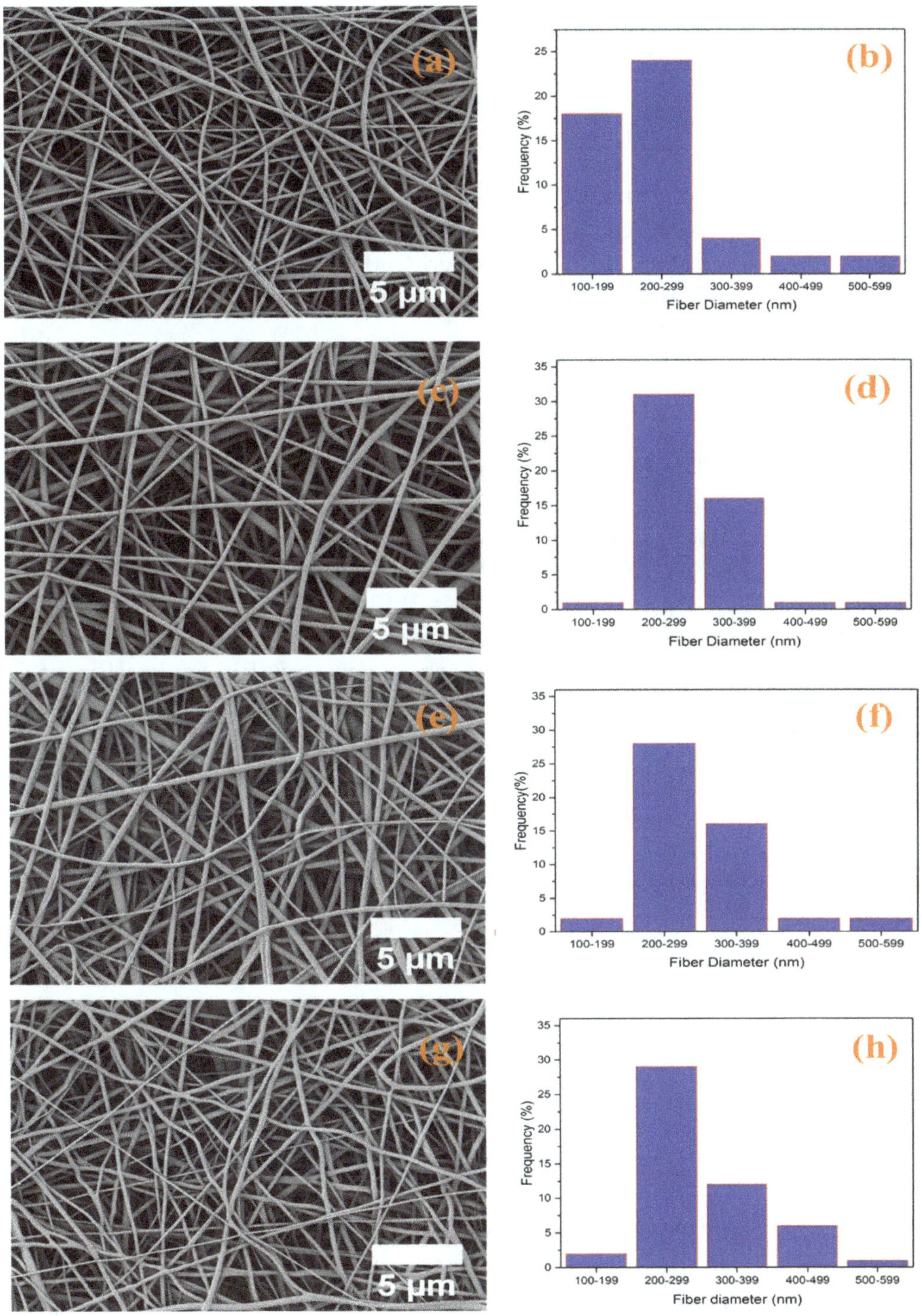

Figure 2. The morphology and fiber diameter distribution of poly(ε-caprolactone) gelatin (PCL-GEL) (**a**,**b**), PCL-GEL/clove essential oil (CLV)1.5 (**c**,**d**), PCL-GEL/CLV3 (**e**,**f**), and PCL-GEL/CLV6 (**g**,**h**) nanofiber mats, respectively.

Table 1. Sample composition, sample label, average fiber diameter, and loading efficiency of nanofiber mats.

Sample Code	PCL (*w/v* %)	GEL (*w/v* %)	CLV (*v/v* %)	Average Fiber Diameter (nm)	Contact Angle(°)	Encapsulation Efficiency (EE) (%)
PCL-GEL	11.2	4.8	-	241 ± 96	37 ± 8	-
PCL-GEL/CLV1.5	11.2	4.8	1.5	285 ± 67	18 ± 3	53 ± 4
PCL-GEL/CLV3	11.2	4.8	3	300 ± 73	21 ± 4	68 ± 11
PCL-GEL/CLV6	11.2	4.8	6	305 ± 82	27 ± 5	73 ± 3

3.2. Wettability

The wettability of the nanofiber mats was analyzed by the sessile drop method. The contact angle values of the samples are shown in Table 1. The incorporation of CLV within the PCL-GEL nanofiber mats resulted in a decreasing contact angle compared to the PCL-GEL nanofiber mats. The contact angle values were 37 ± 8°, 18 ± 3°, 21 ± 4°, and 27 ± 5° for PCL-GEL, PCL-GEL/CLV1.5, PCL-GEL/CLV3, and PCL-GEL/CLV6 nanofiber mats.

3.3. Fourier-Transform Infrared Spectroscopy Analysis

The presence of CLV within the nanofiber mats was analyzed by Fourier-transform infrared spectroscopy (FTIR) (Figure 3). The typical peaks of PCL were at 2942 and 2866 cm^{-1}, corresponding to the asymmetric and symmetric stretching of CH_2 bonds. Further peaks were at 1720, 1240, and 1168 cm^{-1} related to carbonyl stretching as well as both asymmetric and symmetric stretching of C–O–C bonds, respectively [30]. Characteristic GEL peaks were obtained at 1651 cm^{-1} for amide I and N–H deformation at around 1540 cm^{-1} for the amide II [34]. With the addition of CLV, a new peak appeared within the nanofiber mats. The CLV bands were observed at 1514 cm^{-1}, which corresponds to the main component of CLV—eugenol—attributed to the stretching vibration of C=C aromatic bonds [17].

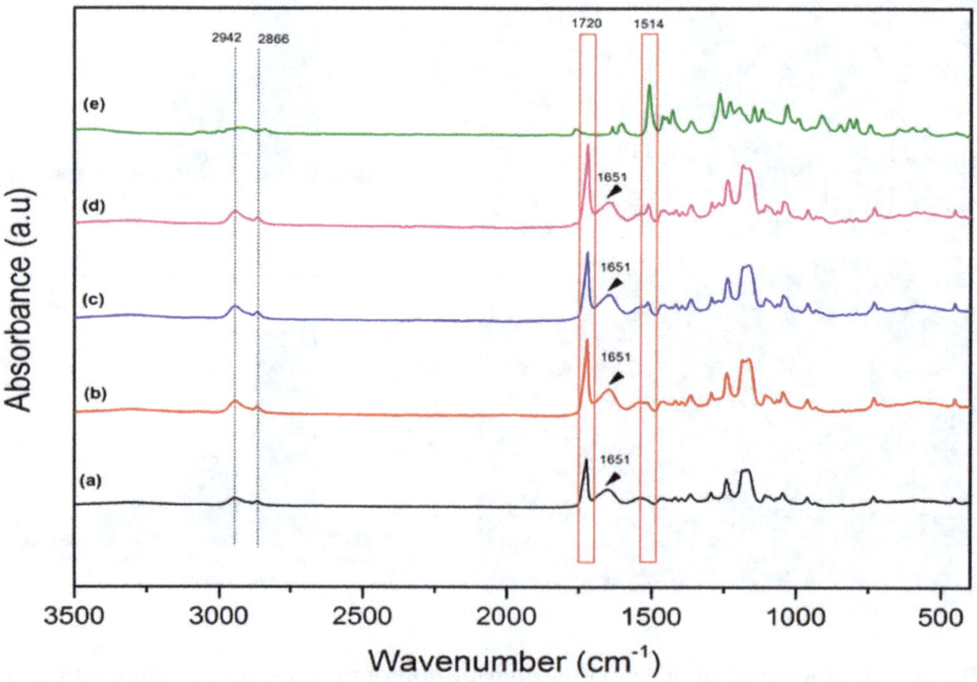

Figure 3. The Fourier-transform infrared spectroscopy (FTIR) spectra of PCL-GEL (**a**), PCL-GEL/CLV1.5 (**b**), PCL-GEL/CLV3 (**c**), and PCL-GEL/CLV6 (**d**) nanofiber mats and pure CLV (**e**).

3.4. *CLV Content in PCL-GEL Nanofiber Mats*

The encapsulation efficiency of CLV in PCL-GEL nanofiber mats was investigated by GC-MS. The effect of the different concentrations of CLV on the percentage of encapsulation efficiency is shown in Table 1. The encapsulation efficiency of PCL-GEL/CLV3 and PCL-GEL/CLV6 nanofiber mats were higher than the PCL-GEL/CLV1.5. However, there were no statistically significant differences between the PCL-GEL/CLV3 and PCL-GEL/CLV6.

3.5. *Antibacterial Assay*

The antibacterial activity of PCL-GEL, PCL-GEL/CLV1.5, PCL-GEL/CLV3, and PCL-GEL/CLV6 nanofiber mats was tested with *S. aureus* (Gram-positive) and *E. coli* (Gram-negative) bacteria. The bacterial viability against both bacteria strains is illustrated in Figure 4. CLV addition improved the antibacterial activity of nanofiber mats compared to PCL-GEL. The highest inhibition effect was observed at 6 h for *S. aureus*, whereas *E. coli* was active up to 24 h. However, there were no significant differences between the PCL-GEL/CLV1.5, PCL-GEL/CLV3, and PCL-GEL/CLV6 nanofiber mats. Moreover, after 24 h incubation, PCL-GEL/CLV3 and PCL-GEL/CLV6 showed lower *E. coli* bacteria viability than the control (CNT) and PCL-GEL. On the other hand, bacteria viability of *S. aureus* PCL-GEL/CLV1.5, PCL-GEL/CLV3, and PCL-GEL/CLV6 nanofiber mats were reduced compared to CNT at 6 h incubation.

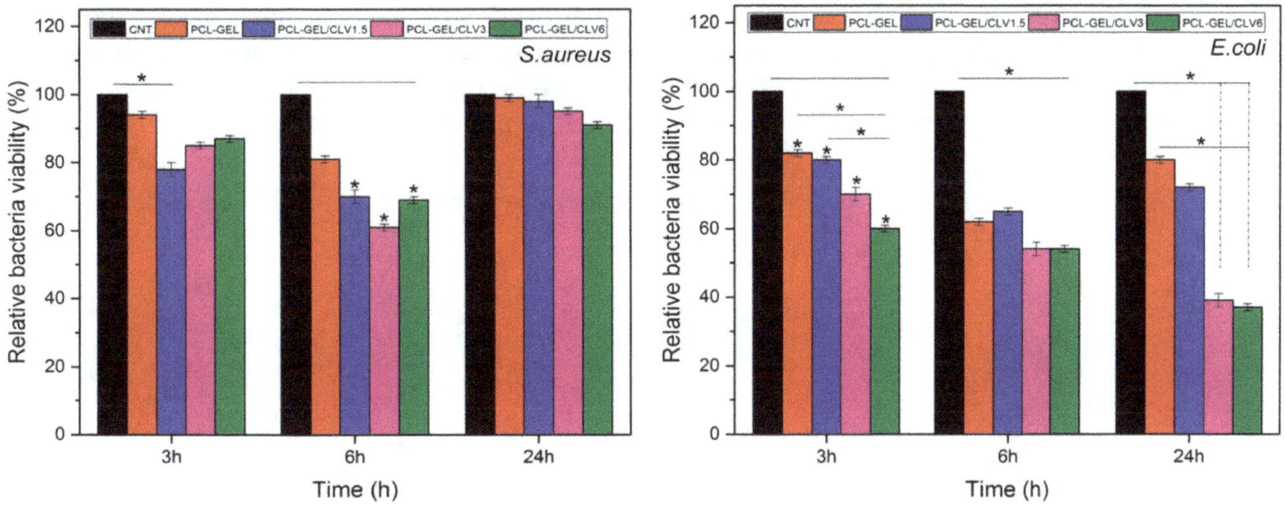

Figure 4. Antibacterial activity of PCL-GEL and CLV-loaded PCL-GEL nanofiber mats after 3, 6, and 24 h incubation with *S. aureus* (Gram-positive) and *E. coli* (Gram-negative) bacteria ($n = 3$, samples in triplicate,* $p < 0.05$).

3.6. *In Vitro Assay*

3.6.1. Cell Viability

The viability and growth of NHDF cells were determined to investigate the in vitro biocompatibility of PCL-GEL, PCL-GEL/CLV1.5, PCL-GEL/CLV3, and PCL-GEL/CLV6 nanofiber mats after 48 h of incubation, as shown in Figure 5. It is shown that there was no apparent difference between the nanofiber mats compared to the control (CNT). Furthermore, there was no significant change in NHDF cell viability with the increase of to CLV concentration in the nanofiber mats ($p < 0.05$). The results demonstrated that PCL-GEL and PCL-GEL/CLV nanofiber mats show no cytotoxicity on NHDF cells.

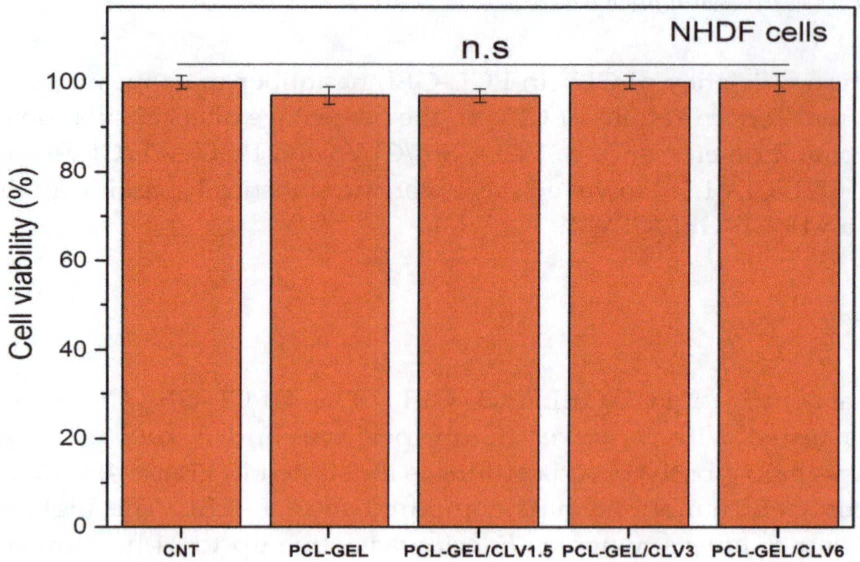

Figure 5. Cell viability percentage of PCL-GEL and CLV-loaded PCL-GEL nanofiber mats after 48 h incubation ($n = 6$, n.s: not significant).

3.6.2. Hematoxylin and Eosin (H&E) Staining

Light microscopy images of H&E-stained NHDF cells cultured with PCL-GEL, PCL-GEL/CLV1.5, PCL-GEL/CLV3, and PCL-GEL/CLV6 nanofiber mats after 48 h are shown in Figure 6. As evident from light microscope images, the cells exhibited phenotypical cell morphology and were firmly attached and well-spread on the well plate. Also, the addition and increasing the CLV did not affect the morphology and spreading of the NHDF cells. Moreover, the cell confluence obtained after each treatment was in agreement with cell viability measured by the WST-8 assay.

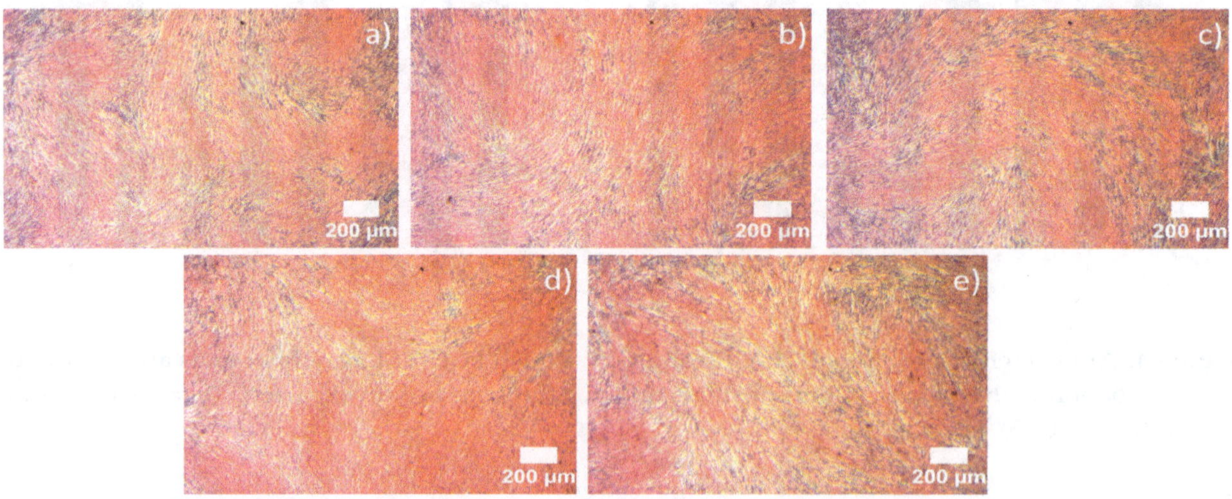

Figure 6. Light microscopy images of hematoxylin and eosin (H&E)-stained NHDF cells cultured with CNT (**a**), PCL-GEL (**b**), PCL-GEL/CLV1.5 (**c**), PCL-GEL/CLV3 (**d**), and PCL-GEL/CLV6 (**e**) nanofiber mats. The H&E staining highlighted the cell nuclei (blue) within the pink cytoplasm.

3.6.3. In Vitro Wound Healing Assay (Scratch Test)

The effect of CLV-loaded into PCL-GEL nanofiber mats to the wound healing activity of NHDF cells was assessed using the in vitro wound healing (scratch) assay. The cell migration into the wound areas and rate of wound closure are presented in Figures 7 and 8, respectively. After 6 h, the percentages of cells in the wound area for the control (CNT), PCL-GEL, PCL-GEL/CLV1.5, PCL-GEL/CLV3, and PCL-GEL/CLV6 nanofiber mats were 41 ± 1, 31 ± 1, 29 ± 3, 30 ± 2, and 16 ± 1%, respectively (Figure 8). However, after 24 h of treatment, in the CNT group complete closure was observed, whereas in PCL-GEL, PCL-GEL/CLV1.5, PCL-GEL/CLV3, and PCL-GEL/CLV6 nanofiber mats, this closure was 86 ± 1, 83 ± 3, 78 ± 2, and 68 ± 1%, respectively. Increasing CLV concentration inhibited NHDF cell migration and proliferation in a dose-dependent manner. On the other hand, there was no significant ($p < 0.05$) difference in wound closure rates between PCL-GEL and PCL-GEL/CLV1.5 at 4, 6, and 24 h.

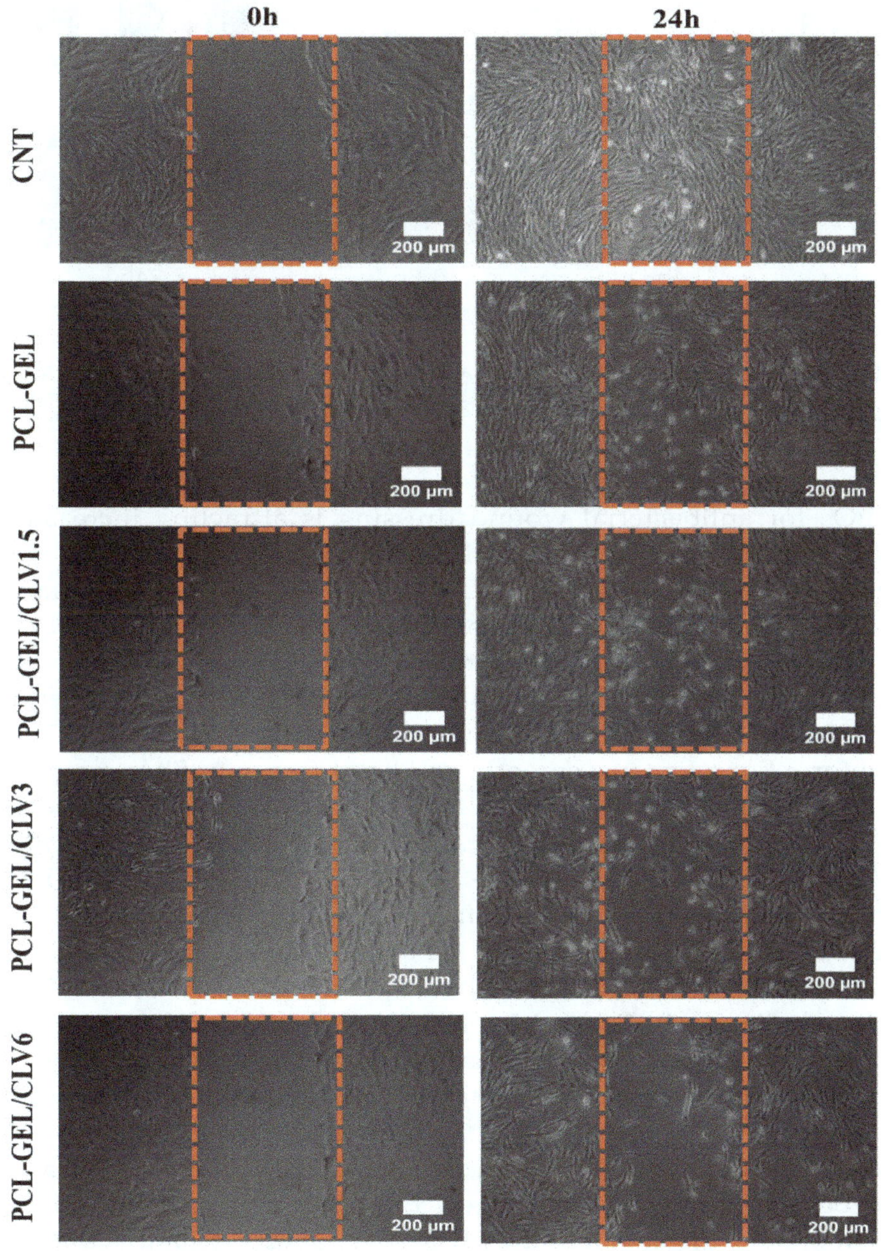

Figure 7. Illustrative micrographs of cell migrating into a scratch area over a 24 h period in CNT, PCL-GEL, PCL-GEL/CLV1.5, PCL-GEL/CLV3, and PCL-GEL/CLV6.

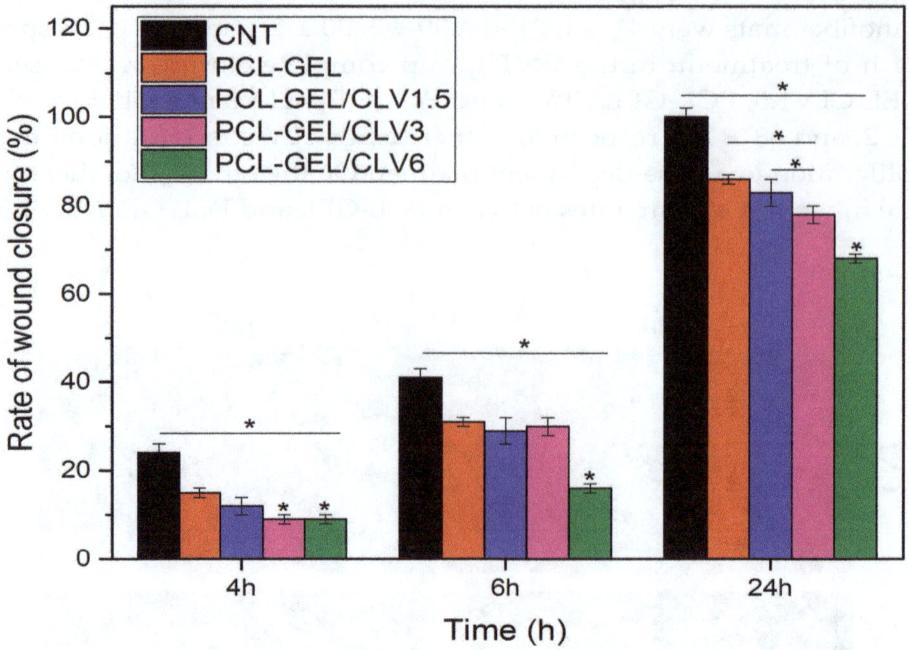

Figure 8. In vitro wound healing assay in the presence of CNT, PCL-GEL, PCL-GEL/CLV1.5, PCL-GEL/CLV3, and PCL-GEL/CLV6 in 24 h ($n = 3$, samples in triplicate, * $p < 0.05$).

4. Discussion

The usage of EOs for antibacterial wound dressing is attracting increasing interest due to their antibacterial, anti-inflammatory, and antioxidant properties. In this study, CLV-loaded PCL-GEL nanofiber mats were produced using benign solvents for antibacterial wound dressings. The concentrations used in the fabrication of nanofiber mats are shown in Table 1. SEM images of the obtained nanofiber mats with and without CLV are depicted in Figure 2. The results indicate that the incorporation of CLV did not affect the fiber formation. However, the average fiber diameter increased by the addition of CLV and increased the CLV amount from 1.5% to 6% (*w*/*v*). It is well known that the fabrication of uniform homogenous, smooth, and bead-free nanofiber morphology depends on electrospinning parameters such as polymer concentration, solution viscosity, electrical conductivity, temperature, and humidity [22]. The lower electrical conductivity of the solution affects the elongation of the jet by the electrical forces and can cause large fiber diameters [35]. The increment of the PCL-GEL/CLV nanofiber diameter could be attributed to the reduction of solution electric conductivity. Aside from this, increasing the solution viscosity led to increased average fiber diameter [36]. In the present study, the addition of CLV could reduce the solution viscosity due to the interaction between CLV and PCL-GEL. In a similar study, García-Moreno et al. [37] reported that the average fiber diameter of poly(vinyl alcohol) (PVA) nanofibers was increased with the encapsulation of fish oil. Mori et al. [38] showed similar results in that various concentrations of candeia essential oil addition increased the average fiber diameter of polylactic acid (PLA) nanostructured mats.

The contact angle measurement, which is a cost-effective and useful method used to investigate the effect of additives on surface properties, has been commonly used to demonstrate the wettability of biomaterials. Furthermore, the increment of the surface wettability enhances the absorption of excess wound exudates, which is important for wound healing applications [39]. In this study, the contact angle measurement was used to determine the effect of CLV on the PCL-GEL nanofiber mats (Table 1). Data obtained in this study indicated that the wettability of PCL-GEL nanofiber mats was increased with CLV addition. This result could be due to the chemical structure of CLV that presents polar phytochemicals and hydrophilic –OH groups. However, increasing the concentrations of CLV, the contact angle of PCL-GEL/CLV1.5, PCL-GEL/CLV3, and PCL-GEL/CLV6 nanofiber mats was slightly increased, which might be due to the loss of free functional groups (amino and hydroxyl groups) on the GEL. According to Liu et al. [40], cinnamon essential oil encapsulated chitosan nanoparticle incorporation in poly (lactic acid) (PLA) composite fibers, increasing the hydrophilic behavior. In another study, Anges Mary and Giri Dev [41] fabricated PCL electrospun matrices incorporated with aloe vera (AV). Their results revealed that the addition of AV decreased the contact angle value compared to pure PCL [41]. Similarly, findings of Ramalingam et al. [27] indicated that PCL/GEL hybrid composite mats comprising natural herbal extract (*Gymnema sylvestre*) had lower contact angle value.

FTIR analysis (Figure 3) revealed the presence of CLV loading in the PCL-GEL nanofiber mats, attributable to the characteristic peak of CLV.

The influence of different CLV ratios in PCL-GEL nanofiber mats on the encapsulation efficiency was examined (Table 1). On the basis of the findings in this study, increasing the CLV content from 1.5% to 3% (*v/v*) increased the encapsulation efficiency. However, the encapsulation efficiency of PCL-GEL/CLV3 and PCL-GEL/CLV6 nanofiber mats were not significantly different. This result could have been due to the capacity of nanofibers, which exhibited a maximum encapsulation efficiency of 73 ± 3%. Recently, clove oil (CO)/chitosan nanoparticles embedded gelatin nanofibers were produced by Cui et al. [20]. The encapsulation efficiency results revealed values that measured ranged from 21.1 ± 0.4% to 39.6 ± 0.8%. Similarly, Tampau et al. [42] reported the fabrication of starch or PCL-based matrices incorporated with carvacrol. The results showed that the encapsulation efficiency of carvacrol in starch or PCL-based matrices increased from 15% to 75% with increasing carvacrol ratios. Moreover, gelatin nanofiber mats encapsulated with orange essential oil were studied by Tavassoli-Kafrani et al. [43] They found that the increment of the orange essential oil ratio in the gelatin nanofibers increased the encapsulation efficiency from 35 ± 0.09% to 69.0 ± 0.22%.

The antibacterial properties of CLV have been investigated using various bacteria such as *E. coli*, *S. aureus*, *Bacillus subtilis*, and *Pseudomonas fluorescens* [13]. The present study investigated the antibacterial activity of CLV-loaded PCL-GEL nanofiber mats against *S. aureus* as Gram-positive bacteria and *E. coli* as Gram-negative bacteria for antibacterial wound dressings. The results indicated that the addition of CLV reduced the bacteria viability for both bacteria strains, as shown in Figure 4. The lowest bacterial viability was observed at 6 h for *S. aureus*, whereas bacterial viability of *E. coli* was reduced at 24 h. This result could have been due to different bacterial characteristics and morphology; for instance: Gram-negative bacteria have a thicker double layer cell membrane than the single membrane of Gram-positive bacteria [5,12]. In a similar study, Fallah et al. [28] reported that the incorporation with curcumin exhibited antibacterial activity against both Gram-positive and Gram-negative bacteria on PCL-GEL fiber mats. Similarly, Figueroa-Lopez et al. [44] produced GEL-coated PCL ultrathin fibers containing black pepper oleoresin (OR). Their results revealed that the viability of *S. aureus* was reduced with the addition of OR. In another study, Ramalingam et al. [27] evaluated the effect of the addition of *Gymnema sylvestre* as a natural herbal in PCL-GEL on the antibacterial performance of these nanofibrous mats. It was found that the antibacterial activity of the samples all increased with the addition of *Gymnema sylvestre*. Furthermore, our results revealed that the highest bacteria inhibition was observed in *E. coli* compared to *S. aureus*. According to Li et al. [45], eugenol loaded PCL-GEL fiber mats are more effective against *S. aureus* compared to *E.coli*; this is in contrast to our studies. The result might have been due to the chemical structure of CLV, which additionally consists of other components such as eugenyl acetate or beta-caryophyllene. In conclusion, the antibacterial activity of CLV-loaded PCL-GEL nanofiber mats confirms the present fibrous structures as promising materials for antibacterial wound dressing.

In the present study, the cell viability of PCL-GEL nanofiber mats with and without CLV was investigated with NHDF cells. The results indicated that there were no significant differences ($p < 0.05$) in cell viability and morphology of the nanofiber mats in comparison to control (Figures 5 and 6). Accordingly, the in vitro cell viability and morphology results demonstrated that PCL-GEL, PCL-GEL/CLV1.5, PCL-GEL/CLV3, and PCL-GEL/CLV6 nanofiber mats are biocompatible. In a related study, Tang et al. [46] produced peppermint and chamomile essential oil-loaded gelatin nanofibers.

Their cytotoxicity results indicated that incorporation of peppermint and chamomile essential oil into gelatin nanofibers did not change the NIH-3T3 fibroblast cell viability [46]. In another study, Hajiali et al. [47] investigated the antibacterial activity and biocompatibility of alginate–lavender nanofibers. The cell viability of lavender-incorporated alginate nanofibers was 91%. It was stated that the addition of lavender oil did not affect the cell viability of human foreskin fibroblast (HFF-1) cells compared to the control group [47]. Similarly, Balasubramanian and Kodam [48] assessed mouse fibroblasts (NIH-3T3) on polyacrylonitrile (PAN)/lavender oil nanofibrous mats. Lavender-loaded nanofibrous mats showed non-cytotoxic behavior for NIH-3T3, which is in agreement with our results [48].

Wound healing is a complex and multiphase process that can be categorized into wounding, hemostasis, inflammation, proliferation, and maturation [49]. During this process, the formation of new tissue and wound healing rate are also affected by external factors [50]. In our study, the potential effect of CLV on wound healing was investigated by an in vitro wound-healing assay. This assay revealed that increasing the CLV concentration reduced the NHDF cell migration and proliferation, whereas the same samples had no adverse effect on the NHDF cell viability. On the other hand, after 24 h measurements, PCL-GEL/CLV1.5 values were not significantly different when compared with PCL-GEL. In the literature, a few studies have been conducted to assess the cell migration effect of EOs. For instance, the dose-dependent wound healing effect of *Eugenia dysenterica* DC leaves were reported by da Silva et al. [51] In a similar study, Léguillier et al. studied keratinocyte cell migration ability at various concentrations of *Calophyllum inophyllum* oil (0.01%, 0.1%, and 1% diluted in olive oil) [52]. Their results proved that the effective dose of EO enhances cell migration [52]. To the best of the authors' knowledge, this is the first study on CLV-loaded PCL-GEL nanofiber mats using cultured NHDF cells to determine the wound closure rate. Therefore, the biological activity of CLV-loaded PCL-GEL nanofiber mats is promising and should be further investigated, quantifying in particular the time-dependent release of the EO and its effect on cell behavior.

5. Conclusions

We evaluated the antibacterial and biological activity of CLV-loaded PCL-GEL nanofiber mats on wound dressings. PCL-GEL and clove oil-loaded PCL-GEL nanofiber mats were successfully fabricated by electrospinning. Our results revealed that bead-free, uniform, and smooth fibers were obtained. However, the addition of CLV increased the average fiber diameter. The wettability study inferred that the addition of CLV decreased the contact angle value compared to PCL-GEL nanofiber mats. The FTIR spectrum suggested that the CLV component is loaded into the PCL-GEL nanofiber mats. Moreover, the cytotoxicity results revealed that the incorporation of CLV on the PCL-GEL nanofiber mats did not demonstrate a toxic effect on NHDF cell viability. Aside from this, the addition of CLV promoted the antibacterial properties against *S. aureus* and *E. coli*. In conclusion, CLV-loaded PCL-GEL nanofiber mats may have a potential in wound healing applications and can be considered as promising biomaterial for avoiding bacterial infections without using antibiotics.

Author Contributions: Conceptualization: I.U. and A.R.B., methodology: I.U. B.S., A.B., W.H.G. and R.D., formal analysis: I.U., S.J.E., B.S., A.B. and W.H.G., investigation: I.U., S.J.E. and A.R.B., resources: A.B. and A.R.B.; data curation: I.U., writing—original draft preparation: I.U., writing—review and editing: I.U., B.S., A.B., W.H.G., R.D. and A.R.B., visualization: I.U., supervision: A.R.B., project administration: A.R.B.

Acknowledgments: The first author is funded by the Deutscher Akademischer Austauschdienst (DAAD) program of Research Grants – Doctoral Programs. The authors want to thank Raminder Singh from the Translational Research Center (TRC) Erlangen for the supply of normal human dermal fibroblasts.

References

1. Edwards, R.; Harding, K.G. Bacteria and wound healing. *Curr. Opin. Infect. Dis.* **2004**, *17*, 91–96. [CrossRef] [PubMed]
2. Macneil, S. Biomaterials for tissue engineering of skin. *Mater. Today* **2008**, *11*, 26–35. [CrossRef]

3. Ramos-e-Silva, M.; Ribeiro de Castro, D.C.M. New dressings, including tissue-engineered living skin. *Clin. Derm.* **2002**, *20*, 715–723. [CrossRef]
4. Dhivya, S.; Vijaya Padma, V.; Santhini, E. Wound dressings-a review. *BioMedicine* **2015**, *5*, 24–28. [CrossRef] [PubMed]
5. Silva, N.C.C.; Fernandes, J.A. Biological properties of medicinal plants: A review of their antimicrobial activity. *J. Venom Anim Toxins Incl. Trop. Dis.* **2010**, *16*, 402–413. [CrossRef]
6. Jaganathan, S.; Mani, M.; Polymers, A.K. Electrospun Combination of Peppermint Oil and Copper Sulphate with Conducive Physico-Chemical properties for Wound Dressing Applications. *Polymers* **2019**, *11*, 586. [CrossRef]
7. Sadri, M.; Arab-Sorkhi, S.; Vatani, H.; Bagheri-Pebdeni, A. New wound dressing polymeric nanofiber containing green tea extract prepared by electrospinning method. *Fibers Polym.* **2015**, *16*, 1742–1750. [CrossRef]
8. Bakkali, F.; Averbeck, S.; Averbeck, D.; Idaomar, M. Biological effects of essential oils – A review. *Food Chem. Toxicol.* **2008**, *46*, 446–475. [CrossRef]
9. Velluti, A.; Sanchis, V.; Ramos, A.J.; Egido, J.; Marın, S. Inhibitory effect of cinnamon, clove, lemongrass, oregano and palmarose essential oils on growth and fumonisin B1 production by Fusarium proliferatum in maize grain. *Int. J. Food Microbiol.* **2003**, *89*, 145–154. [CrossRef]
10. Prabuseenivasan, S.; Jayakumar, M.; Ignacimuthu, S. In vitro antibacterial activity of some plant essential oils. *Bmc Complement. Altern. Med.* **2006**, *6*, 39. [CrossRef]
11. Jirovetz, L.; Buchbauer, G.; Stoilova, I.; Stoyanova, A.; Krastanov, A.; Schmidt, E. Chemical composition and antioxidant properties of clove leaf essential oil. *J. Agric. Food Chem.* **2006**, *54*, 6303–6307. [CrossRef] [PubMed]
12. Teixeira, B.; Marques, A.; Ramos, C.; Neng, N.R.; Nogueira, J.M.F.; Saraiva, J.A.; Nunes, M.L. Chemical composition and antibacterial and antioxidant properties of commercial essential oils. *Ind. Crop. Prod.* **2013**, *43*, 587–595. [CrossRef]
13. Chaieb, K.; Hajlaoui, H.; Zmantar, T.; Kahla-Nakbi, A.B.; Rouabhia, M.; Mahdouani, K.; Bakhrouf, A. The chemical composition and biological activity of clove essential oil, Eugenia caryophyllata (Syzigium aromaticum L. Myrtaceae): A short review. *Phytother. Res.* **2007**, *21*, 501–506.
14. Khunkitti, W.; Veerapan, P.; Hahnvajanawong, C. In vitro bioactivities of clove buds oil (Eugenia caryophyllata) and its effect on dermal fibroblast. *Int. J. Pharm. Pharm. Sci.* **2012**, *4*, 556–560.
15. Prashar, A.; Locke, I.C.; Evans, C.S. Cytotoxicity of clove (Syzygium aromaticum) oil and its major components to human skin cells. *Cell Proliferation* **2006**, *39*, 241–248. [CrossRef]
16. Asbahani, A.; Miladi, K.; Badri, W.; Sala, M.; Addi, E.H.A.; Casabianca, H.; Mousadik, A.; Hartmann, D.; Jilale, A.; Renaud, F.N.R.; et al. Essential oils: From extraction to encapsulation. *Int. J. Pharma.* **2015**, *483*, 220–243. [CrossRef]
17. Wang, L.; Liu, F.; Jiang, Y.; Chai, Z.; Li, P.; Cheng, Y.; Jing, H.; Leng, X. Synergistic antimicrobial activities of natural essential oils with chitosan films. *J. Agric. Food Chem.* **2011**, *59*, 12411–12419. [CrossRef]
18. Pereira dos Santos, E.; Nicácio, P.H.M.; Coêlho Barbosa, F.; Nunes da Silva, H.; Andrade, A.L.S.; Lia Fook, M.V.; de Lima Silva, S.M.; Farias Leite, I. Chitosan/Essential Oils Formulations for Potential Use as Wound Dressing: Physical and Antimicrobial Properties. *Materials* **2019**, *12*, 2223. [CrossRef]
19. Alam, P.; Ansari, M.J.; Anwer, M.K.; Raish, M.; Kamal, Y.K.T.; Shakeel, F. Wound healing effects of nanoemulsion containing clove essential oil. *Artif. CellsNanomed. Biotechnol.* **2017**, *45*, 591–597. [CrossRef]
20. Cui, H.; Bai, M.; Rashed, M.M.A.; Lin, L. The antibacterial activity of clove oil/chitosan nanoparticles embedded gelatin nanofibers against *Escherichia coli* O157:H7 biofilms on cucumber. *Int. J. Food Microbiol.* **2018**, *266*, 69–78. [CrossRef]
21. Verma, C.; Rohit, P.S.; Anjum, S.; Gupta, B. Novel Approach for Nanobiocomposites by Nanoencapsulation of Lecithin-Clove oil within PVA Nanofibrous Web. *Mater. Today Proc.* **2019**, *15*, 183–187. [CrossRef]
22. Sill, T.; von Recum, H.A. Electrospinning: Applications in drug delivery and tissue engineering. *Biomaterials* **2008**, *29*, 1989–2006. [CrossRef] [PubMed]
23. Martins, A.; Reis, R.L.; Neves, N.M. Electrospinning: Processing technique for tissue engineering scaffolding. *Int. Mater. Rev.* **2008**, *53*, 257–274. [CrossRef]
24. Wang, L.; Abedalwafa, M.; Wang, F.; Li, C. Biodegradable poly-epsilon-caprolactone (PCL) for tissue engineering applications: A review. *Rev. Adv. Mater. Sci.* **2013**, *34*, 123–140.

25. Gaspar-Pintiliescu, A.; Stanciuc, A.-M.; Craciunescu, O. Natural composite dressings based on collagen, gelatin and plant bioactive compounds for wound healing: A review. *Int. J. Biol. Macromol.* **2019**, *138*, 854–865. [CrossRef]
26. Yao, R.; He, J.; Meng, G.; Jiang, B.; Wu, F. Electrospun PCL/Gelatin composite fibrous scaffolds: Mechanical properties and cellular responses. *J. Biomater. Sci. Polym. Ed.* **2016**, *27*, 824–838. [CrossRef]
27. Ramalingam, R.; Dhand, C.; Leung, C.M.; Ezhilarasu, H.; Prasannan, P.; Ong, S.T.; Subramanian, S.; Kamruddin, M.; Lakshminarayanan, R.; Ramakrishna, S.; et al. Poly-ε-caprolactone/gelatin hybrid electrospun composite nanofibrous mats containing ultrasound assisted herbal extract: Antimicrobial and cell proliferation study. *Nanomaterials* **2019**, *9*, 462. [CrossRef]
28. Fallah, M.; Bahrami, S.H.; Ranjbar-Mohammadi, M. Fabrication and characterization of PCL/gelatin/curcumin nanofibers and their antibacterial properties. *J. Ind. Text.* **2016**, *46*, 562–577. [CrossRef]
29. Chemat, F.; Vian, M. Green extraction of natural products: Concept and principles. *Int. J. Mol. Sci* **2012**, *13*, 8615–8627. [CrossRef]
30. Liverani, L.; Boccaccini, A.R. Versatile production of poly (epsilon-caprolactone) fibers by electrospinning using benign solvents. *Nanomaterials* **2016**, *6*, 75. [CrossRef]
31. Engel, W.; Bahr, W.; Schieberle, P. Solvent assisted flavour evaporation–a new and versatile technique for the careful and direct isolation of aroma compounds from complex food matrices. *Eur. Food Res. Technol.* **1999**, *209*, 237–241. [CrossRef]
32. Bemelmans, J.M.H. Review of Isolation and Concentration Techniques Progress in flavour research. *Appl. Sci.* **1976**, *8*, 79–98.
33. Liang, C.C.; Park, A.Y.; Guan, J.L. In vitro scratch assay: A convenient and inexpensive method for analysis of cell migration *in vitro*. *Nat. Protoc.* **2007**, *2*, 329. [CrossRef] [PubMed]
34. Ghasemi-Mobarakeh, L.; Prabhakaran, M.P.; Morshed, M.; Nasr-Esfahani, M.H.; Ramakrishna, S. Electrospun poly(ε-caprolactone)/gelatin nanofibrous scaffolds for nerve tissue engineering. *Biomaterials* **2008**, *29*, 4532–4539. [CrossRef] [PubMed]
35. Garg, K.; Bowlin, G.L. Electrospinning jets and nanofibrous structures. *Biomicrofluidics* **2011**, *5*, 013403. [CrossRef] [PubMed]
36. Cramariuc, B.; Cramariuc, R.; Scarlet, R.; Manea, L.R.; Lupu, I.G.; Cramariuc, O. Fiber diameter in electrospinning process. *J. Electrostat.* **2013**, *71*, 189–198. [CrossRef]
37. García-Moreno, P.J.; Guadix, A.; Guadix, E.M.; Jacobsen, C. Physical and oxidative stability of fish oil-in-water emulsions stabilized with fish protein hydrolysates. *Food Chem.* **2016**, *203*, 124–135. [CrossRef]
38. Mori, C.L.; Passos, N.A.D.; Oliveira, J.E.; Altoé, T.F.; Mori, F.A.; Mattoso, L.H.C.; Tonoli, G.H.D. Nanostructured polylactic acid/candeia essential oil mats obtained by electrospinning. *J. Nanomater.* **2015**, *16*, 33. [CrossRef]
39. Xu, L.C.; Siedlecki, C.A. Effects of surface wettability and contact time on protein adhesion to biomaterial surfaces. *Biomaterials* **2007**, *28*, 3273–3283. [CrossRef]
40. Liu, Y.; Wang, S.; Zhang, R.; Lan, W.; Qin, W. Development of poly(lactic acid)/chitosan fibers loaded with essential oil for antimicrobial applications. *Nanomaterials* **2017**, *7*, 194. [CrossRef]
41. Agnes Mary, S.; Giri Dev, V.R. Electrospun herbal nanofibrous wound dressings for skin tissue engineering. *J. Text. Inst.* **2015**, *106*, 886–895. [CrossRef]
42. Tampau, A.; González-Martinez, C.; Chiralt, A. Carvacrol encapsulation in starch or PCL based matrices by electrospinning. *J. Food Eng.* **2017**, *214*, 245–256. [CrossRef]
43. Tavassoli-Kafrani, E.; Goli, S.A.H.; Fathi, M. Encapsulation of Orange Essential Oil Using Cross-linked Electrospun Gelatin Nanofibers. *Food Bioprocess Technol.* **2018**, *11*, 427–434. [CrossRef]
44. Figueroa-Lopez, K.J.; Castro-Mayorga, J.L.; Andrade-Mahecha, M.M.; Cabedo, L.; Lagaron, J.M. Antibacterial and barrier properties of gelatin coated by electrospun polycaprolactone ultrathin fibers containing black pepper oleoresin of interest in active food biopackaging applications. *Nanomaterials* **2018**, *8*, 199. [CrossRef] [PubMed]
45. Li, Z.; Zhou, P.; Zhou, F.; Zhao, Y.; Ren, L.; Yuan, X. Antimicrobial eugenol-loaded electrospun membranes of poly(ε-caprolactone)/gelatin incorporated with REDV for vascular graft applications. *Colloids Surf B Biointerfaces* **2018**, *162*, 335–344. [CrossRef] [PubMed]
46. Tang, Y.; Zhou, Y.; Lan, X.; Huang, D.; Luo, T.; Ji, J.; Mafang, Z.; Miao, X.; Wang, H.; Wang, W. Electrospun Gelatin Nanofibers Encapsulated with Peppermint and Chamomile Essential Oils as Potential Edible Packaging. *J. Agric. Food Chem.* **2019**, *67*, 2227–2234. [CrossRef]

47. Hajiali, H.; Summa, M.; Russo, D.; Armirotti, A.; Brunetti, V.; Bertorelli, R.; Athanassiou, A.; Mele, E. Alginate-lavender nanofibers with antibacterial and anti-inflammatory activity to effectively promote burn healing. *J. Mater. Chem. B* **2016**, *4*, 1686–1695. [CrossRef]
48. Balasubramanian, K.; Kodam, K.M. Encapsulation of therapeutic lavender oil in an electrolyte assisted polyacrylonitrile nanofibres for antibacterial applications. *RSC Adv.* **2014**, *4*, 54892–54901. [CrossRef]
49. Rieger, K.A.; Birch, N.P.; Schiffman, J.D. Designing electrospun nanofiber mats to promote wound healing-a review. *J. Mater. Chem. B* **2013**, *1*, 4531–4541. [CrossRef]
50. Reinke, J.M.; Sorg, H. Wound repair and regeneration. *Eur. Surg. Res.* **2012**, *49*, 35–43. [CrossRef]
51. Da Silva, S.M.M.; Costa, C.R.R.; Gelfuso, G.M.; Guerra, E.N.S.; De Medeiros Nóbrega, Y.K.; Gomes, S.M.; Pic-Taylor, A.; Fonseca-Bazzo, Y.M.; Silveira, D.; De Oliveira Magalhães, P. Wound healing effect of essential oil extracted from eugenia dysenterica DC (Myrtaceae) leaves. *Molecules* **2019**, *24*, 2. [CrossRef]
52. Léguillier, T.; Lecsö-Bornet, M.; Lémus, C.; Rousseau-Ralliard, D.; Lebouvier, N.; Hnawia, E.; Nour, M.; Aalbersberg, W.; Ghazi, K.; Raharivelomanana, P.; et al. The wound healing and antibacterial activity of five ethnomedical Calophyllum inophyllum oils: An alternative therapeutic strategy to treat infected wounds. *PLoS ONE* **2015**, *10*, e0138602. [CrossRef]

Development and Evaluation of Alginate Membranes with Curcumin-Loaded Nanoparticles for Potential Wound-Healing Applications

Mónica C. Guadarrama-Acevedo [1,†], Raisa A. Mendoza-Flores [1,†], María L. Del Prado-Audelo [1,2], Zaida Urbán-Morlán [1], David M. Giraldo-Gomez [3], Jonathan J. Magaña [4], Maykel González-Torres [5,6], Octavio D. Reyes-Hernández [7], Gabriela Figueroa-González [8], Isaac H. Caballero-Florán [1,9], Carla D. Florán-Hernández [4], Benjamín Florán [9], Hernán Cortés [4] and Gerardo Leyva-Gómez [1,*]

[1] Departamento de Farmacia, Facultad de Química, Universidad Nacional Autónoma de México, Ciudad Universitaria, Circuito Exterior S/N, Del. Coyoacán, Ciudad de México 04510, México
[2] Laboratorio de Posgrado en Tecnología Farmacéutica, FES-Cuautitlán, Universidad Nacional Autónoma de México, Cuautitlán Izcalli 54740, México
[3] Departamento de Biología Celular y Tisular, Facultad de Medicina, Universidad Nacional Autónoma de México (UNAM), Edificio "A" 3er piso, Circuito Interior, Avenida Universidad 3000, Ciudad Universitaria, Coyoacán, Ciudad de México 04510, México
[4] Laboratorio de Medicina Genómica, Departamento de Genética, Instituto Nacional de Rehabilitación Luis Guillermo Ibarra Ibarra, Ciudad de México 14389, México
[5] CONACyT-Laboratorio de Biotecnología, Instituto Nacional de Rehabilitación Luis Guillermo Ibarra Ibarra, Ciudad de México 14389, México
[6] Instituto Tecnológico y de Estudios Superiores de Monterrey, Campus Ciudad de México 14380, México
[7] Laboratorio de Biología Molecular del Cáncer, UMIEZ, Facultad de Estudios Superiores Zaragoza, Universidad Nacional Autónoma de México, Ciudad de México 09230, México
[8] CONACyT-Laboratorio de Genómica, Dirección de Investigación, Instituto Nacional de Cancerología. Av. San Fernando 22, Tlalpan, Sección XVI, Ciudad de México 14080, México
[9] Departamento de Fisiología, Biofísica & Neurociencias, Centro de Investigación y de Estudios Avanzados del Instituto Politécnico Nacional, Ciudad de México 07360, México
* Correspondence: gerardoleyva@hotmail.com
† Mónica C. Guadarrama-Acevedo and Raisa A. Mendoza-Flores equally contributed as first authors to the present work.

Abstract: Non-biodegradable materials with a low swelling capacity and which are opaque and occlusive are the main problems associated with the clinical performance of some commercially available wound dressings. In this work, a novel biodegradable wound dressing was developed by means of alginate membrane and polycaprolactone nanoparticles loaded with curcumin for potential use in wound healing. Curcumin was employed as a model drug due to its important properties in wound healing, including antimicrobial, antifungal, and anti-inflammatory effects. To determine the potential use of wound dressing, in vitro, ex vivo, and in vivo studies were carried out. The novel membrane exhibited the diverse functional characteristics required to perform as a substitute for synthetic skin, such as a high capacity for swelling and adherence to the skin, evidence of pores to regulate the loss of transepidermal water, transparency for monitoring the wound, and drug-controlled release by the incorporation of nanoparticles. The incorporation of the nanocarriers aids the drug in permeating into different skin layers, solving the solubility problems of curcumin. The clinical application of this system would cover extensive areas of mixed first- and second-degree wounds, without the need for removal, thus decreasing the patient's discomfort and the risk of altering the formation of the new epithelium.

Keywords: wound dressing; polymeric membrane; nanoparticles; curcumin; alginate; pluronic F68; drug skin permeation; Franz cells; tape stripping

1. Introduction

Human skin exerts a pivotal function as a protection barrier against diverse exogenous noxious factors; however, it is exposed and undergoes diverse types of injuries, including burns, ulcers, trauma, lacerations, and acute or chronic wounds, which may compromise its integrity [1].

In this regard, when skin is damaged, a specialized and highly regulated dynamic process immediately takes place: wound healing [2]. The main goal of wound healing is to restore tissue integrity and to achieve homeostasis; however, this process may be complicated by distinct intrinsic and extrinsic factors [2]. Thus, in order to accelerate wound healing, a variety of wound dressings have been designed.

Irrespective of the type of wound, the main function of dressings is to aid in the repair of the wound through the reduction of pain and inflammation, to protect the damaged tissue from pathogenic agents, and to enhance cell differentiation and proliferation [3]. Although there several types of dressings which are commercially available, many of these present some drawbacks, such as an inefficient absorption of exudates, poor protection against infections by microbes, the lack of ability to maintain humidity, and the triggering of allergic effects [4]. In addition, several dressings may adhere to the wound and require constant changes, which may interfere with the granulation process and delay the healing course.

Therefore, in recent years, there has been increasing interest in asymmetric membranes as an alternative for designing wound dressings [5]. These types of membranes possess multiple advantages, such as structural similarity with the skin, an ability to absorb exudates due to their porous structure, and improved cell adhesion and proliferation [6,7]. Different polymers have been employed for their development, including chitosan, hyaluronic acid, collagen, poly vinyl alcohol (PVA), polycaprolactone (PCL), and alginate [8]. In particular, alginate is a biopolymer extracted from seaweed and has shown several unique properties, such as biodegradability, good hydrophilicity, and good biocompatibility [4]. Alginate has exhibited potential for improving wound healing due to its hemostatic properties; moreover, it may reduce microbial infections, enhance the absorption of exudates, and decrease allergic reactions [9]. These features render alginate an interesting option for wound dressings. In addition, alginate membranes possess the advantage that they may be functionalized with bioactive compounds that enhance their healing properties.

In this regard, curcumin is a natural compound that possesses a plethora of biological activities, including antimicrobial, antifungal, anti-inflammatory, and antioxidant effects [10–12]. In addition, curcumin improves wound healing, enhances epithelial regeneration, and increases the proliferation of fibroblasts [13,14]. Thus, curcumin could be a suitable pharmacological agent for the elaboration of wound dressings. However, curcumin exhibits low bioavailability and is unstable in neutral and alkaline aqueous solutions, as well as in hydrophilic topical preparations [12,15]. These drawbacks could be overcome by a nanoparticle formulation that permits the controlled and gradual release of the compound.

Therefore, the objective of this study was to design and develop a novel wound dressing comprising an alginate membrane and PCL nanoparticles loaded with curcumin and stabilized with Pluronic® F-68 (CNp) for possible application in wound healing. The wound dressing was physicochemically characterized, and in vivo and ex vivo permeation assays were performed.

2. Materials and Methods

2.1. Materials

For CNp fabrication, we used PCL (Mn 80,000 g/mol), Pluronic® F-68, and trehalose dihydrate, which were purchased from Sigma-Aldrich® (Merck KGaA, Darmstadt, Germany), whereas methanol, ethyl acetate, and curcumin were supplied by Spectrum® (Spectrum Laboratory Products, CA, USA). For membrane elaboration and characterization, we employed sodium alginate [(SA) (300–700 cps 1.0%, RV, 20 rpm, 25 °C], glycerol (Gly), propylene glycol (Prop), and Tween 80, which were purchased from Droguería Cosmopolita (Mexico City, Mexico). PVA, Pluronic® F-127, acetone, and phosphate buffered saline (PBS) solution were supplied by Sigma-Aldrich® (Merck KGaA, Darmstadt, Germany). Kollidon® 30 [Polyvinylpyrrolidone k 30; (PVP k30)] was obtained from BASF (USA). Ethyl acetate was acquired from Distribuidora Química Alvi (State of Mexico, Mexico). Methanol was purchased from Fermont (Nuevo León, Mexico). All other chemicals and reagents were of at least analytical-grade quality.

2.2. Preparation of PCL Nanoparticles Loaded with Curcumin (CNp)

CNp were prepared by the emulsification–diffusion method, as previously described by Quintanar-Guerrero, et al. [16]. Briefly, the organic saturated phase and aqueous saturated phase were obtained by the saturation of an ethyl acetate and distilled water mixture at a 1:1 ratio. After that, 2% (*w*/*v*) solution of PCL was prepared by dissolving 400 mg of PCL in 20 mL of the organic saturated phase; once PCL was dissolved, 100 mg of curcumin was added. At the same time, 5% (*w*/*v*) of Pluronic® F-68 solution was prepared using an aqueous saturated phase as solvent. In order to obtain an emulsion, both solutions were mixed at a 1:2 ratio with a high-speed homogenizer (Ultra Turrax T18; IKA®) at 14,000 rpm for 10 min at room temperature. Then, 160 mL of water was added to the emulsion to generate polymer aggregation, and the system was maintained under the same conditions for 10 min. The organic solvent was evaporated by a rotary vacuum (Heidolph®, Schwabach, Germany), and the nanoparticle suspension obtained was centrifuged at 15,557 *g* for 30 min at 25 °C. Finally, the pellet was dissolved in distilled water. In order to assess the thermal stability and the properties of the nanoparticles, CNp were frozen and lyophilized at −49 °C, 0.05 mBar for 24 h, employing 5% *w*/*v* trehalose dihydrate as a cryoprotectant.

2.3. Physicochemical Characterization of CNp

2.3.1. Particle Size and Zeta Potential Assessment

The particle size and distribution (polydispersity index, PDI) of the CNp were evaluated by dynamic light scattering. On the other hand, to determine the Zeta potential of CNp, laser Doppler velocimetry was employed. CNp dispersions were assessed five times at 25 °C in a Zetasizer (Malvern Instrument ZS90; Malvern, UK).

2.3.2. Atomic Force Microscopy (AFM)

CNp size and geometry were analyzed by atomic force microscopy (AFM) with a scanning probe microscope (JSPM-4210, JEOL®, Tokyo, Japan). In brief, the CNp dispersion was obtained after centrifugation, and the pellet resuspension was diluted to 1:100 with distilled water. A drop was placed on a coverslip, allowing it to dry at room temperature. The coverslip with the drop was held in place with carbon tape, and room-temperature conditions were utilized to assess the samples.

2.3.3. Drug Loading and Entrapment Efficiency of CNp

To calculate entrapment efficiency (EE) and drug loading (DL), the CNp dispersion was centrifuged at 15,557 *g* for 40 min; then, the sediment was resuspended in ethyl acetate and the absorbance was measured by UV–Vis spectrophotometry at 420 nm (DLAB®, SP-UV1000, Beijing, China). The amount of curcumin was obtained by interpolation in a calibration curve (R^2 coefficient = 0.99985).

The percentages of EE and DL were calculated from the equations below:

$$\%\ \text{EE} = \frac{\text{CN}}{\text{IC}} \times 100 \quad (1)$$

$$\%\ \text{DL} = \frac{\text{CN}}{\text{N}} \times 100 \quad (2)$$

where CN = the amount of curcumin in nanoparticles, IC = the initial amount of curcumin, and N = the number of nanoparticles.

2.4. Preparation of Polymer Gels and Membranes

Four membrane formulations based on SA (M1, M2, M3, and M4) (See Table 1) were prepared using the solvent casting method as published by Karki et al. [17]. First, SA and the polymer were dissolved separately in injectable water by stirring at 35 °C. After dissolution, they were mixed with each other by mechanical stirring. Then, the plasticizer (or a plasticizer mixture) was added by stirring at room temperature until a homogeneous gel was obtained. In order to eliminate bubbles from the gel, it was centrifuged at 636 *g* for 20 min at room temperature (BIOBASE, BKC-TH18II, Shandong, China).

Table 1. Formulation of alginate membranes with different polymers as plasticizers. PVA: poly vinyl alcohol; PVP: polyvinylpyrrolidone; CNp: polycaprolactone (PCL) nanoparticles loaded with curcumin.

Formulation Code	SA (% *w/v*)	Polymer		Plasticizer	
		PVA (%*w/v*)	PVP (%*w/v*)	Gly (%*w/v*)	Prop (%*v/v*)
	4	2	—	10	—
M2	4	2	—	10	12
M3	4	—	2	10	—
M4	4	—	2	10	12
CNp-M4	4	—	2	10	12

In order to obtain the membranes, 10 g of each gel, prepared with the previously mentioned methodology, was poured into a Teflon cast 12 cm in diameter and left to dry into an oven (OAKTON Stable Temp, IL, USA) at 75.0 ± 0.5 °C for 3 h.

2.4.1. Preparation of Nanoparticle-Coated Alginate Membranes (CNp-M4)

The methodology described previously was followed to prepare our nanoparticle-coated alginate membrane (CNp-M4), but the vehicle utilized was a dispersion of CNp to obtain 0.01% *w/v* of curcumin instead of injectable water. In order to prepare the membranes, the gel obtained was poured into a Teflon cast and left to dry in an oven at 40.0 ± 0.5 °C for 4 h.

2.5. Physicochemical Characterization of Membranes

2.5.1. Swelling Test

Samples of M1, M2, M3, M4, and CNp-M4 membranes were cut to a size of 1 × 1 cm and weighed on pre-weighed aluminum trays. The samples were divided into five blocks, corresponding to different times as follows: 5, 10, 20, 30, and 60 min. The membranes on the trays were placed on a flat surface, and 750 μL of PBS 1X pH 7.4 was added to each sample.

Once the established time had elapsed, the trays were turned vertically for 2 min on absorbent paper, allowing the draining and absorbption of the excess of PBS. After that time, the membranes in the trays were weighed again [18]. The assessment was performed in triplicate for each of the different times.

The swelling percentage (%S) was calculated using the following formula [19]:

$$\%S = \frac{M_s - M_d}{M_d} \times 100 \quad (3)$$

where M_s and M_d are the weight of the swollen membrane and dried membrane, respectively.

2.5.2. Mechanical Test

Tensile strength (TS) and the elongation at a break (%E) of M1, M2, M3, M4, and CNp-M4 were determined using a Sintech $\frac{1}{2}$ testing machine (MTS, USA), which was equipped with a 100-N load cell at a crosshead speed of 2.4 mm s^{-1}. Three samples of each formulation were cut into a dumbbell shape with a width of 10 mm and an effective length of 40 mm between the clamps at the beginning of the measurement. The thickness of each sample was measured using a Vernier at five different points before testing, and the average of these was employed for TS calculation. The load (Lb) and displacement (mm) of each film were recorded during the stretching. TS and %E were calculated by Equations (4) and (5), as published by Karki et al. [17]:

$$TS = \frac{F}{A} \quad (4)$$

$$\%E = \frac{D}{L} \times 100 \quad (5)$$

where TS is reported in MPa, F is the maximum load (N) required to break the film, and A is the initial cross-sectional area in mm^2. In Equation (5), D is the displacement of the film elongation at the rupture and L is the initial length.

2.5.3. Thermogravimetric Analysis (TGA)

The thermal stability of the membranes (M4, CNp-M4), CNp, and curcumin was evaluated through TGA, employing a Hi-Res TGA 2950 Thermogravimetric Analyzer (Modulated TA Instruments, New Castle, DE, USA). In brief, 5 mg of each sample was analyzed starting at room temperature and increasing to 500 °C at a heating rate of 10 °C/min under a nitrogen atmosphere.

2.5.4. Differential Scanning Calorimetry (DSC)

The thermal properties of the membranes (M4, CNp-M4), CNp, and curcumin were determined with the DSC 2910 (Modulated TA Instruments, DE, USA). Lyophilized samples were placed in hermetic aluminum cells and evaluated starting at room temperature and increasing to 250 °C at a heating rate of 10 °C/min under a nitrogen atmosphere.

2.5.5. pH Values

The pH values of M1, M2, M3, M4, and CNp-M4 polymer gels was measured through a pH meter. The samples were put into contact with the electrode until a constant value was obtained. The pH meter was previously calibrated against standard solutions to ensure the highest level of accuracy.

2.5.6. Structure and Morphology of M4 and CNp-M4 Membranes

In order to analyze the structure and morphology of the membranes, samples were cut in a circular shape 1 cm in diameter and in a longitudinal section and were analyzed using a scanning electron microscope (Jeol-JCM 6000, MA, USA) at 100× and 220× magnification; then, photographs were taken in four different fields.

The pore diameter and membrane width were measured using a software package (ImageJ, MD, USA), and the average was calculated. Pore number was counted field-by-field, and the average was determined.

In order to evaluate the transparency of M4 and CNp-M4 membranes, samples were cut into a circular shape 3 cm in diameter and these were placed over an image (before swelling); then, they were observed and photographed. Afterward, 1 mL of PBS 1X was added to the samples, and after 20 min (swelling process), photographs were taken of the samples.

2.5.7. In Vitro Release Study of Drug Dispersion, CNp and CNp-M4 Membrane

To evaluate the curcumin release profile from the CNp and CNp-M4 membrane, the direct dispersion method was applied. For the drug and CNp dispersion, a certain amount of curcumin (and the equivalent in nanoparticles) was dissolved into PBS solution (pH 7.4, Pluronic® F-127 2% *w*/*v*), divided into sets of three tubes each, and placed in a shaker incubator, maintaining this at 37 °C. For the CNp-M4 membrane, disks 1 cm in diameter were placed in tubes with the PBS solution under the conditions previously described. At the defined times of 0, 0.25, 0.5, 1, 2, 4, 6, 24, and 48 h, one set of tubes was removed from shaking and centrifuged at 18,514 *g* for 30 min. The curcumin released in the supernatant was quantified by UV-Vis spectrophotometry at 420 nm.

The results of the release tests of CNp and CNp-M4 membrane were analyzed by mathematical models such as zero-order, first-order, the Higuchi model, and the Korsmeyer–Peppas model to predict the drug release mechanism.

2.6. Permeation Assays

2.6.1. Ex Vivo Permeation Assay

Porcine skin was obtained from the back of pig ears within 12 h after slaughter. The pig ears were cut into circular sections 3 cm in diameter. The excess of fat was removed with surgical scissors, and the samples were washed with saline solution. The samples were divided into three groups: drug dispersion with 0.01% *w*/*v* of curcumin (2 mL; $n = 3$), CNp dispersion with 0.01% *w*/*v* of curcumin (2 mL; $n = 3$), and CNp-M4 membranes (3 cm in diameter; $n = 3$).

The experiments were conducted in 12 independent Franz cells with a diffusion area of 7.07 cm^2. The freshly excised skin was placed into Franz cells, and the stratum corneum remained in contact with the donor compartment, with the dermis facing the receptor compartment. This was filled with 30 mL of 0.1 M PBS solution (pH 7.4) with 2.5% of Tween 80 and maintained under constant stirring at 400 rpm.

Franz cells were immersed in a water bath at a constant temperature of 37.0 ± 0.5 °C. At predetermined times (1, 2, 3, 4, 5, 6, 7, 8, 22, 24, 26, 28, and 30 h), 1000 µL of medium was removed from the receptor compartment and replaced with 1000 µL of fresh receptor medium.

At the end of the test, the skin samples were carefully removed from the Franz cells to conduct the tape-stripping test, following the in vivo permeation assay methodology (described in Section 2.6.2). All tapes were placed in a flask with 40 mL of acetone and mechanically stirred for 15 h. Subsequently, each skin sample was fragmented into small pieces using surgical scissors. The curcumin was extracted with 25 mL of ethyl acetate:methanol at a ratio of 9:1. The extract was centrifuged at 10,174 *g* for 10 min. All samples were analyzed by UV-visible spectrophotometry at a wavelength of 420 nm.

2.6.2. In Vivo Permeation Assay

To evaluate the in vivo permeation of the CNp-M4 membrane through the stratum corneum, the tape-stripping technique was employed. Four healthy Mexican males aged 22–36 years were recruited as volunteers. The individuals had neither a history of skin disorders nor had used cosmetic products on their forearms 24 h prior to the test. Written informed consent was obtained from each volunteer before each study.

Four sites (3 × 3 cm) were demarcated: two on the right forearm and two on the left forearm. Before administering the treatment, the sites were cleaned with cotton impregnated with water. Three treatments were administered to each volunteer. The CNp dispersion with 0.01% of curcumin (2 mL) and the drug dispersion at the same concentration were contained within a glass cylinder on the left forearm. The CNp-M4 membrane (3 cm in diameter) was put on the right forearm, and 1.75 mL of distilled water was added onto the surface of the membrane. The last site on the right forearm was used for the blank. The treatments were in contact with the skin for 6 h [20]. Once the time had elapsed, the membrane was removed with steel nippers. The skin was subjected to 15 successive tape strips (Scotch® 3M®), previously cut into 3 × 3 cm squares. In each case, the site was pressed uniformly by sliding a spatula over the surface of the tape five times; then, it was removed by pulling it with steel nippers from the lower right to the upper left end. The blank site was subjected to the same procedure. Each tape was immersed in 15 mL of acetone in a different amber glass bottle with a lid. All of the bottles were placed under mechanical agitation for 15 h; subsequently, the samples were filtered to remove the glue particles. The quantification of curcumin was performed by UV–visible spectrophotometry at a wavelength of 420 nm. Each sample was analyzed in triplicate.

3. Results and Discussion

3.1. *Physicochemical Characterization of CNp*

3.1.1. Particle Size and Zeta Potential Assessment

CNps were obtained, and their mean particle size and PDI were 148.3 ± 1.9 nm and 0.044 ± 0.020, respectively. These values were expected to improve dermal permeation [21], since nanoparticles below 500 nm have a larger surface area-to-volume ratio, which ensures direct contact with the stratum corneum and skin appendages [6,7]. Moreover, the PDI value was below 0.1, which indicates that the small size measured in the sample is reliable and monodisperse [22].

On the other hand, CNp exhibited a zeta potential value of −7.32 ± 0.03 mV. In this regard, zeta potential is commonly employed to measure the charge in the nanoparticles and/or electrostatic repulsion [1], and the literature indicates that nanoparticles are stable in suspension with a zeta potential above ±30 mV [23]. Despite the CNp zeta potential value not being in this range, it should be considered that Pluronic® F-68 was added as a stabilizer of nanoparticles, which provides them with stability by means of a repulsion effect through a steric mechanism [24]. Likewise, CNp possesses a negative charge, which is related to the carboxylic end group of PCL [25]; thus, negatively charged nanoparticles could permeate adequately in conjunction with the negative charges existing on the skin [26].

3.1.2. Atomic Force Microscopy (AFM)

The morphology and size of CNp were evaluated by AFM. In agreement with the particle-size and zeta-potential assessments, the nanoparticles demonstrated a spherical shape and a size of approximately 200 nm with no agglomeration (Figure 1) [27]. These results support the idea that the small size of CNp could improve the dermal permeation of curcumin, which would increase its anti-inflammatory, antimicrobial, and wound-healing activities [6,12].

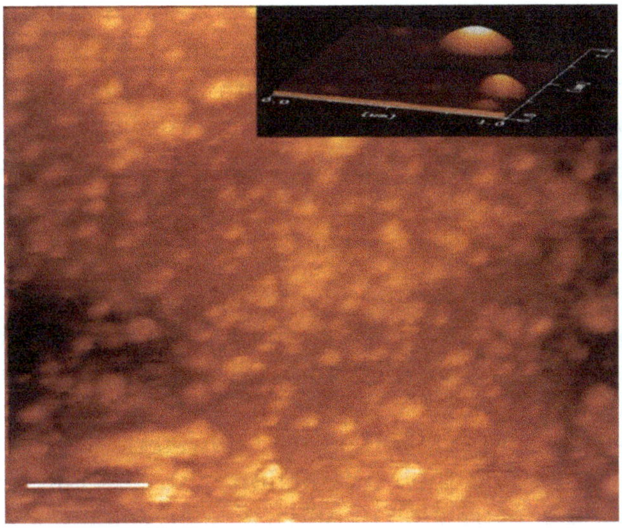

Figure 1. Atomic force microscopy (AFM) topography images of the CNp. The size bar is 1 μm.

3.1.3. Drug Loading and Entrapment Efficiency of Nanoparticles

In order to determine the amount of curcumin entrapped inside the CNp, the DL and EE were determined. The CNp showed DL and EE values of 4.9 ± 0.7% and 96.01 ± 0.95%, respectively. It is known that the emulsification diffusion method ensures high encapsulation efficiencies (generally >70%) [28]. On the other hand, DL depends on nanoparticle structure and methodology [29], whereas both DL and EE depend on the interactions between the drug, the matrix, and the medium [29].

3.2. Physicochemical and Mechanical Characterization of Nanoparticle-Coated Alginate Membranes as Wound Dressings

3.2.1. Swelling Test

From a practical point of view, the membranes should absorb the exudate from the wound and at the same time provide a moist environment that promotes healing. For this reason, the percentage of swelling of five different formulations was determined by weight difference (Figure 2).

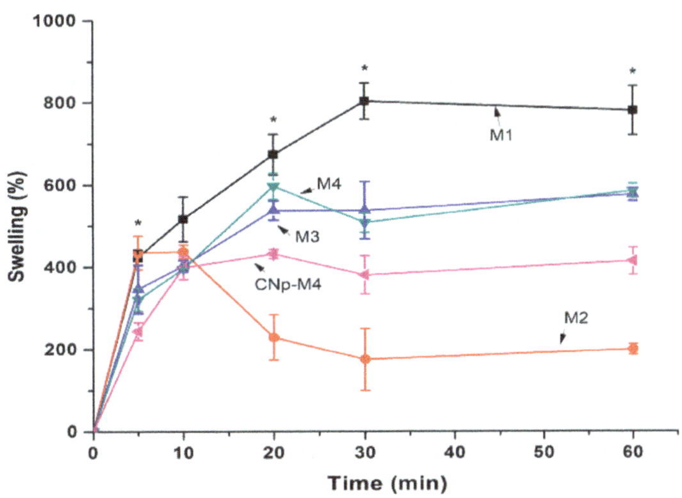

Figure 2. Percentage of swelling in alginate membranes as a function of time. Effect on swelling capacity by the addition of PVA + glycerin (**M1**), PVA + glycerin + propylene glycol (**M2**), PVP + glycerin (**M3**), PVP + glycerin + propylene glycol (**M4**), and CNp + PVP + glycerin + propylene glycol (**CNp-M4**) (mean ± SE; $n = 3$). There were significant differences when ANOVA was applied at 5, 20, 30, and 60 min ($p < 0.05$).

Figure 2 depicts a difference at a time of 20 min, when propylene glycol is added to the formulation with PVA (M2) in comparison to M1; however, there is no significant difference between using or not using propylene glycol in the formulation combined with PVP (M3 and M4, respectively). In order to determine the differences in the percentage of swelling according to each formulation as a function of time, an ANOVA was performed. It was demonstrated that both the formulation and the time during which the membrane was exposed to PBS exerted a statistically significant effect on swelling with a 95% confidence level.

The formulation with the highest swelling value was M1, at 30 min (802.8 ± 76.0%), while the addition of propylene glycol (M2) decreased the swelling percentage after 10 min. On the other hand, M2 showed the lowest value in the swelling test before dissolving. The addition of propylene glycol to the polyvinyl alcohol mixture could increase the intermolecular interactions between both excipients via hydrogen bonds in the –OH groups, favored by a wide steric disposition, but could decrease the entry capacity of water molecules and their interaction with alginate by saturation, decreasing the swelling ability. In the case of the interaction of propylene glycol and PVP, the situation could be the opposite. The interaction of both excipients is lower, resulting in a lower swelling capacity of the alginate; i.e., the excipient that determines the majority of the response. This phenomenon is confirmed with the profile observed for CNp-M4 in relation to M4.

Namely, when water enters the polymer matrix, the chains begin to relax, giving rise to the opening of the polymer networks. This promotes the penetration of more water; however, in the last stages of swelling, the diffusion coefficient is diminished because the chains are completely relaxed and near equilibrium [30].

The membranes began to dissolve after being exposed to PBS for a longer period of time. According to the composition of the medium, polymers undergo degradation and erosion processes. When a polymer degrades, the chains are cleaved into oligomers and subsequently monomers. The continuous loss of monomers will eventually lead to the phenomenon of erosion, which progressively changes the microstructure of the membrane through the formation of pores [31]. The combination of these processes could favor the possible application of our M4 and CNp-M4 membranes as wound dressings, because it would not be necessary to remove them from the application site, avoiding harm through injury and discomfort to the patient.

Moreover, the level of exudate from a wound (for example, an ulcer) can vary from absent (dry ulcer) to minimally exuding (<5 mL fluid per 24 h), to moderately exuding (5 to 10 mL fluid per 24 h), and finally to highly exuding (>10 mL fluid per 24 h) [32]. In this regard, the measurement of the swelling capacity of a wound dressing developed with alginate could be classified as dressings of low absorbance (alginate wound dressing that absorbs less than 6 g of liquid per g of dressing, or less than 12 g/100 cm^2), and dressings of high absorbency (an alginate wound dressing that absorbs 6 g or more liquid per g of dressing, or 12 g or more/100 cm^2) [33]. With this consideration, CNp-M4 possesses a value of 17.48 g/100 cm^2, corresponding to high absorbency and similar to several commercial products.

3.2.2. Mechanical Test

Wound dressings must be resistant and flexible for ease of handling [17]. Thus, the mechanical properties of the membranes are depicted in Figure 3. Formulations with PVA (M1 and M2) did not demonstrate a significant difference in %E with 73.54 ± 0.87% and 74.90 ± 1.67%, respectively. TS was similar for M1, M2, and M3 samples with 1.32 ± 0.02, 1.34 ± 0.01, and 1.96 ± 0.05 MPa, respectively. By way of comparison, M1 and M2 membranes exhibited a lower TS and %E than the remaining formulations, probably due to PVA being a polymer that has been characterized as possessing poor elasticity, a rigid membrane, and low hydrophilic characteristics [34].

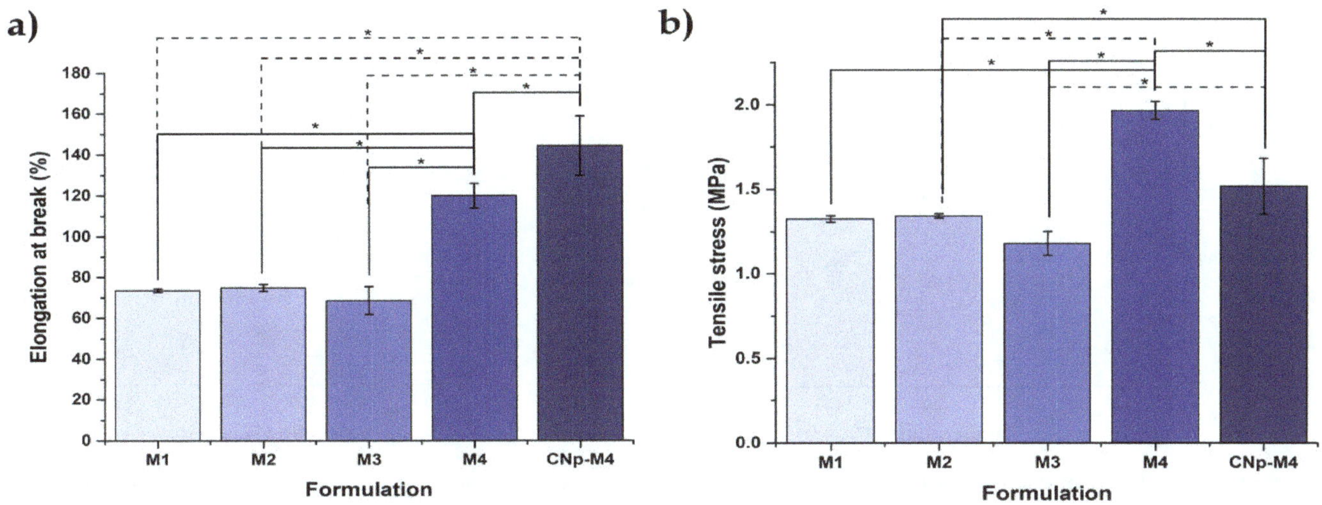

Figure 3. Effect of plasticizers on the mechanical properties of alginate membranes. Effect on mechanical properties by the addition of PVA + glycerin (M1), PVA + glycerin + propylene glycol (M2), PVP + glycerin (M3), PVP + glycerin + propylene glycol (M4), and CNp + PVP + glycerin + propylene glycol (CNp-M4), respectively. (**a**) Elongation at break; (**b**) tensile stress, (mean ± SD; $n = 3$). * indicates $p < 0.05$ as statistically significant.

The %E and TS of M3 were 68.63 ± 6.75% and 1.18 ± 0.07 MPa, respectively; these values significantly increased with the addition of propylene glycol (M4), to 120.01 ± 5.97% and 1.96 ± 0.05 MPa, respectively. M4 exhibited the highest values in the assay and showed a significant difference with respect to the remaining formulations without CNp. This may be explained, at least in part, by the properties of propylene glycol, which is a plasticizer with a small molecular weight that is able to create multiple H-bonds with PVP and SA chains into a package and, consequently, aid in the formation of cross-linked networks [35].

Therefore, because of its greater swelling capacity and better mechanical properties, the M4 membrane (a mixture of sodium alginate, PVP, and propylene glycol) was chosen for the incorporation of CNp.

On the other hand, the mechanical properties of M4 were modified when CNp dispersion was added to the formulation. The %E of CNp-M4 showed the highest value, with 144.39 ± 14.52%; in contrast, TS decreased to 1.52 ± 0.16 MPa. This could be due to the addition of CNp dispersion to the formulation decreasing the number of hydrogen bonds between the polymer molecular chains; as a result, less strength is necessary to break the membrane [36]. In comparison, CNp-M4 showed the highest %E, which could be due to the effect of Pluronic® F-68. The latter is a surfactant that decreases the pore number, providing a membrane with a homogeneous structure; thus, it is more resistant to changes, rendering higher elasticity properties.

3.2.3. Thermogravimetric Analysis (TGA)

It is important to determine the thermal properties of a substance, because these provide useful information for their identification and the characterization of materials. In Figure 4, thermograms of curcumin, CNp, M4, and CNp-M4 membranes are presented. For curcumin, mass loss was observed at 173 °C by TGA (Figure 4a); due to the degradation of turmeric powder, water loss was not observed, possibly due to its high hydrophobicity [37]. The weight loss of CNp started at approximately 90 °C, corresponding to dehydration, and there was a second plateau from 280 to 350 °C, suggesting a better thermal stability for curcumin when it is inside PCL nanoparticles than when alone. However, CNp lost more weight in a smaller temperature range.

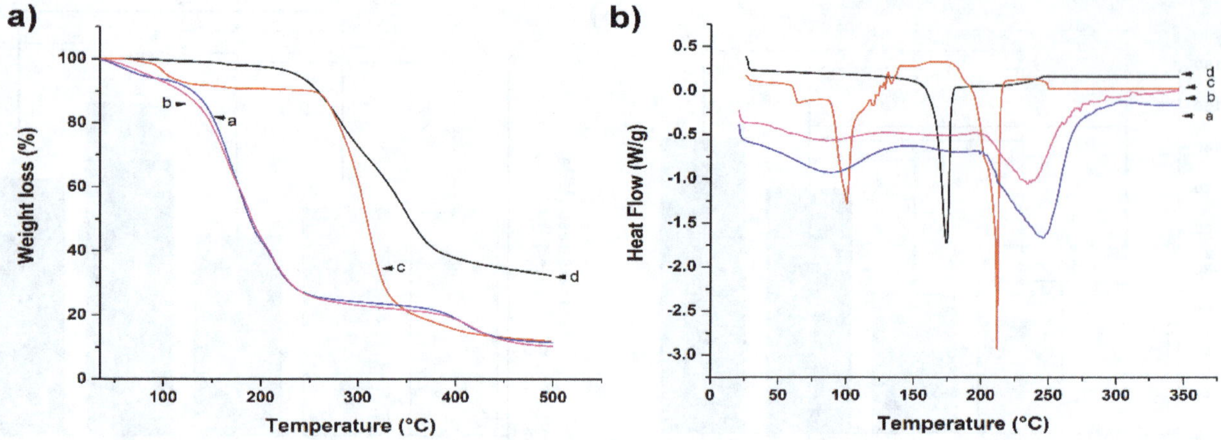

Figure 4. Thermal analysis of nanoparticle-coated alginate membrane using (**a**) thermogravimetric analysis (TGA) and (**b**) differential scanning calorimetry (DSC). The thermal properties of the M4 membrane, CNp-M4 membrane, CNp, and curcumin are represented as a, b, c, and d, respectively.

On the other hand, in the M4 membrane, the first mass loss occurred between 90 and 240 °C, whereas for the CNp-M4 sample, weight loss began between 100 and 240 °C. This could be due to the evaporation of water traces, the degradation of propylene glycol, PVP, glycerin (150-220 °C), and turmeric powder [38]. In the case of the CNp-M4 membrane, it presented a slighter weight loss compared to the M4 membrane. The second mass loss of both samples was between 270 and 425 °C; in this stage, the decomposition of the functional groups of SA polymer chains is presented. Finally, the last plateau in M4 and CNp-M4 membranes started at 425 °C, which corresponds to the degradation of the SA backbone [19]. In the same manner, the CNp-M4 membrane thermogram revealed a lower weight-loss temperature compared with that of CNp; this is probably because membrane formulation is a mixture that contains more substances than CNp. This is similar to the thermal behavior exhibited by curcumin and CNp.

3.2.4. Differential Scanning Calorimetry (DSC)

DSC is a technique used to determine the quantity of heat either absorbed or released when substances undergo physical or chemical changes [39]. In Figure 4b, DSC thermograms of curcumin, CNp, M4 membrane as vehicle, and CNp-M4 membrane are presented. The melting point of curcumin was found to be 174 °C (Table 2), which was expected with regard to the literature [40]. Furthermore, three thermal events were observed in the CNp: at 63.5; 101, and 212 °C. The first thermal event could correspond to the melting point of PCL (61 °C) [41], while events at 101 and 212 °C may indicate the presence of trehalose, which was employed as a cryoprotectant to lyophilize the CNp [42]. Interestingly, the melting point of curcumin was not detected in the CNp sample; this could be due to the high EE of curcumin inside PCL nanoparticles as a molecular dispersion.

Table 2. Thermal events of curcumin, CNp, and alginate membranes by DSC.

Sample	T_{m1} (°C)	T_{m2} (°C)	T_{m3} (°C)
Curcumin	174	—	—
CNp	63.5	101	212
M4	87	249	—
CNp-M4	87	233	—

On the other hand, both M4 and CNp-M4 membranes revealed two thermal events. The first peak was around 87 °C for both formulations, whereas the second peak was around 233 °C for the M4 membrane and 249 °C for the CNp-M4 membrane. The latter peaks were due to the presence of SA in the formulation. A thermal peak prior to 100 °C was observed for both samples, possibly due to the presence of water in the membranes.

3.2.5. pH Determination

The pH values of all the polymer gels were 5.78 ± 0.06, 5.76 ± 0.03, 5.65 ± 0.01, 5.97 ± 0.05 and 5.68 ± 0.03 for M1, M2, M3, M4, and CNp-M4, respectively. All of these values are acceptable because pH wound dressings must be neither acid nor alkaline in order to avoid skin irritation. Moreover, membrane pH is important to regulate the wound-healing process. The natural pH of the skin is within a range of 5–6, depending on the person, while the pH of the chronic wound oscillates in an alkaline range between pH 7 and 8, which increases susceptibility to wound infection.

3.2.6. Structure and Morphology of M4 and CNp-M4 Membranes

An ideal scaffold is expected to have a suitable microstructure (number of pores and pore size controlled) in order to transport nutrients, cells, metabolites, gases, and signaling molecules [43]. In this respect, pores were observed in the top of the membrane structure, which did not span the membrane (Figure 5a). However, it should be expected that the addition of water to the membranes (for example, from the wound exudate) promotes the total formation of pores through these. This would allow skin transpiration and an optimal environment for the wound.

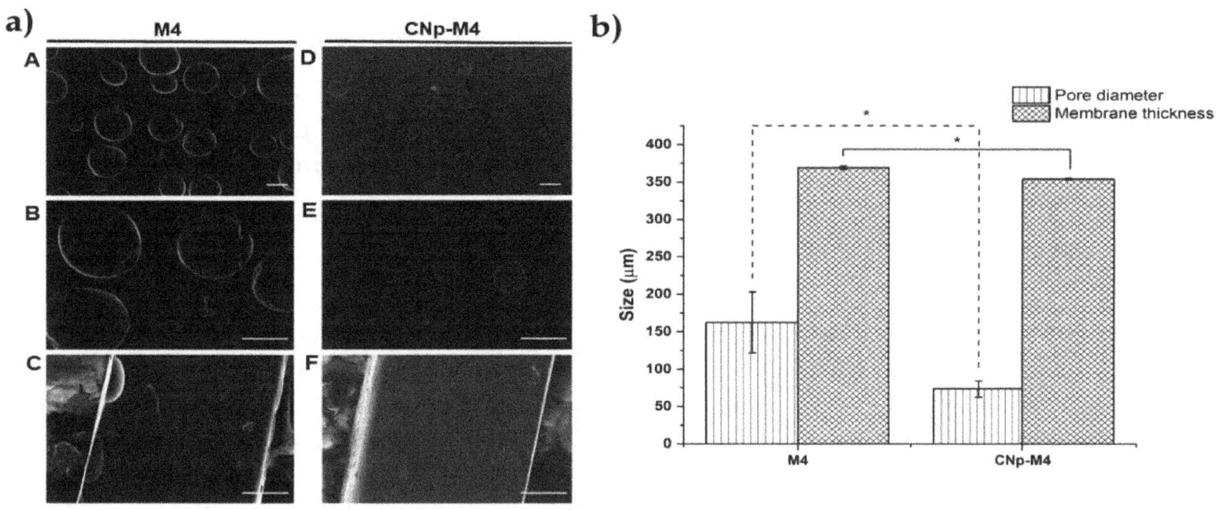

Figure 5. Morphology and porosity of alginate membranes. (**a**) Micrographs by scanning electronic microscopy of the alginate membrane surface (A, B, D, and E) and membrane thickness (C and F). Magnification of 100× for A, D; 220× in B, C, E and F; the scale bar is 100 μm; (**b**) pore diameter and membrane thickness of M4 and CNp-M4 membranes, mean ± SE, $n = 3$. * indicates that $p < 0.05$ is statistically significant.

On the other hand, the mean pore numbers in M4 and CNp-M4 membranes found in each 0.199 mm^2 were 4 and 2, respectively. The pore diameter in the M4 membrane was 162.25 ± 40.75 μm, while for CNp-M4 membranes, this was 73.43 ± 11.04 μm (Figure 5b). Moreover, M4 membranes were significantly thicker and more homogenous in structure than CNp-M4 membranes. These features could be due to the fact that CNp-M4 membranes have CNp dispersion in their formulation, which contains Pluronic® F-68, a nonionic surfactant used as a nanoparticle coating that decreases tensile surface in the polymer gel, thus reducing the number and size of the pores formed in the membranes [43].

Finally, transparency is an expected feature in our alginate membranes used as wound dressings, in order to observe the possible wound-healing process without removing the dressing. M4 and CNp-M4 membranes revealed a transparent feature prior to swelling, while CNp-M4 membranes demonstrated a translucent feature during the swelling process (Figure 6). Although the latter was not completely transparent, it was possible to see through it.

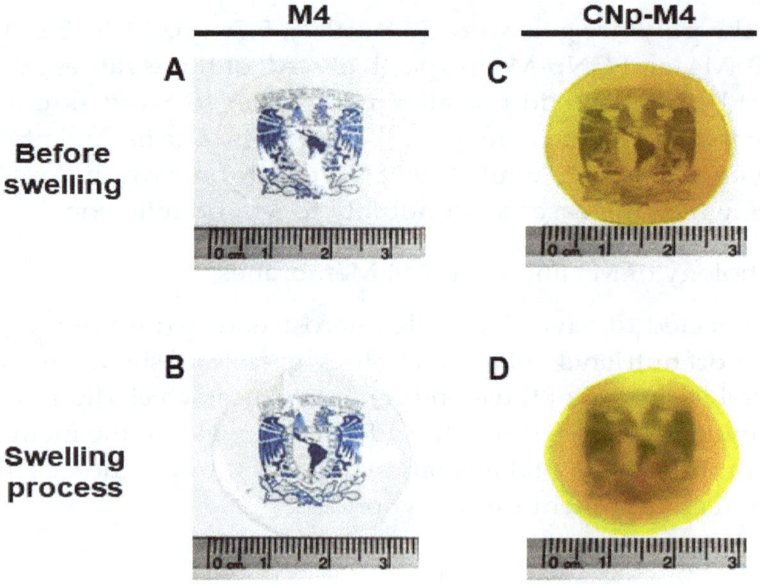

Figure 6. Alginate membranes (M4) before swelling and during the swelling process in PBS medium (**A**,**B**, respectively), and alginate membranes with curcumin nanoparticles (CNp-M4) before swelling and during the swelling process in PBS medium (**C**,**D**, respectively). Scale in centimeters.

3.2.7. In Vitro Release Study of Drug Dispersion, CNp and CNp-M4

To analyze the mechanism of drug release from the nanoparticles (CNp) and from the nanoparticles inside the membrane (CNp-M4), an in vitro release study was performed via the dispersion method and is presented in Figure 7. The curcumin release from CNp (red line, circle symbol) showed a low burst effect at 2 h; this behavior could be related to the presence of the curcumin released from the nanoparticles, as well as to the curcumin outside the nanoparticle, inside the border-zone matrix-stabilizer. After that, the release profile exhibited a linear behavior, with nearly 60% of the curcumin released after 48 h of study. Interestingly, in the release profile for CNp-M4 (blue line, triangle symbol), the burst effect was not evident, and a faster release than CNp (80% of curcumin released at 48 h) was found. These behaviors may be due to the interaction among the membrane excipients, the solvents, and the nanoparticles. To elaborate the CNp-M4 membrane (Section 2.4.1), the nanoparticles are in contact with water, and the hydrolysis of CNp could be stimulated. In addition, some excipients, such as glycerin and propylene glycol, are co-solvents that could improve the prior solubilization of curcumin. As can be observed, the release from both the CNp and CNp-M4 membrane was considerably slower than the drug dispersion release (black line, square symbol).

In order to investigate the mechanism of curcumin release from CNp and CNp-M4, different mathematical models were applied (Table 3). The CNp data were fixed with the Higuchi model (A = 0.0852, B = −0.0459, R^2 = 0.9551), according to those previously reported [44]. This model describes the release of the drug by diffusion from the nanoparticle core into the external solution. On the other hand, the release from CNp-M4 could be explained with the Korsmeyer–Peppas model, due to the highest squared-correlation-coefficient value being obtained with this method (A = 0.3119, B = −0.5609, R^2 = 0.9536). This model combines the diffusion and erosion mechanisms of the nanoparticles as the explanation for drug release.

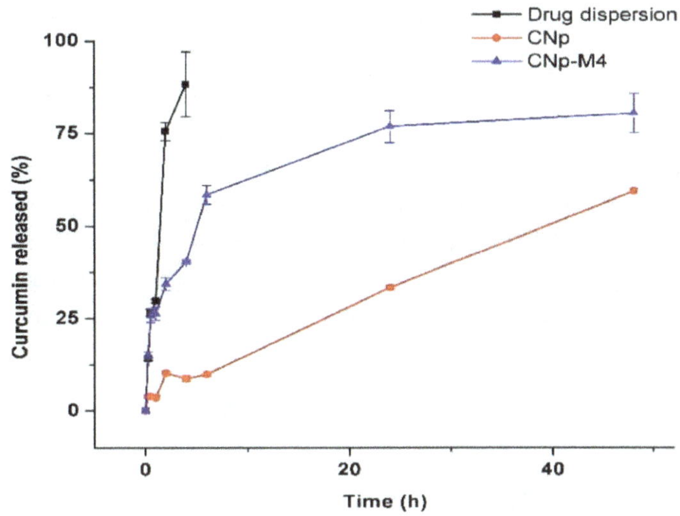

Figure 7. Release profile of curcumin from the drug dispersion, CNp and CNp-M4 membrane in PBS pH 7.4 (0.1 M, Pluronic® F-127 2% *w/v*) at 37 °C. Each point represents the mean ± SE, *n* = 3.

Table 3. Squared of the correlation coefficient (R^2) and coefficients obtained after the linear regression of release data from CNp and CNP-M4 utilizing four mathematical models.

Mathematical Model	Equation	CNp			CNp-M4		
		R^2	A	B	R^2	A	B
Zero-order	$Q_t = Q_0 + K_0 t$	0.842	0.5264	4.7385	0.7358	1.2362	31.432
First-order	$\text{ln}Q_t = \text{lo}Q_0 + K_1 t$	0.8436	−0.0066	−2.3991	0.8453	−0.0303	−3.1975
Higuchi	$Q_t = K_H t^{1/2}$	0.9551	0.0852	−0.0459	0.8939	0.1017	0.194
Korsmeyer–Peppas	$\frac{Q_t}{Q_\infty} = K_K t^n$	0.9037	0.5422	−1.2655	0.9536	0.3119	−0.5609

Q_t: amount of drug released in time t; Q_0: initial amount of drug in the dosage form; Q_∞: total amount of drug dissolved when the dosage form is exhausted; K_0, K_1, K_H, K_K: release rate constants; R^2: squared correlation coefficient. y = ax ± b is an equation obtained after regression: a, slope and b, linear coefficient.

3.3. Curcumin Permeation Assays

3.3.1. Ex Vivo Permeation

An ideal system for potential use in chronic diseases with a slow healing process, such as wounds or psoriasis, should exhibit sustained drug release in order to allow permeation through the skin [20,45]. In this regard, the alginate membranes developed in our study possess polymeric networks as a structure, as well as the curcumin encapsulated in PCL nanoparticles dispersed within these networks. These features will allow the slow release of curcumin.

An ex vivo permeation study was conducted to determine the distribution of the drug and CNp throughout the stratum corneum, epidermis, and dermis, and to verify whether curcumin can pass through the skin and reach blood circulation after the administration of CNp-M4 and CNp formulations. With respect to the aqueous dispersion of curcumin (Figure 8), due to the high lipophilic character of the drug, a high accumulation was observed in some superficial layers of the stratum corneum (10.04 ± 1.73 μg/cm^2). Interestingly, permeation comprises a considerable amount, even from the application of a curcumin dispersion in water, which involves solid particle clusters. This means that the drug particles engage in a dissolution process with the oily components of the stratum corneum, leading to their brief permeation in the superficial region. Although the values are high, there is a higher efficiency of permeation with CNp (14.80 ± 1.61 μg/cm^2). In the region of the dermis, with a hydrophilic character, the permeated amount of the drug dispersion decreases considerably due to its highly limited solubility in aqueous media (2.40 ± 0.46 μg/cm^2); this is nearly one third in relation to the CNp value (6.99 ± 0.27 μg/cm^2). No detection was recorded for the dispersion of the drug that could completely permeate the skin. According to Figure 8, a significant difference was observed between CNp dispersion and CNp-M4 membrane treatments, with the highest permeation values observed for CNp. The CNp-M4 membrane treatment revealed the highest amount of curcumin retained in the epidermis and dermis—that is, 5.7 μg/cm^2 (1.620 ± 0.051% of the total concentration of curcumin)—and the lowest concentration was found in the stratum corneum (SC), at 0.65 μg/cm^2 (0.140 ± 0.006%). On the other hand, in the CNp dispersion treatment, curcumin was found mostly in the SC; that is, 14.8 μg/cm^2 (2.62 ± 0.49%) [26], the highest curcumin value in the entire assay.

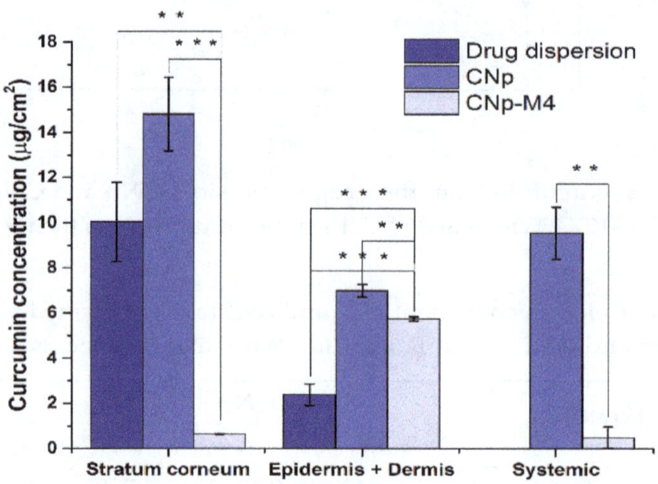

Figure 8. Ex vivo permeation of curcumin after 30 h of treatment with drug dispersion, CNp dispersion, or CNp-M4 membrane. Stratum corneum-bound particles (obtained from 15 tape strips), epidermis + dermis (surface on which dosed skin was handled after 30 h), and systemic (receptor compartment), mean ± SE, $n = 4$; ** indicates $p < 0.01$ and *** indicates $p < 0.001$ as statistically significant.

There was also a significant difference in the amount of curcumin that crossed through the skin (which, in an in vivo model, means reaching the systemic circulation), since the concentration derived from the CNp-M4 membrane was significantly lower than CNp (0.32% and 2.04% respectively; p-value = 0.0019).

The aqueous system of CNp dispersion permitted the curcumin to permeate through the dermis and completely cross the skin. Moreover, CNps have a negative charge; negatively charged nanoparticles permeate the skin more rapidly than positively charged nanoparticles. The skin is predominately negatively charged, and the electrostatic interaction of positive particles with the negatively charged molecules in the skin matrix slows particle diffusion [26]. However, curcumin from CNp-M4 membranes diffuses more slowly through the skin than that from CNp. These observations may be due to the fact that, in the CNp dispersion, water was used as the medium. Water affects the absorption rates of different substances through the stratum corneum, which is in a constant state of partial hydration under normal conditions. Thus, when immersed in water, dead keratinocytes quickly absorb it, resulting in the pruning effect of the skin [45]. Furthermore, water in contact with skin creates a flow gradient toward the skin's inner layers, since the inside of the stratum corneum is more hydrated than the surface [46]. On the other hand, the CNp-M4 membrane does not have a liquid medium in the interface that allows the nanoparticles to flow easily into the deep layers, such as water in the case of the CNp dispersion. Despite this, for the CNp-M4 membrane, a modulated release is expected because of the degree of swelling of the membrane in response to the presence of exudate. The swelling would permit the relaxation of the polymer chains and the release from the CNp. Otherwise, diffusion from a solid state (CNp-M4) into a semi-solid state (the skin) would be expected. Therefore, the CNp-M4 membrane represents a prolonged release system.

In addition, the skin possesses furrows, in which a considerable amount of curcumin is retained, which could not be extracted with the application of adhesive tapes [47]. This curcumin was quantified until mechanical disaggregation. This could explain why the epidermis and dermis had the highest concentration of the drug.

On the other hand, particle size is an important factor in obtaining the desired therapeutic effect, because nanoparticles with a small size can more easily permeate the physiological barriers; moreover, due to their greater surface, release of the drug is favored [48]. Thus, it should be expected that CNps, with their small size (148.3 nm), and the surfactant effect of Pluronic® F-68 can permeate intercellularly and through hair follicles, favoring accumulation for several hours. In the same way, due to the contact of nanoparticles with the corneocytes of the skin, as well as the prolonged release thereof, a large amount of curcumin was found to be retained in the dermis [24,27]. Although after 30 h the majority of curcumin remained in the stratum corneum when CNp dispersion was applied, the monitoring of the permeation at longer times could allow the observation of a prolonged release system [49]. Therefore, the CNp-M4 membrane is proposed as a functional prolonged release system for drug delivery in chronic diseases; however, it would be necessary to perform a more prolonged test to observe the diffusion of the drug at a greater proportion.

3.3.2. Permeation Assay in Vivo

In order to evaluate the in vivo skin permeation of curcumin from the CNp-M4 membrane, CNp dispersion [20], and drug dispersion, a quantification of the curcumin deposited in the stratum corneum by UV–Vis spectrophotometry was performed. The results are presented in Figure 9, according to the work of Goto et al. [50].

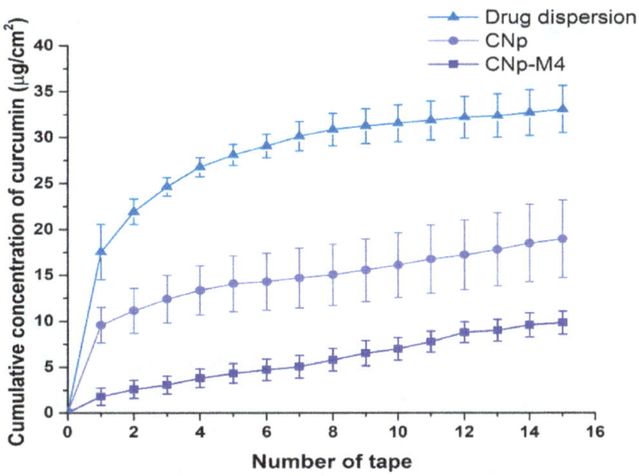

Figure 9. Cumulative concentration of curcumin quantified in the stratum corneum of healthy volunteers. Drug extraction from 15 adhesive tapes applied to the treatment site after placing a CNp-M4 membrane, CNp dispersion, or drug dispersion for 6 h (mean ± SE; $n = 4$).

Higher permeation values were observed for the drug dispersion in water compared to the CNp and CNp-M4 membrane, at least in the superficial layers of the stratum corneum, where the tape stripping technique is applied. The higher values of drug permeation could correspond to the high lipophilicity value of the drug, structural symmetry, and low molecular weight. These values coincide with Figure 8: greater drug deposition on the stratum corneum surface, a lower proportion in the dermis due to an inadequate hydrophilic–lipophilic balance, and no recorded quantity that completely permeates the skin. At 6 h after the application of the drug dispersion, CNp-M4 membrane, and CNp dispersion, the curcumin measured in the stratum corneum reached 33.08 ± 2.57, 9.82 ± 4.23, and 18.96 ± 1.25 µg/cm^2, respectively [25]. CNp-M4 remained well adhered during the study, even up to 48 h in other volunteers (data not shown). As can be noted, a greater amount of curcumin was observed in the stratum corneum when the CNp dispersion treatment was applied, compared with the

CNp-M4 membrane. This is because, in the CNp-M4 membrane, the nanoparticles must be released from the polymeric matrix. This result suggests our formulation as a system of prolonged release that may be useful for long treatments, such as that for a wound (for example, for 7–14 days of application until closure of the lesion). It is noteworthy that the smallest variation observed in permeation values with the CNp-M4 treatment reveals a system that allows better gradual control release. Moreover, these nanoparticles also possess a stabilizer on the outside, Pluronic® F-68, which interacts through hydrogen bonds with the -OH groups of plasticizers and polymers used in the formulation. Thus, when the water makes contact with the membrane, the external part of the polymers swells and promotes the drug—in this case, CNp—to flow outward, permitting its release [51].

With respect to the CNp dispersion, the nanoparticles are free in the medium; thus, they interact more easily with the stratum corneum. Curcumin is encapsulated and uniformly distributed in the PCL nanoparticles, forming nanospheres [52]. The release of curcumin from these latter will depend on the solubility of the drug, the diffusion of curcumin through the matrix of the nanoparticles, thedesorption of curcumin from PCL, the erosion or degradation of the matrix of the nanoparticles, and on the combination of the erosion and diffusion processes [23]. It is also known that, under physiological conditions, a random cleavage of PCL ester bonds occurs, which produces a destabilization of the polymer matrix of the CNp, inducing the release of curcumin [25].

Finally, many studies have reported an accumulation of nanoparticles in hair follicles and the pilosebaceous glands in ex vivo skin experiments [49]. In the same manner, it has been reported that there is better permeation of the drug into the skin, as well as greater absorption in areas with high hair-follicle density. The hair follicle can become a reservoir of substances comparable to the stratum corneum [53]. This means that drugs will penetrate better through the skin of a person with greater amounts of hair follicles. This may explain slight variations in the results obtained, together with variability among individuals (age, body mass, color, and skin moisturization).

4. Conclusions

In this study, the development of a new wound dressing for possible application in wound healing was demonstrated. The wound dressing comprises an alginate membrane and PCL nanoparticles stabilized with Pluronic® F-68 with curcumin inside. This new system was designed with a mixture of aqueous plasticizers to confer high-strength mechanical properties. The characterization of the formulation exhibited that it possesses a high absorbency capacity for the removal of possible exudates, transparency for monitoring the wound bed, the presence of pores with controlled dimensions that could facilitate the transpiration of the wound as a synthetic skin substitute, and the gradual release of the drug according to the ex vivo and in vivo studies. In addition, the high adherence of the wound dressing should be noted even in dry skin, as well as its degradation at later times. Therefore, all of these advantages reveal our wound dressing as a good option for wound healing without the need for its removal from the patient.

Author Contributions: Conceptualization, G.L.-G.; methodology, M.C.G.-A., R.A.M.-F., and M.L.D.P.-A.; validation, I.H.C.-F., C.D.F.-H., and B.F.; formal analysis, M.C.G.-A., R.A.M.-F., M.L.D.P.-A., and G.L.-G.; investigation, M.C.G.-A., R.A.M.-F., and G.L.-G.; resources, M.C.G.-A., R.A.M.-F., M.L.D.P.-A., and G.L.-G.; data curation, M.C.G.-A., R.A.M.-F., M.L.D.P.-A., Z.U.-M., H.C., and G.L.-G.; writing—original draft preparation, M.C.G.-A., R.A.M.-F., M.L.D.P.-A., Z.U.-M., H.C., and G.L.-G.; writing—review and editing, M.C.G.-A., R.A.M.-F., Z.U.-M., D.M.G.-G., J.J.M., M.G.-T., O.D.R.-H., G.F.-G., I.H.C.-F., C.D.F.-H., B.F., H.C., and G.L.-G.; visualization, G.L.-G.; supervision, M.L.D.P.-A., Z.U.-M., H.C., and G.L.-G.; project administration, M.L.D.P.-A. and G.L.-G.; funding acquisition, G.L.-G.

References

1. Eming, S.A.; Brachvogel, B.; Odorisio, T.; Koch, M. Regulation of angiogenesis: Wound healing as a model. *Prog. Histochem. Cytochem.* **2007**, *42*, 115–170. [CrossRef] [PubMed]
2. Demidova-Rice, T.N.; Hamblin, M.R.; Herman, I.M. Current Methods for Drug Delivery, Part 1: Normal and Chronic Wounds: Biology, Causes, and Approaches to Care. *Adv. Skin Wound Care* **2013**, *25*, 304–314. [CrossRef] [PubMed]

3. Axibal, E.; Brown, M. Surgical Dressings and Novel Skin Substitutes. *Dermatol. Clin.* **2019**, *37*, 349–366. [CrossRef] [PubMed]
4. Aderibigbe, B.A.; Buyana, B. Alginate in wound dressings. *Pharmaceutics* **2018**, *10*, 42. [CrossRef] [PubMed]
5. Morgado, P.I.; Aguiar-Ricardo, A.; Correia, I.J. Asymmetric membranes as ideal wound dressings: An overview on production methods, structure, properties and performance relationship. *J. Memb. Sci.* **2015**, *490*, 139–151. [CrossRef]
6. Mi, F.L.; Wu, Y.B.; Shyu, S.S.; Chao, A.C.; Lai, J.Y.; Su, C.C. Asymmetric chitosan membranes prepared by dry/wet phase separation: A new type of wound dressing for controlled antibacterial release. *J. Memb. Sci.* **2003**, *212*, 237–254. [CrossRef]
7. Priya, S.G.; Gupta, A.; Jain, E.; Sarkar, J.; Damania, A.; Jagdale, P.R.; Chaudhari, B.P.; Gupta, K.C.; Kumar, A. Bilayer Cryogel Wound Dressing and Skin Regeneration Grafts for the Treatment of Acute Skin Wounds. *ACS Appl. Mater. Interfaces* **2016**, *8*, 15145–15159. [CrossRef]
8. Miguel, S.P.; Moreira, A.F.; Correia, I.J. Chitosan based-asymmetric membranes for wound healing: A review. *Int. J. Biol. Macromol.* **2019**, *127*, 460–475. [CrossRef]
9. Sood, A.; Granick, M.S.; Tomaselli, N.L. Wound Dressings and Comparative Effectiveness Data. *Adv. Wound Care* **2014**, *3*, 511–529. [CrossRef]
10. Aggarwal, B.B.; Harikumar, K.B. Potential therapeutic effects of curcumin, the anti-inflammatory agent, against neurodegenerative, cardiovascular, pulmonary, metabolic, autoimmune and neoplastic diseases. *Int. J. Biochem. Cell Biol.* **2009**, *41*, 40–59. [CrossRef]
11. Augustyniak, A.; Bartosz, G.; Čipak, A.; Duburs, G.; Horáková, L.; Łuczaj, W.; Majekova, M.; Odysseos, A.D.; Rackova, L.; Skrzydlewska, E.; et al. Natural and synthetic antioxidants: An updated overview. *Free Radic. Res.* **2010**, *44*, 1216–1262. [CrossRef]
12. Del Prado-Audelo, M.L.; Caballero-Florán, I.H.; Meza-Toledo, J.A.; Mendoza-Muñoz, N.; González-Torres, M.; Florán, B.; Cortés, H.; Leyva-Gómez, G. Formulations of curcumin nanoparticles for brain diseases. *Biomolecules* **2019**, *9*, 56. [CrossRef]
13. Sidhu, G.S.; Singh, A.K.; Thaloor, D.; Banaudha, K.K.; Patnaik, G.K.; Srimal, R.C.; Maheshwari, R.K. Enhancement of wound healing by curcumin in animals. *Wound Repair Regen.* **1998**, *6*, 167–177. [CrossRef]
14. Thangapazham, R.L.; Sharad, S.; Maheshwari, R.K. Skin regenerative potentials of curcumin. *Biofactors* **2013**, *39*, 141–149. [CrossRef]
15. Yallapu, M.M.; Jaggi, M.; Chauhan, S.C. Curcumin nanoformulations: A future nanomedicine for cancer. *Drug Discov. Today* **2012**, *17*, 71–80. [CrossRef]
16. Quintanar-guerrero, D.; Allémann, E.; Fessi, H.; Doelker, E.; Allémann, E.; Fessi, H.; Doelker, E. Preparation Techniques and Mechanisms of Formation of Biodegradable Nanoparticles from Preformed Polymers. *Drug Dev. Ind. Pharm.* **1998**, *24*, 1113–1128. [CrossRef]
17. Karki, S.; Kim, H.; Na, S.; Shin, D.; Jo, K.; Lee, J. Thin films as an emerging platform for drug delivery. *Asian J. Pharm. Sci.* **2016**, *11*, 559–574. [CrossRef]
18. Golafshan, N.; Rezahasani, R.; Tarkesh Esfahani, M.; Kharaziha, M.; Khorasani, S.N. Nanohybrid hydrogels of laponite: PVA-Alginate as a potential wound healing material. *Carbohydr. Polym.* **2017**, *176*, 392–401. [CrossRef]
19. Song, Y.; Jiang, Z.; Gao, B.; Wang, H.; Wang, M.; He, Z.; Cao, X.; Pan, F. Embedding hydrophobic MoS2nanosheets within hydrophilic sodium alginate membrane for enhanced ethanol dehydration. *Chem. Eng. Sci.* **2018**, *185*, 231–242. [CrossRef]
20. Mao, K.; Fan, Z.; Yuan, J.; Chen, P.; Yang, J.; Xu, J. Skin-penetrating polymeric nanoparticles incorporated in silk fibroin hydrogel for topical delivery of curcumin to improve its therapeutic effect on psoriasis mouse model. *Colloids Surf. B Biointerfaces* **2017**, *160*, 704–714. [CrossRef]
21. Kamar, S.S.; Abdel-Kader, D.H.; Rashed, L.A. Beneficial effect of Curcumin Nanoparticles-Hydrogel on excisional skin wound healing in type-I diabetic rat: Histological and immunohistochemical studies. *Ann. Anat.* **2019**, *222*, 94–102. [CrossRef]
22. Clayton, K.N.; Salameh, J.W.; Wereley, S.T.; Kinzer-Ursem, T.L. Physical characterization of nanoparticle size and surface modification using particle scattering diffusometry. *Biomicrofluidics* **2016**, *10*, 1–14. [CrossRef]
23. Singh, R.; Lillard, J.W., Jr. Nanoparticle-based targeted drug delivery. *Exp. Mol. Pathol.* **2009**, *86*, 215–223. [CrossRef]

24. Moghimi, S.M.; Hunter, A.C. Good Review on Poloxamers and Poloxamines in Pharma. *Elsevier* **2000**, *18*, 412–420.
25. Ramanujam, R.; Sundaram, B.; Janarthanan, G.; Devendran, E.; Venkadasalam, M.; John Milton, M.C. Biodegradable Polycaprolactone Nanoparticles Based Drug Delivery Systems: A Short Review. *Biosci. Biotechnol. Res. Asia* **2018**, *15*, 679–685. [CrossRef]
26. Kraeling, M.E.K.; Topping, V.D.; Keltner, Z.M.; Belgrave, K.R.; Bailey, K.D.; Gao, X.; Yourick, J. In vitro percutaneous penetration of silver nanoparticles in pig and human skin. *Regul. Toxicol. Pharmacol.* **2018**, *95*, 314–322. [CrossRef]
27. Quintanar-Guerrero, D.; de la Luz Zambrano-Zaragoza, M.; Gutierrez-Cortez, E.; Mendoza-Munoz, N. Impact of the emulsification-diffusion method on the development of pharmaceutical nanoparticles. *Recent Pat. Drug Deliv. Formul.* **2012**, *6*, 184–194. [CrossRef]
28. Pinto Reis, C.; Neufeld, R.J.; Ribeiro, A.J.; Veiga, F.; Nanoencapsulation, I. Methods for preparation of drug-loaded polymeric nanoparticles. *Nanomed. Nanotechnol. Biol. Med.* **2006**, *2*, 8–21. [CrossRef]
29. Judefeind, A.; de Villiers, M.M. *Nanotechnology in Drug Delivery*; de Villiers, M.M., Aramwit, P.S., Kwon, G., Eds.; Springer US: New York, NY, USA, 2009; ISBN 9780387776675.
30. Singh, B.; Pal, L. Radiation crosslinking polymerization of sterculia polysaccharide-PVA-PVP for making hydrogel wound dressings. *Int. J. Biol. Macromol.* **2011**, *48*, 501–510. [CrossRef]
31. Göpferich, A. Mechanisms of polymer degradation and erosion. *Biomaterials* **1996**, *17*, 103–114. [CrossRef]
32. GD, M. Quantifying wound fluids for the clinician and researcher. *Ostomy Wound Manag.* **1994**, *40*, 66–69.
33. Parikh, D.V.; Fink, T.; Delucca, A.J.; Parikh, A.D. Absorption and swelling characteristics of silver (I) antimicrobial wound dressings. *Text. Res. J.* **2011**, *81*, 494–503. [CrossRef]
34. Kamoun, E.A.; Kenawy, E.S.; Chen, X. A review on polymeric hydrogel membranes for wound dressing applications: PVA-based hydrogel dressings. *J. Adv. Res.* **2017**, *8*, 217–233. [CrossRef]
35. Shi, S.; Peng, X.; Liu, T.; Chen, Y.N.; He, C.; Wang, H. Facile preparation of hydrogen-bonded supramolecular polyvinyl alcohol-glycerol gels with excellent thermoplasticity and mechanical properties. *Polymer* **2017**, *111*, 168–176. [CrossRef]
36. Wang, R.-M.; Zheng, S.-R.; Zheng, Y.-P. Matrix materials. In *Polymer Matrix Composites and Technology*; Elsevier: Amsterdam, The Netherlands, 2011; pp. 101–548.
37. Sun, B.; Tian, Y.; Chen, L.; Jin, Z. Food Hydrocolloids Linear dextrin as curcumin delivery system: Effect of degree of polymerization on the functional stability of curcumin. *Food Hydrocoll.* **2018**, *77*, 911–920. [CrossRef]
38. Campus, K.; Kanchanaburi, M.L.; Road, S. Nanocomposites Based on Cassava Starch and Chitosan-Modified Clay: Physico-Mechanical Properties and Biodegradability in Simulated Compost Soil. *J. Braz. Chem. Soc.* **2017**, *28*, 649–658.
39. Aghazadeh, M.; Karim, R.; Abdul Rahman, R.; Sultan, M.T.; Johnson, S.K.; Paykary, M. Effect of Glycerol on the Physicochemical Properties of Cereal Starch Films. *Food Technol. Econ. Eng. Phys. Prop.* **2018**, *36*, 403–409. [CrossRef]
40. Shrotriya, S.; Ranpise, N.; Satpute, P.; Vidhate, B. Skin targeting of curcumin solid lipid nanoparticles-engrossed topical gel for the treatment of pigmentation and irritant contact dermatitis. *Artif. Cells Nanomed. Biotechnol.* **2018**, *46*, 1471–1482. [CrossRef]
41. Kossack, W.; Kremer, F. Banded spherulites and twisting lamellae in poly–ε–caprolactone. *Colloid Polym. Sci.* **2019**, *297*, 771–779. [CrossRef]
42. Verhoeven, N.; Neoh, T.L.; Furuta, T.; Yamamoto, C.; Ohashi, T.; Yoshii, H. Characteristics of dehydration kinetics of dihydrate trehalose to its anhydrous form in ethanol by DSC. *Food Chem.* **2012**, *132*, 1638–1643. [CrossRef]
43. Bueno, C.Z.; Moraes, Â.M. Development of Porous Lamellar Chitosa-Alginate Membranes: Effect of Different Surfactants on Biomaterial Properties. *J. Appl. Polym. Sci.* **2011**, *122*, 624–631. [CrossRef]
44. Del Prado-Audelo, M.L.; Magaña, J.J.; Mejía-Contreras, B.A.; Borbolla-Jiménez, F.V.; Giraldo-Gomez, D.M.; Piña-Barba, M.C.; Quintanar-Guerrero, D.; Leyva-Gómez, G. In vitro cell uptake evaluation of curcumin-loaded PCL/F68 nanoparticles for potential application in neuronal diseases. *J. Drug Deliv. Sci. Technol.* **2019**, *52*, 905–914. [CrossRef]
45. Blattner, C.M.; Coman, G.; Blickenstaff, N.R.; Maibach, H.I. Percutaneous absorption of water in skin: A review. *Rev. Environ. Health* **2014**, *29*, 175–180. [CrossRef]

46. Tagami, H.; Kanamaru, Y.; Inoue, K.; Suehisa, S.; Iwatsuki, K.; Yoshikuni, K.; Yamada, M. Water sorption-desorption test of the skin in vivo for functional assessment of the stratum corneum. *J. Invest. Dermatol.* **1982**, *78*, 425–428. [CrossRef]
47. Van der Molen, R.; Spies, F.; van´t Noordende, J.M.; Boelsma, E.; Mommaas, A.M.; Koerten, H.K. Tape stripping of human stratum corneum yields cell layers that originate from various depths because of furrows in the skin. *Arch. Dermatol. Res.* **1997**, *289*, 514–518. [CrossRef]
48. Kucukturmen, B.; Oz, U.C.; Bozkir, A. In Situ Hydrogel Formulation for Intra-Articular Application of Diclofenac Sodium-Loaded Polymeric Nanoparticles. *Turk. J. Pharm. Sci.* **2017**, *14*, 56–64. [CrossRef]
49. Zhang, N.; Said, A.; Wischke, C.; Kral, V.; Brodwolf, R.; Volz, P.; Boreham, A.; Gerecke, C.; Li, W.; Neffe, A.T.; et al. Poly[acrylonitrile-co-(N-vinyl pyrrolidone)] nanoparticles—Composition-dependent skin penetration enhancement of a dye probe and biocompatibility. *Eur. J. Pharm. Biopharm.* **2017**, *116*, 66–75. [CrossRef]
50. Goto, N.; Morita, Y.; Terada, K. Deposits from Creams Containing 20% (w/w) Urea and Suppression of Crystallization (Part 2): Novel Analytical Methods of Urea Accumulated in the Stratum Corneum by Tape stripping and Colorimetry. *Chem. Pharm. Bull.* **2016**, *64*, 1092–1098. [CrossRef]
51. Langer, R. New Methods of Drug Delivery. *Science* **1990**, *249*, 1527–1533. [CrossRef]
52. Urrejola, M.C.; Soto, L.V.; Zumarán, C.; Peñaloza, P.; Álvarez, B.; Fuentevilla, I.; Haidar, Z.S. Sistemas de Nanopartículas Poliméricas II: Estructura, Métodos de Elaboración, Características, Propiedades, Biofuncionalización y Tecnologías de Auto-Ensamblaje Capa por Capa (Layer-by-Layer Self-Assembly). *Int. J. Morphol.* **2018**, *36*, 1463–1471. [CrossRef]
53. Lademann, J.; Richter, H.; Teichmann, A.; Otberg, N.; Blume-Peytavi, U.; Luengo, J.; Weiß, B.; Schaefer, U.F.; Lehr, C.M.; Wepf, R.; et al. Nanoparticles—An efficient carrier for drug delivery into the hair follicles. *Eur. J. Pharm. Biopharm.* **2007**, *66*, 159–164. [CrossRef]

14

In Vivo Biocompatibility of Electrospun Biodegradable Dual Carrier (Antibiotic + Growth Factor) in a Mouse Model—Implications for Rapid Wound Healing

Charu Dwivedi [1,2], Himanshu Pandey [2,3], Avinash C. Pandey [2], Sandip Patil [4], Pramod W. Ramteke [1,*], Peter Laux [5], Andreas Luch [5] and Ajay Vikram Singh [5,6,*]

1. Department of Biological Sciences, Sam Higginbottom University of Agriculture, Technology and Sciences, Allahabad 211007, India; charucas0505@gmail.com
2. Nanotechnology Application Centre, Faculty of Science, University of Allahabad, Allahabad 211002, India; himanshu.nac@gmail.com (H.P.); prof.avinashcpandey@gmail.com (A.C.P.)
3. Department of Pharmaceutical Sciences, Faculty of Health Sciences, Sam Higginbottom University of Agriculture, Technology & Sciences, Allahabad 211007, India
4. E-Spin Nanotech Pvt Ltd., Kanpur 208016, India; espinnanotech@gmail.com
5. Department of Chemical and Product Safety, German Federal Institute for Risk Assessment (BfR), Max-Dohrn-Strasse 8-10, 10589 Berlin, Germany; peter.laux@bfr.bund.de (P.L.); andreas.luch@bfr.bund.de (A.L.)
6. Physical Intelligence Department, Max Planck Institute for Intelligent Systems, 70569 Stuttgart, Germany

* Correspondence: avsingh@is.mpg.de or Ajay-Vikram.Singh@bfr.bund.de (A.V.S.); pwramteke@gmail.com (P.W.R.)

Abstract: Tissue engineering technologies involving growth factors have produced one of the most advanced generations of diabetic wound healing solutions. Using this approach, a nanocomposite carrier was designed using Poly(D,L-lactide-*co*-glycolide) (PLGA)/Gelatin polymer solutions for the simultaneous release of recombinant human epidermal growth factor (rhEGF) and gentamicin sulfate at the wound site to hasten the process of diabetic wound healing and inactivation of bacterial growth. The physicochemical characterization of the fabricated scaffolds was carried out using scanning electron microscopy (SEM) and X-ay diffraction (XRD). The scaffolds were analyzed for thermal stability using thermogravimetric analysis and differential scanning calorimetry. The porosity, biodegradability, and swelling behavior of the scaffolds was also evaluated. Encapsulation efficiency, drug loading capacity, and in vitro drug release were also investigated. Further, the bacterial inhibition percentage and detailed in vivo biocompatibility for wound healing efficiency was performed on diabetic C57BL6 mice with dorsal wounds. The scaffolds exhibited excellent wound healing and continuous proliferation of cells for 12 days. These results support the applicability of such systems in rapid healing of diabetic wounds and ulcers.

Keywords: tissue engineering; growth factor; diabetic; wound healing; nanocomposite

---

1. Introduction

Wound healing or tissue repair is a complex multistep process comprising a multitude of cells, cytokines, extracellular matrix (ECM) molecules, blood cells, and a number of other factors [1]. Disturbances at proliferation or inflammation phases of wound healing lead to perturbations in the process [2]. Chronic wounds, such as those in diabetic patients, present worldwide health challenges as well as an economic burden. The existing therapies exhibit unsatisfactory results and despite treatment of these chronic wounds, which involves tight glucose control and meticulous wound care, the prognosis for their healing is quite poor and finally leads to morbidity [3,4]. Microorganisms are naturally present on the wound bed without any detrimental effects to the normal wound healing process since the number of bacteria is quite low. Since diabetes lowers the normal immunity of the body, such patients are more prone to infection in wounds [5]. Hence, chronic wounds, such as leg ulcers, foot ulcers, and pressure ulcers, are more prone to such microbial infections due to the presence of multiple microbial populations consisting of *S. aureus* [6], *P. aeruginosa* [7], coliform bacteria [8], *Streptococcus* spp., and *Enterococcus* spp. [9]. During injury, foreign bodies including pathogenic microbes can enter deep into the wounds causing chronic inflammatory responses and, thereby, delaying healing of the wounds. The patient may develop a more serious deep-wound infection, and require amputation due to the occurrence of anaerobic bacteria in diabetic foot ulcers and may also lead to abscess or granuloma formation [10,11].

Generally, the process of wound healing is driven by many cellular mediators including various growth factors which are proteinaceous molecules playing a key role in tissue repair and wound care [12]. One of the major obstacles in the treatment method involving growth factors is that the encapsulated growth factor tends to be released in a non-controllable manner due to its physical association with the drug reservoir systems [13]. Moreover, the growth factors are either easily degraded by proteinases or removed by exudate before reaching the wound bed. Until now, only platelet-derived growth factor-BB (PDGF-BB) has successfully passed clinical trials [1]. Epidermal growth factor (EGF) is a low-molecular-weight polypeptide and plays a significant role in wound healing as it stimulates proliferation, differentiation, and survival of cells [14]. Hence, recombinant human epidermal growth factor (rhEGF) was selected as the bioactive agent for immobilization on the nanofibrous scaffolds. It acts by binding with high affinity to epidermal growth factor receptor (EGFR) on the cell surface and stimulating the intrinsic protein-tyrosine kinase activity of the receptor. The tyrosine kinase activity, in turn, initiates a signal transduction cascade that results in a variety of biochemical changes within the cell—a rise in intracellular calcium levels, increased glycolysis and protein synthesis, and increases in the expression of certain genes including the gene for EGFR—that ultimately lead to DNA synthesis and cell proliferation [15].

In the recent scenario, due to their comprehensive assortment of implementations in the world of biomedicine, nanomaterials have emerged as potent tools for clinicians and researchers in different biomedical and allied fields of human life [16–18]. Nanomaterials possess notable virtues, such as high reactivity, large surface-to-mass ratio, and ultra-small size making them highly useful in biomedical applications [19,20].

In view of these strategies, current tissue engineering approaches are centered around the fabrication of three dimensional (3D) nanoscaffolds or ECM analogs that should conform to multifactorial requirements, for example, those associated with tissue repair [16]. Such scaffolds tune the biomimetic nature of the ECM, possess large surface area to volume ratio, are able to facilitate diffusion (as a result of high porosity), and have tunability of physical properties simultaneously providing a local release of different biomolecules to address successful tissue regeneration [21]. Numerous studies have been done to fabricate potentially applicable scaffold materials for tissue engineering and wound healing applications. Electrospun nanofibrous scaffolds have been successfully used in site-specific delivery of many bioactive molecules and for the treatment of various infections and cancers. Such scaffolds allow for the release of loaded biomolecules in therapeutic dosage and have a negligible influence on drug activity and possess well-controlled drug release rate [22,23]. One of the smart property of these scaffolds is that they possess physical resemblance with ECM and are easy to implement due to their superior mechanical durability, flexibility in surface functionalities, and interconnected and readily controlled secondary structures [24]. Polymers had been a choice material for the fabrication of nanofibrous scaffolds. Synthetic biodegradable polymers, such as poly(3-caprolactone), polyethylene oxide, poly(L-lactide-*co*-3-caprolactone) (PLCL), polylactic acid, poly(lactide-*co*-glycolide), and polyglycolic acid (PGA), Poly(vinyl alcohol (PVA), Polyvinyl chloride

(PVC), Poly-L-lactic acid (PLLA), nylon, gelatin, polyurethane, etc., have proven useful in the preparation of nanofibrous scaffolds. Researches have proved these scaffolds to be biocompatible and to enhance cell functions in vitro [25,26].

Cell functions include the growth, differentiation, and metabolism of cells via interaction with specific cell-surface receptors [27]. Polymers like Poly (D,L-lactide-*co*-glycolide) (PLGA) have been extensively used for application in drug-delivery, surgical implants, and tissue engineering scaffolds owing to their biodegradability and biocompatibility [28,29]. Further, it is imperative that the wound is free from infection-causing microbes and all factors which inhibit its natural healing process [30]. The addition of antibacterial agents into electrospun fibers has been a thrust area of research for clinicians especially as antibiotic-resistant bacteria strains increasingly emerge [31]. Gentamicin sulfate is a bactericidal aminoglycoside antibiotic that is widely used for the treatment of bacterial infections [32]. Electrospun nanofibers could increase the drug efficiency and drug solubility in aqueous solution due to their high surface-to-volume ratio. They could provide a controlled drug delivery to the site of action in the body in an optimal concentration-versus-time profile. A multitude of nanomaterials conjugated with vancomycin has been designed to enhance the pharmacokinetics and pharmacodynamics of the antibiotic molecule [31,33–36].

In this work, we fabricated a novel biomimetic drug and rhEGF delivery system by the electrospinning of PLGA/Gelatin solutions containing Gentamicin Sulfate (GS) and further immobilizing the scaffolds with rhEGF. The purpose of this work is to support diabetic wound healing and to eliminate microbial infections while releasing gentamicin and rhEGF in a controlled fashion. To our knowledge, synchronous release of drug and growth factor from electrospun scaffolds has not been investigated and we did not find any paper which discusses it. In the present scenario, controlled release of antibiotic and growth factor was achieved, and the dual delivery system allows for efficient and for the treatment of wounds in diabetic patients.

2. Experimental

2.1. Materials

Poly (D,L-lactide-*co*-glycolide) (LA/GA 85/15) (Gangwal Chemicals Pvt. Ltd., Mumbai, India), gentamicin sulfate (FDC India Ltd., Mumbai, India), streptozotocin (Sisco Research Laboratories Pvt. Ltd., Bhiwandi, India), nutrient broth and nutrient agar (Merck Specialities Pvt. Ltd. Mumbai, India), 2,2,2-trifluoroethanol, suberic acid bis(*N*-hydroxy-succinimide ester) (NHS), 1,6-diaminohexane and 2,2-dihydroxyindane-1,3-dione (ninhydrin) (Loba Chemie Pvt. Ltd. Mumbai, India) and rhEGF (Life Technologies India Pvt. Ltd., New Delhi, India). All other chemicals and reagents were of analytical grade as purchased.

2.2. Fabrication of GS-Loaded Composite PLGA/Gelatin Nanoscaffolds

Composite PLGA/Gelatin nanoscaffolds were fabricated as described in our previous study [21,37]. Schematic Figure 1 demonstrates the procedure for the fabrication of electrospun nanofibrous scaffolds, their immobilization with the growth factors (rhEGF and Gentamicin sulfate (GS) and their application on wounds of diabetic mice for in vivo test. Poly (D,L-lactide-*co*-glycolide) was used with LA/GA in the ratio 85/15 due to the fact that it takes an average degradation time of 5 to 6 weeks [38]. Briefly, two different composite polymer solutions of 10% PLGA/Gelatin (wt. ratio 70:30 and 50:50, respectively) in 2,2,2-trifluoroethanol were prepared. Thereafter, 5 mg/mL gentamicin sulfate and 0.2 mL of PEG-400 was added to each of the prepared polymer solutions, and were electrospun into nanofibrous scaffolds using an electrospinning setup. The electrospinning was operated at the flow rate of 0.6 mL/h, and a high voltage (16 kV) was applied to the tip of the needle (0.9 mm inner hole diameter) attached to the syringe. The ultrafine aligned nanofibers were collected by a rotating the disc wrapped with a piece of aluminum foil with a horizontal distance of 10 cm from the needle tip. The obtained electrospun nanofibrous scaffolds were dried at room temperature under vacuum for 24 h to remove organic solvent and moisture. The scaffolds were stored at −20 °C for further analysis.

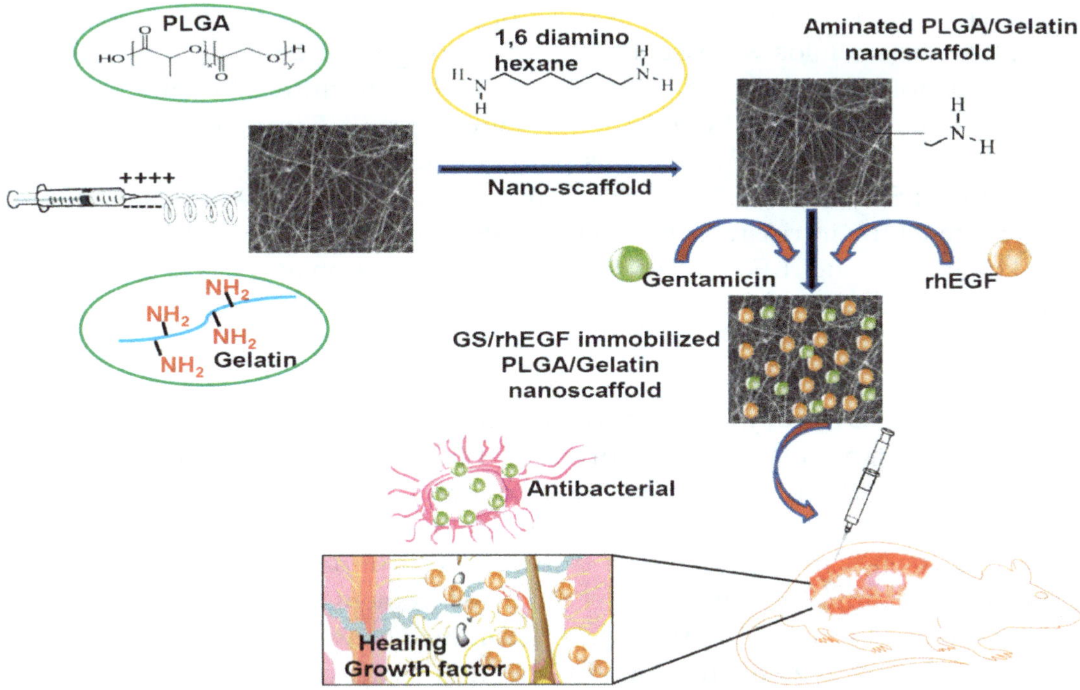

Figure 1. Process of fabrication of aminolyzed Poly(D,L-lactide-*co*-glycolide) (PLGA)/Gelatin nanoscaffolds and subsequent application on diabetic wounds.

2.3. Post-treatment of Composite Nanoscaffolds via Covalent Immobilization of rhEGF

The growth factor rhEGF was immobilized on the surface of the prepared nanoscaffolds by the covalent immobilization technique [21]. Before immobilization, the scaffolds were aminolyzed to introduce amine groups into the surface of the prepared scaffolds. Henceforth, the scaffold pieces (20 mm in diameter) were soaked into a 10% (*w*/*v*) solution of 1,6-hexanediamine prepared in isopropanol and were incubated at room temperature for 3 h and subsequently washed in PBS (phosphate-buffered saline, pH 7.4) five times. Then the scaffolds were rinsed with 70% ethanol and PBS. Thereafter, they were immersed in 10 mL PBS containing 0.08 mmol NHS with gentle agitation for 4 h at room temperature. The scaffolds were again rinsed gently five times with PBS to remove residual solvents and make sure that scaffolds are not removed from the substrate (Supplementary Material: Figure S1) five times with PBS. Finally, the activated scaffolds were soaked into 10 µg/mL rhEGF solutions in PBS with gentle shaking for 12 h at 4 °C. Then the rhEGF-immobilized composite nanoscaffolds were washed with PBS and freeze-dried.

2.4. Surface Topography and Properties

The surface topography and size of the composite nanofibrous scaffolds was examined by a Hitachi-4800 scanning electron microscope (SEM) (Hitachi India Pvt. Ltd, Mumbai, India). Before examination, the samples were adhered to SEM studs, and coated with 5 nm thin gold film using a sputter-coater (EMITECH K550X, EMITECH ENGINEERING (INDIA) PRIVATE LIMITED, Mumbai, India) for 4 min at 30 mA. The fibers were quantified using DiameterJ tool in imageJ (https://imagej.net/DiameterJ) and plot was generated into origin software.

2.5. Quantitative Analysis of rhEGF-Immobilized Composite Nanoscaffolds

The amine groups present on the surface of 1,6-hexanediamine treated nanoscaffolds (diameter 15 mm) were determined using ninhydrin assay [39,40]. Ninhydrin solution (1.0 M) was prepared in ethanol and each scaffold was immersed into this solution for 1 min. Then, the scaffolds were transferred to a glass vial that was heated for 15 min at 70 °C. The scaffolds were then dissolved in 2 mL tetrahydrofuron and isopropanol each and mixed with the solution. The absorbance was measured at 560 nm using a Lambda 25 UV–Vis spectrophotometer (Perkin-Elmer, New York, NY, USA). The amine groups on the scaffolds were quantified by plotting a standard curve of 1,6-hexanediamine solutions in isopropanol in the range of 5 to 25 μg/mL. To determine the amount of immobilized rhEGF, the fluorescence intensity of the tryptophan group of rhEGF immobilized on the nanofibrous scaffolds was measured. The rhEGF assay was performed using a fluorescence spectrophotometer (Perkin Elmer Model–LS 45, Perkin Elmer, New York, NY, USA) at 280 nm excitation and 342 nm emission wavelength as the intrinsic tryptophan fluorescence. The amount of immobilized rhEGF was determined by subtracting rhEGF residual intensity in solution at the end of the immobilization process from the initial amount of rhEGF in the solution.

2.6. Thermal Analysis

The thermal properties of composite nanoscaffolds were determined using thermogravimetric analysis (TGA) and differential scanning calorimetry (DSC). TGA was performed in an automatic thermal analyzer system Thermogravimetry/Differential Thermal Analysis (TG/DTA) (Diamond TG/DTA 8.0, Perkin-Elmer, Perkin Elmer India Ltd., Noida, India). Sealed samples were healed in an aluminum pan at 20.00 °C/min from 50.00 °C to 900.00 °C under a constant nitrogen flow rate of 150 mL/min through the sample chamber. The DSC measurements were carried out in an automatic thermal analyzer system (Diamond TG/DTA 8.0, Perkin-Elmer, New York, NY, USA) in the temperature range from −50 °C to 300 °C at a heating rate of 15 °C /min under a nitrogen atmosphere.

2.7. X-Ray Diffraction

The crystalline structure of composite nanoscaffolds was characterized by Spinner PW3064 XPERT-PRO diffraction (XRD) system using Cu Kα radiation with continuous scanning at 40 mA, 45 kV. The scan was performed from 5° to 60° (2θ). The plane spacing of different diffraction planes (d_{hkl}) can be calculated from the Bragg's Law (Equation (1)):

$$d_{hk} = \lambda/2 \sin\theta \;\hat{} \tag{1}$$

where λ is the wavelength of the copper anode source (λ = 1.54 Å), and θ stands for the diffraction angle of each indexed diffraction plane.

2.8. Degree of Swelling and Porosity.

The degree of swelling of nanoscaffolds was calculated by immersing them in phosphate buffer saline (pH 7.4) for 24 h at room temperature [21]. After 24 h, the nanoscaffolds were removed, and the excess buffer solution was wiped with filter paper and weighed. The weights were recorded, and the swelling index was calculated using Equation (2) as given below.

$$\text{Degree of swelling } (\%) = \frac{W - W_O}{W_O} \times 100 \tag{2}$$

where, W = weight of scaffolds after immersion and Wo = weight of scaffolds before immersion: The porosity of the composite nanoscaffolds was measured using the gravimetric method [21]. The thicknesses of the nanoscaffolds were measured using microcallipers, and then their apparent density ($\rho_{scaffold}$) and porosity(ε) were calculated according to the Equation (3).

$$\varepsilon = 1 - \frac{\rho_{scaffold}}{\rho_{material}} \tag{3}$$

where, $\rho_{scaffold}$ is the density of scaffold and $\rho_{material}$ is the density of bulk PLGA

2.9. Water Contact Angle Measurement

The water contact angle measurements were performed using an FTA1000 (First Ten Ångstroms Inc., Manchester, UK) instrument. An average obtained from at least five measurements of the contact angle was obtained with MilliQ water (volume ~3 nano-liters, FirstTenÅngstroms Inc., Noida, India) on different nanoscaffolds composite spots. For statistical validation of results, each measurement of a particular contact angle was recorded in 150 images taken within 5 s with a Pelco Model PCHM 575-4 camera (standard deviation ~2°, unless otherwise stated). Images analysis was performed by the FTA Windows Mode 4 software.

2.10. In Vitro Biodegradability Studies

To evaluate the in vitro biodegradability of composite nanoscaffolds, degradation studies were performed over a period of 14 days in phosphate buffer saline solution (PBS; pH 7.4) [21,41]. Degradation, as the percentage of weight loss (W_L) was calculated on 3rd, 7th, 10th, and 14th day using Equation (4).

$$W_L(\%) = \frac{W - W_O}{W_O} \times 100 \tag{4}$$

where W_O is initial weight and W is weight after degradation:

2.11. Drug-Polymer Profile

Drug assay was carried out to determine the drug entrapment efficiency of the composite nanoscaffolds as reported in our previous study [21]. Drug loaded nanoscaffolds were placed in phosphate buffer saline (pH 7.4) and centrifuged at 8000 rpm for 5 min. A 3 mL of ninhydrin reagent was added to the supernatant, and the absorbance was measured using a Lambda 25 UV−vis spectrophotometer (Perkin-Elmer, New York, NY, USA) at 566 nm. The amount of drug in the sample was calculated using the standard curve prepared from PBS. The drug entrapment efficiency was calculated by comparing the amount of drug used to prepare the scaffolds according to Equation (5).

$$\text{Drug entrapment efficiency } (\%) = \frac{\mathrm{M}}{\mathrm{M_O}} \times 100 \tag{5}$$

where, M = mass of entrapped drug and $\mathrm{M_O}$ = mass of drug used in the formulation. The drug loading capacity is the ratio of the mass of bound drug to the mass of the scaffold and was calculated using Equation (6).

$$\text{Drug loading capacity } (\%) = \frac{F}{W} \times 100 \tag{6}$$

2.12. In Vitro Drug Release Studies

The release of gentamicin sulfate from composite nanoscaffolds was studied at different pH values. It is well known that the pH values have a significant impact on the assembly and organization of nanoscaffolds by affecting the surface charge density of weak electrolytes. It also has an effect on the degree of ionization of weak polyelectrolytes [42]. The membrane diffusion technique was used for the in-vitro release studies of gentamicin sulfate from composite nanoscaffolds, as described in our previous study [21,41]. The studies were conducted within a temperature controlled incubator (37 ± 0.5 °C) using PBS (150 mM, pH 7.4) under gentle mixing.

The nanoscaffolds were incubated in 5 mL of aqueous buffer solution with pH 3, 7.4, and 9, respectively. Aliquots of 1.0 mL of the diffusion medium were withdrawn at certain incubation time points and were replaced with an equal quantity of a fresh diffusion medium. Samples were quantitatively analyzed using Systronics 10 UV–Vis spectrophotometer at 566.0 nm, after treatment with ninhydrin reagent against the mixture of diffusion medium and ninhydrin reagent as blank.

2.13. *In Vitro Antibacterial Activity Testing*

Antibacterial activity of composite nanoscaffolds was evaluated against *Staphylococcus aureus*, a Gram-positive bacteria in liquid medium [21,24]. *Staphylococcus aureus* was obtained from the Microbiology department, Sam Higginbottom Institute of Agriculture, Technology and Sciences, Allahabad. The bacterial culture was grown in nutrient broth, and when the absorbance reached 0.1 to 0.2 at 625 nm, 5 mL of the culture was taken in test tubes, and the drug loaded nanoscaffolds were submerged in them. GS powder was taken as a positive control while the tube without scaffold was taken as negative control. Another tube with cotton gauze was set as another negative control. The samples were incubated on a shaker at 200 rpm for 24 h at 37 °C. After that, the absorbance at 625 nm was monitored using UV−vis spectroscopy. All experiments were performed in triplicate, and only the average values were reported. The percentage of bacterial inhibition was calculated from Equation (7).

$$\text{Bacterial inhibition}(\%) = \frac{I_C - I_S}{I_C} \times 100 \quad (7)$$

where Ic and Is are the average absorbance readings of the control group and the experimental group, respectively.

The assessment was conducted based on the disc agar diffusion method [21,24]. Nutrient agar plates were prepared by autoclaving the nutrient agar media and pouring onto petri dishes and air-dried. A 100 μL aliquot of bacteria reconstituted in nutrient broth and previously subcultured was spread onto an agar plate. The GS-free and GS-containing nanoscaffolds were cut into circular discs (15 mm in diameter) and placed on the top of the agar plate. The plates were incubated at 37 °C for 24 h. If inhibitory concentrations were reached, there would be no growth of the bacteria, which could be seen as a clear zone around the scaffold specimens. The zone was then recorded as an indication of inhibition against the bacterial species.

2.14. *In Vivo Wound Healing Studies in Diabetic Mice*

In vivo studies were performed in accordance with the Institutional Animal Ethics Committee (IAEC) constituted as per directions of the Committee for the Purpose of Control and Supervision of Experiments on Animals (CPCSEA), under the Ministry of Animal Welfare Division, Government of India, New Delhi. The approval from the Institutional Animal Ethical Committee of Bundelkhand University, Jhansi, was taken before the experimental work (BU/Pharm/IAEC/13/29). Five groups of Female C57BL/6 mice weighing (14–15 g) were selected, each group having 6 mice. All animals were allowed to adapt to cages for 3 days, after which they were fasted overnight. Streptozotocin (STZ) was freshly dissolved in (0.1 M, pH 4.5) citrate buffer and non-insulin-dependent diabetes mellitus was induced in overnight fasted mice by a single intraperitoneal injection of Streptozotocin (40 mg/kg bodyweight). Blood glucose levels were measured 4 days after STZ injection, and only mice with fasting blood glucose levels greater than 200 mg/dL were considered to be diabetic and were used in the experiment. Wounds in the diabetic mice were created by following the excision wound model, whereby their dorsal hairs were shaven, and an excision made with scissors and tweezer on the back of the animal. The wound areas were sterilized with povidone iodide. All treatments started 4 days after STZ injection. For determination of wound healing activity, the following treatments were applied after creating wounds on five groups—Group 1 (C)—no treatment (negative control), Group 2 (G)—pure GS solution (positive control), Group 3 (P)—PLGA/Gelatin 70:30 scaffold without GS and rhEGF, Group 4 (PG)—PLGA/Gelatin 70:30 scaffold loaded with GS and rhEGF both and Group 5 (PG)—PLGA/Gelatin 70:30 scaffold loaded with GS only. The treatments were applied to aseptically treated wounds to determine the therapeutic effects on the wounds. After each treatment interval, the scaffolds were removed with tweezers. The wounds were photographed on day 1 and the treatment regime repeated on day 4, 8, and 12. The percentage reduction of the wound area was calculated using Equation (8) below.

$$\text{Wound area } (\%) = \frac{A}{A_i} \times 100 \quad (8)$$

where, A_i is the initial wound area, and A is the wound area after a fixed time interval.

2.15. Statistical Analysis

Data are expressed as means ± standard deviation. For the statistical validation of data, three independent experiments (n = 3) were performed in triplicates. Statistical analysis was conducted using a paired *t*-test or an unpaired, two-tailed Student's *t*-test. A *p*-value of <0.05 was considered to be statistically significant.

3. Results and Discussion

3.1. Surface Topography and Properties of Composite Nanoscaffolds

The morphologies of the PLGA/Gelatin 70:30 and PLGA/Gelatin 50:50 nanofibrous scaffolds as depicted by SEM micrographs are shown in Figure 2A,B, respectively.

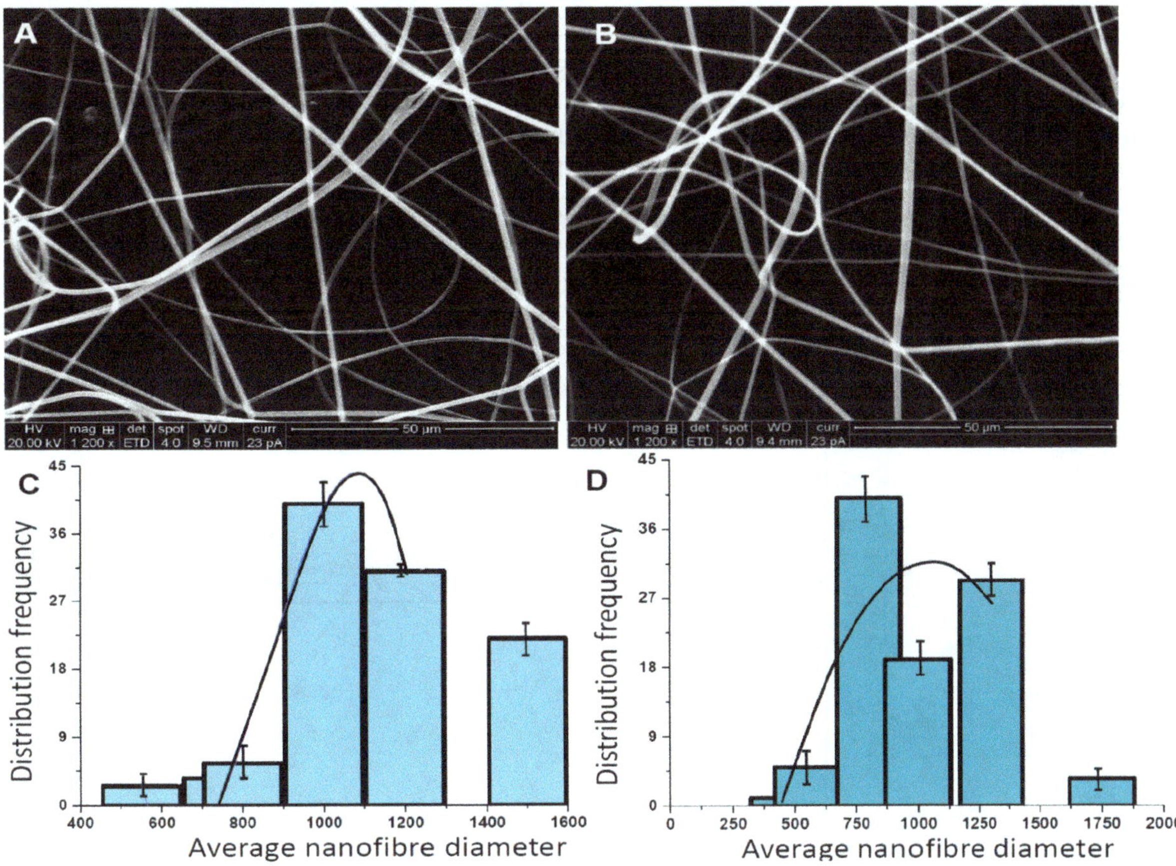

Figure 2. Physical Characterization. Scanning electron microscopy (SEM) micrographs of (**A**) PLGA/Gelatin 70:30 (**B**) PLGA/Gelatin 50:50 nanofibrous scaffolds and (**C**) Average fiber size distribution in PLGA/Gelatin 70:30 and (**D**) PLGA/Gelatin 50:50 nanofibrous scaffolds. The results are expressed as the median ± standard deviation obtained from analysis of 20 to 25 images for each electrospun polymer film (the black curve is drawn to shows the Gaussian distribution of frequency).

The corresponding average fiber diameters are shown as a bar plot in Figure 2C,D, respectively. The graph indicates that there is a random distribution of fibers in both, PLGA/Gelatin 70:30 and 50:50 nanoscaffolds. The average fiber diameter in PLGA/Gelatin 70:30 is slightly higher than 50:50 (~750 nm to 900 nm). The fibers exhibit ECM like interconnectivity, and no bead formation was observed. As gelatin adds viscosity to the solution, both types of fibers were smooth and without any breakage. The probability of fiber breakage increases with increasing gelatin content since an increase in gelatin content decreases the viscosity of the polymeric solution. The calculated average diameters of PLGA/Gelatin 70:30 and PLGA/Gelatin 50:50 nanofibers were 589.6 nm and 566.0 nm, respectively. As the concentration of gelatin increased, the diameter of the nanofibers decreased. This may be attributed to the fact that on increasing the gelatin content, the viscosity of the composite solution decreased, and the amino acids of the gelatin improved the self-repulsion and stretching force due to the increasing charge density of the jet during the electrospinning process. This resulted in the smaller fiber diameter [43]. The overall structure of the fibers mimics that of the ECM.

3.2. Quantitative Analysis of rhEGF-Immobilized Nanoscaffolds

The number of amine groups (µg per scaffold) on scaffolds treated with ninhydrin was quantified using the standard curve, and the results are shown in Figure 3A. It can be inferred from the graph that the quantified amount of amine groups were 25 µg and 30 µg per scaffold in PLGA/Gelatin 70:30 and PLGA/Gelatin 50:50 nanoscaffolds, respectively. The presence of amine groups in both the scaffolds clearly indicates the success of aminolysis. The results obtained from fluorescence spectrophotometry confirmed the presence of rhEGF on the surface of the nanofibrous scaffolds. The rhEGF-conjugated PLGA/Gelatin 50:50 and PLGA/Gelatin 70:30 nanoscaffolds had 7.46 µg and 2.92 µg of rhEGF, respectively, per scaffold when 10 µg of rhEGF was employed for a chemical reaction. Thus, the rhEGF immobilization efficiencies reached 74.6% and 29.2% for PLGA/Gelatin 50:50 and PLGA/Gelatin 70:30 nanofibrous scaffolds, respectively. It could be attributed to the fact that since the number of amine groups per scaffold was higher in PLGA/Gelatin 50:50 scaffolds, they were able to immobilize a greater amount of rhEGF than the PLGA/Gelatin 70:30 nanofibrous scaffolds.

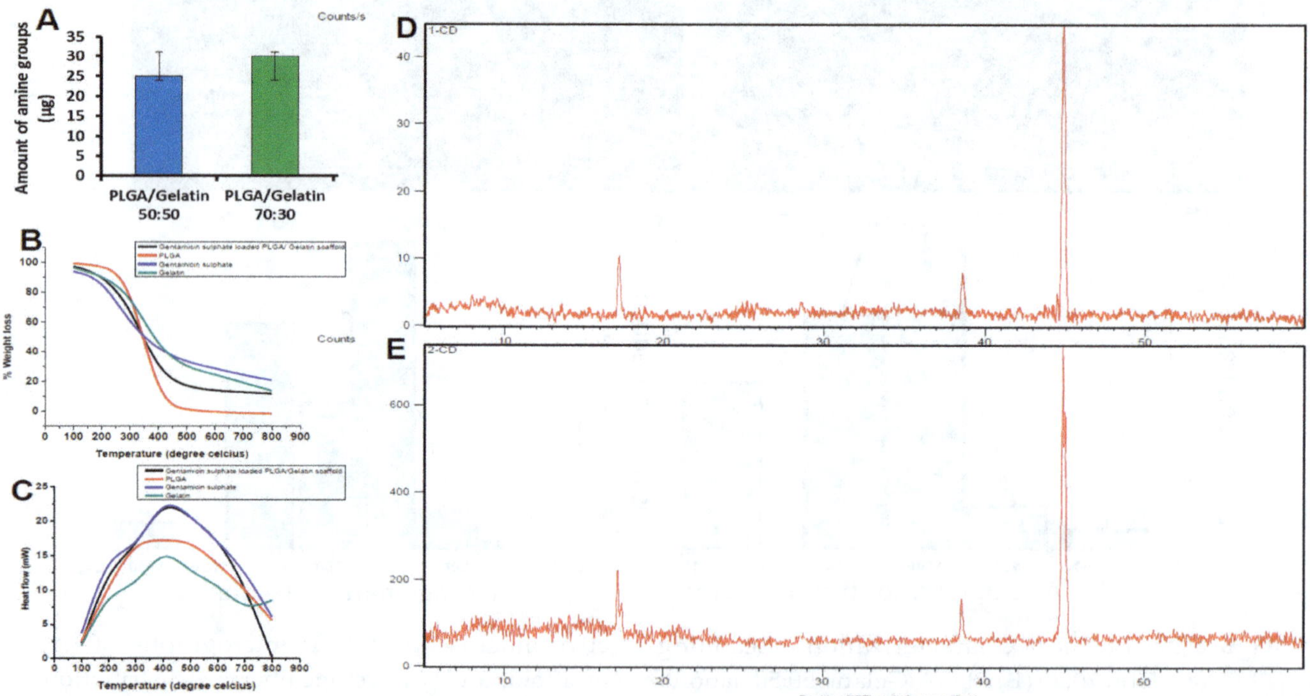

Figure 3. Biochemical characterization. (**A**) 2,2-dihydroxyindane-1,3-dione (ninhydrin) assay applied to 1,6 hexanediamine treated nanofibrous scaffolds (the results are expressed as the median ± standard deviation). (**B**) Thermogravimetric analysis (TGA) curves of PLGA, Gentamicin sulfate loaded PLGA 70:30 nanofibrous scaffolds, Gentamicin sulfate and Gelatin. (**C**) Differential scanning calorimetry (DSC) curves of PLGA, Gentamicin sulfate loaded PLGA nanofibrous scaffolds, Gentamicin sulfate and Gelatin. (**D**) X-Ray diffraction (XRD) spectra of (**A**) PLGA/gelatin 70:30 and (**E**) PLGA/gelatin 50:50 nanofibrous scaffolds.

3.3. Thermal Analysis

The thermal properties of composite nanoscaffolds and other supplements were characterized using TGA and DSC. TGA curves are shown in Figure 3B. The results from the TGA showed two significant weight losses for the gentamicin sulfate at 220 °C and 330 °C. The TGA curves of raw PLGA showed weight losses at 210 °C and 400 °C. In contrast, the TGA curve of gentamicin loaded PLGA/gelatin 70:30 nanofibrous scaffolds showed single significant weight loss at about 260 °C, respectively. As the weight loss of gentamicin sulfate and pure PLGA started at lower temperature compared to the gentamicin sulfate loaded scaffolds, it showed better thermal stability of the composite scaffolds in comparison to gentamicin sulfate or pure polymer alone. Due to the formation of covalent bonds between gentamicin and PLGA/gelatin scaffolds, the labile oxygen containing functional group availability was decreased. Less than 2% weight loss occurred below 200 °C. In addition, the slow weight loss of about 40% below 260 to 350 °C that may be due to the loss of residual functional group on the gentamicin-loaded scaffolds. These observations were missing in the negative control without the gentamicin.

The DSC thermograms of PLGA/Gelatin 70:30 nanofibrous scaffolds are shown in Figure 3C. A peak was observed at the temperature of 210 °C on the DSC thermogram of pure gentamicin sulfate powder, corresponding to the melting point of 210 °C. Another peak was seen at 410 °C, which was due to the reaction between the gentamicin sulfate structures, i.e., degradation of gentamicin sulfate. In the pure PLGA polymer, no sharp peak was observed which may be attributed to the amorphous nature of the PLGA. Whereas, the DSC curve of gelatin showed a peak at 405 °C. In contrast, in the DSC curves of gentamicin loaded PLGA/gelatin 70:30 nanofibrous scaffolds, the peak occurred at 430 °C. This clearly demonstrates that the stability of the drug is enhanced due to encapsulation of the drug between polymeric chains.

3.4. X-Ray Diffraction Analysis

The nanofibrous scaffolds are able to form a stable colloidal layered structure in aqueous solution, that facilitates drug encapsulation. The encapsulation of drug within the PLGA/Gelatin interlayer space may result in a change in the interlayer distance, that can be determined by XRD technology. The XRD patterns of the PLGA/gelatin 70:30 and PLGA/gelatin 50:50 scaffolds after gentamicin sulfate encapsulation are shown in Figure 3D,E, respectively. All the three types of nanofibrous scaffolds displayed patterns lacking any distinct peaks indicating that they are fully amorphous materials. In amorphous materials, X-rays will be scattered in many directions leading to a large bump distributed in a wide range (2 Theta) instead of high intensity narrower peaks. Appearance of the broad peaks in the $2\theta = 5–40°$ region was attributed to the amorphous nature of the PLGA. The absence of any distinct peaks of crystalline gentamicin sulfate in the XRD spectra indicates that the drug is no longer present as crystalline material, but had been totally converted to an amorphous state. The XRD data suggested that the incorporation of gentamicin sulfate within polymers is primarily via the drug intercalation within the polymer interlayer space.

It is also possible that a small portion of gentamicin sulfate can be adsorbed onto the polymer surface via hydrogen bonding or other weak forces. The XRD spectrum of the scaffolds displayed two peaks at 19.3° and 23.5° which were located at the same position with the PEG 400. The sharp XRD peaks indicate the crystallization of PEG in the scaffolds.

3.5. Degree of Swelling and Porosity Analysis

The gentamicin sulfate loaded PLGA/Gelatin 70:30 and PLGA/ Gelatin 50:50 nanofibrous scaffolds were analyzed to determine the swelling behavior by incubating them in PBS (pH 7.4) for 24 h at 37 °C. The results are represented graphically in Figure 4A. The swelling ratios of the PLGA/Gelatin 70:30 and PLGA/ Gelatin 50:50 nanofibrous scaffolds were 421.33 ± 8.22% and 445.33 ± 4.99%, respectively. The swelling index of cotton gauze was only 280.00 ± 8.64%. It can be inferred from these results that the higher swelling index of PLGA/ Gelatin 50:50 scaffolds was due to more concentration of gelatin as compared to the PLGA/Gelatin 70:30 scaffolds, as gelatin improves the hydrophilicity of the scaffold. This may be due to the amine and carboxylic functional groups present in the gelatin structure [44]. The obtained swelling index enables the prepared scaffolds to be used as wound dressings for absorbing excess exudates even from deep wounds with high amounts of exudates [44,45].

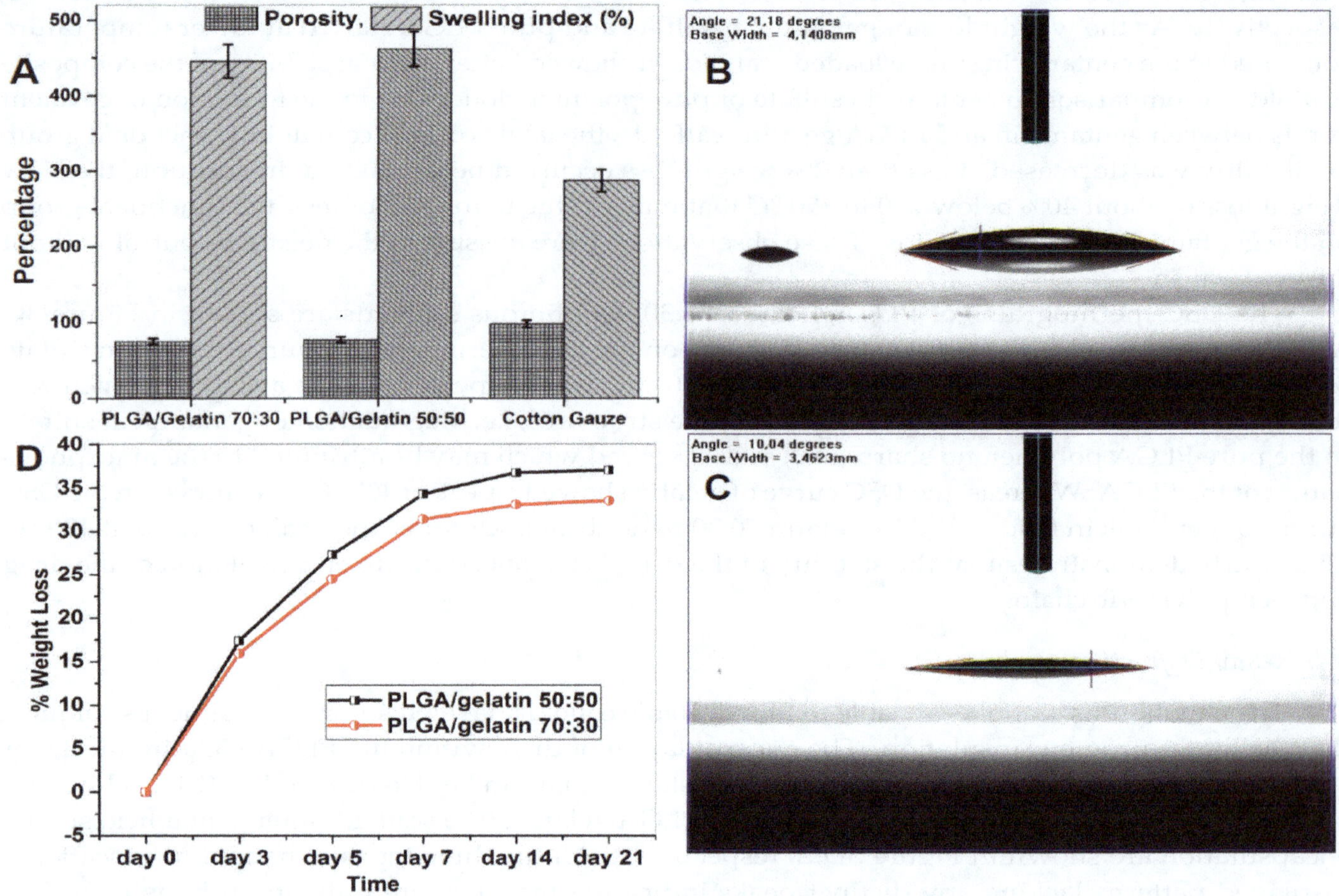

Figure 4. Scaffold stability and wettability analysis. (**A**) Comparison of swelling index and porosities of electrospun PLGA/gelatin 70:30 and 50:50 nanofibrous scaffolds (the results are expressed as the median ± standard deviation from five samples). (**B**) Water Contact Angle Value for PLGA/Gelatin 50:50 Nanofibrous Scaffold. (**C**)Water Contact Angle Value for PLGA/Gelatin 70:30 Nanofibrous Scaffold. (**D**) Biodegradability characteristics of PLGA/gelatin 50:50 and PLGA/gelatin 70:30 nanofibrous scaffolds.

Porosity is a very important criteria for the application of nanofibrous scaffolds in tissue engineering and wound healing practices because the microscale and nanoscale porous structure are most suitable for convenient passage and exchange of nutrients and gases, that are important for cellular growth and tissue regeneration [46]. Porosity should be in the range of 60 to 90% for cellular penetration and efficient tissue regeneration [47]. In the present work, porosity was calculated by the gravimetric method and the results are represented graphically in Figure 4A. The porosities of PLGA/Gelatin 50:50 and PLGA/Gelatin 70:30 nanofibrous scaffolds were 74.1% and 77%, respectively. In contrast, the porosity of cotton gauze was 102%. The possible reason could be that the increased gelatin content decreased the fiber diameter, which caused the decreased porosity of scaffolds.

3.6. Water Contact Angle Measurements

Generally, if the water contact angle is smaller than 90°, the solid surface is considered hydrophilic and wettable, and if the water contact angle is larger than 90°, the solid surface is considered hydrophobic and not wettable. Figure 4B,C, respectively show that the water contact angle values for PLGA/Gelatin 70:30 and PLGA/Gelatin 50:50 nanofibrous scaffolds were 10.04° and 21.18°, respectively. Hence, it could be concluded that the water contact angles of both the scaffolds was much lesser than 90°. Therefore, the surface of the scaffolds could be considered highly hydrophilic. Moreover, the water contact angle of PLGA/Gelatin 50:50 nanofibrous scaffolds were lower than that of PLGA/Gelatin 70:30 nanofibrous scaffolds due to more amount of Gelatin on the former as compared to the latter.

3.7. In Vitro Biodegradability Studies

The in vitro biodegradation studies of the PLGA/Gelatin 70:30 and PLGA/Gelatin 50:50 nanofibrous scaffolds were performed in Phosphate Buffer Saline (PBS; pH 7.4). The scaffolds were placed in a 24-well plate containing 1 mL of PBS in each well and were incubated in vitro at 37 °C for different periods of time (3, 5, 7, 14 days). Figure 4D shows the percent weight losses. A rapid 27.33 ± 1.15% and 24.4 ± 1.82% mass loss was observed in electrospun PLGA/gelatin 50:50 and PLGA/gelatin 70:30 nanofibrous scaffolds, respectively, in first 5 days. After 7 days, the degradability of both scaffolds was decreased which was due to more PLGA in the remaining composition of scaffolds. Since gelatin easily dissolves in water at a temperature of 40 °C, and, hence, by increasing the content of gelatin, the biodegradability of the PLGA/gelatin 50:50 scaffolds was greater as compared to PLGA/gelatin 70:30 scaffolds. In contrast, PLGA nanofibrous scaffolds and cotton gauze used as control did not exhibit any weight loss during the 14 days of incubation.

3.8. Drug Loading Capacity and Drug Entrapment Efficiency

Drug loading capacity is the ratio of the mass of bound drug to the mass of the scaffold, whereas, the drug entrapment efficiency is the ratio of the mass of drug released to the mass of total drug added. The mass of gentamicin sulfate loaded per 20 mg of the scaffolds was investigated by UV-Vis spectrophotometry. The results are summarized in Table 1. It was found to be 174.24 μg and 161.68 μg for PLGA/Gelatin 70:30 and PLGA/Gelatin 50:50 nanofibrous scaffolds, respectively. On the other hand, the entrapment efficiency was found to be 87.12% and 80.26% for PLGA/Gelatin 70:30 and PLGA/Gelatin 50:50 nanofibrous scaffolds, respectively. The comparatively higher entrapment efficiency may be due to the fact that PLGA, being a high molecular weight polymer, and the molecular weight further supplemented by gelatin, is able to absorb a comparatively greater amount of active substances. As shown herein, more than 80% entrapment efficiency ensures more than 150 μg of gentamicin sulfate delivered to the wound site for in-situ release. These results are in line with therapeutically used dosages of gentamicin sulfate 100 μg or more, immobilized on the synthetic carrier for successful treatment of infection in mouse model [48].

Table 1. Drug loading capacity and drug entrapment efficiency of nanofibrous scaffolds.

Nanofibrous Scaffold	Drug Loading Capacity (μg)	Drug Entrapment Efficiency (%)
PLGA/Gelatin 50:50	161.68 ± 13.2	80.26 ± 6.9
PLGA/Gelatin 70:30	174.24 ± 19	87.12 ± 8.1

3.9. In Vitro Drug Release Studies

The gentamicin sulfate release curves from PLGA/Gelatin 70:30 and PLGA/Gelatin 50:50 nanofibrous scaffolds were studied at different pH values, and the release curves are illustrated in Figure 5A,B. The studies from each type of scaffolds revealed constant drug release and no burst effect was observed. It indicates that the drug was homogeneously dispersed in the polymeric matrix and there was no significant amount of drug adsorbed onto the surface of nanofibers. Figure 5A shows the release of gentamicin sulfate from PLGA/Gelatin 70:30 nanofibrous scaffold. At pH 7.4, gentamicin sulfate was released slowly from the PLGA/Gelatin 70:30 nanofibrous scaffold and only 36.64 ± 0.51% of the total bound gentamicin sulfate was released in 12 h. However, 91.46 ± 0.61% and 75.43 ± 0.82%

of the drug was released in acidic and basic conditions, respectively, after 12 h. Figure 5B illustrates the release of gentamicin sulfate from PLGA/Gelatin 50:50 nanofibrous scaffold. At pH 7.4, gentamicin sulfate was released slowly from the PLGA/gelatin 50:50 nanofibrous scaffold and only 44.97 ± 0.14% of the total bound gentamicin sulfate was released in 12 h. However, 93.33 ± 0.82% and 76.03 ± 0.75% of the drug was released in acidic and basic conditions, respectively, after 12 h. The release at pH 3 and pH 9 is much higher than that released at pH 7.4. This is so because the hydrogen bonding interaction between gentamicin sulfate and the nanofibrous scaffolds is strongest at the neutral pH. Whereas, at pH 3 and 9, there is a comparatively weaker hydrogen bonding interaction, so the higher amount of gentamicin sulfate was released at pH 3 and 9. There was a higher percentage release of gentamicin sulfate at pH 3 compared to pH 9 because the hydrogen bonding interaction formed under basic conditions was stronger than that under acidic conditions.

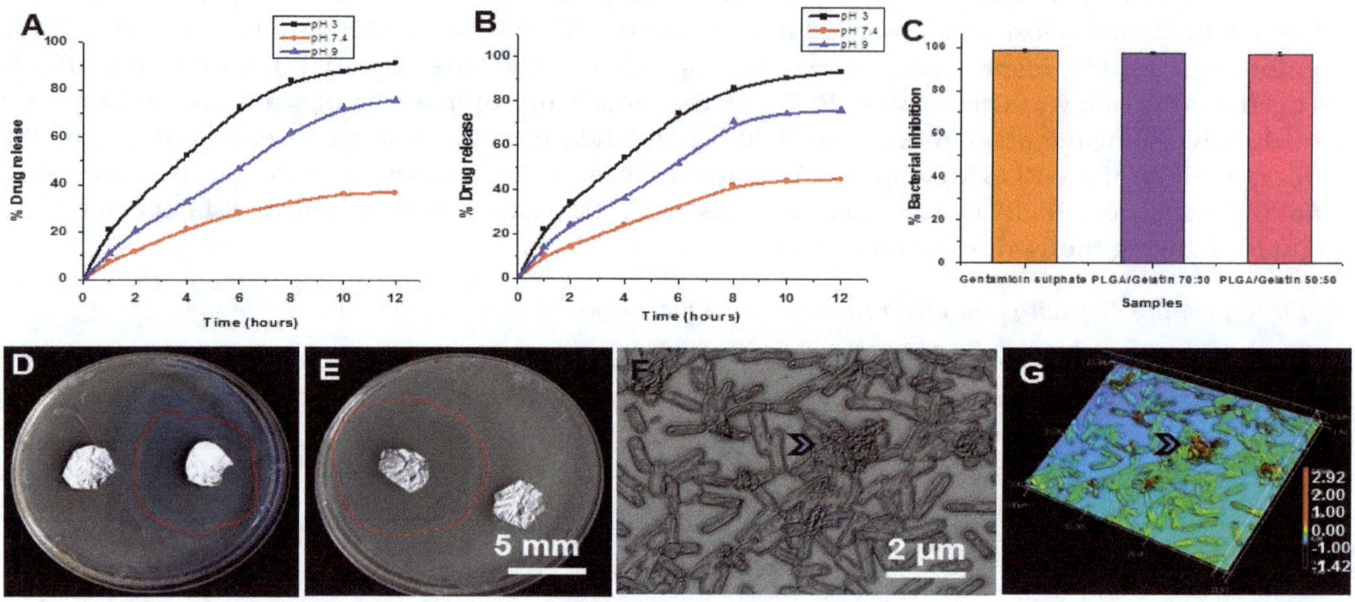

Figure 5. In vitro antibacterial assay. (**A,B**) Release profile of gentamicin sulfate on PLGA/Gelatin 70:30 (A) and 50:50 (B) nanofibrous scaffolds at three different pH values. (**C**) Growth inhibition of *Staphylococcus aureus* after treatment with PLGA/Gelatin 70:30, PLGA/Gelatin 50:50 nanofibrous scaffolds and Gentamicin sulfate powder in aqueous media. The results are expressed as the median ± standard deviation from five independent experiments performed in triplicate (n = 5). (**D**) Antibacterial activity of gentamicin sulfate loaded PLGA/ Gelatin 70:30 nanofibrous scaffolds against *Staphylococcus aureus* on LB Agar semisolid media. (**E**) Antibacterial activity of gentamicin sulfate loaded PLGA/Gelatin 50:50 nanofibrous scaffolds against *Staphylococcus aureus* (dotted red line show zone of inhibitions-ZOI around test sample, next to control). (**F,G**) Optical and laser scanning micrograph from bacterial cells seeded on Gentamicin Sulfate (GS)/PLGA/Gelatin (50:50) surfaces show sunken morphology of bacterial cells trapped in a network of nanofibers scaffolds (arrow heads).

3.10. *In Vitro Antibacterial Activity*

The in vitro antibacterial activity of the gentamicin sulfate loaded PLGA/Gelatin 70:30 and PLGA/Gelatin 50:50 nanofibrous scaffolds were explored against *Staphylococcus aureus* M 0092 in aqueous medium. *S. aureus* bacteria are commonly found in diabetic wounds and used as a pathogenic bacterial model for in vitro antibacterial efficacy [49]. Figure 5C illustrates the results of the antibacterial activity assays. The negative control, which was the tube with cotton gauze, completely failed to inhibit bacterial growth. Gentamicin sulfate powder, which was used as the positive control exhibited 98.73 ± 0.68% inhibition of the bacterial growth at the concentration of 5 mg/mL. The PLGA/Gelatin 70:30 and PLGA/Gelatin 50:50 nanofibrous scaffolds showed 97.39 ± 0.62% and 97.20 ± 0.99% inhibition of bacterial growth, respectively. This may be attributed to the active diffusion of the drug molecules from the scaffolds into the liquid medium, thus, inhibiting the growth of bacteria. These results are promising, since the antibacterial activity of the PLGA/Gelatin 70:30 and PLGA/Gelatin 50:50 nanofibrous scaffolds are comparable to that of the pure gentamicin powder, which presents them as a perfect drug releasing vehicle. Thus, the developed nanofibrous scaffolds could be used as a potential wound dressing material that would successfully eliminate infections, thereby, accelerating wound healing.

The antibacterial activity of the PLGA/Gelatin 70:30 and PLGA/Gelatin 50:50 nanofibrous scaffolds was also analyzed over a solid medium. Figure 5C,D shows the digital photographs of the zone of inhibition on nutrient agar plates. The gentamicin sulfate loaded PLGA/Gelatin 50:50 and PLGA/Gelatin 70:30 nanofibrous scaffolds had "zone of inhibition" values of 40 mm (Figure 5B) and 41 mm (Figure 5C), respectively. These results suggested that each nanofibrous scaffold had a good bacterial inhibition efficacy under the studied conditions. In contrast, PLGA/Gelatin nanofibrous scaffolds without gentamicin sulfate encapsulation did not inhibit the bacterial growth, suggesting that the bacterial inhibition effect is solely related to the encapsulated Gentamicin sulfate drug. Hence, the gentamicin sulfate loaded nanofibrous scaffolds were bactericidal to the testing microorganism due to the strong antibacterial ability of gentamicin sulfate. The results indicate that gentamicin sulfate loaded scaffolds possess efficient antibacterial property and can be effectively used in the treatment of wound healing or dermal bacterial infections, thereby, proving a potential application for use as a drug delivery and as a wound dressing agent [50].

We also studied the morphologies and biovolume of bacterial cells seeded on two nanofibrous scaffold supplemented with GS using laser scanning microscope to quantify surface and biovolume (Figure 5F–G and Supplementary Figure S2A–E). As seen in optical and 3D height profile images, the bacterial cells are entangled into fibers, which affect bacterial cells surface into sunken morphology, reducing their biovolume compare with untreated control cells showing flagella and normal morphology (arrow, Figure 5F–G and Figure S1C).

3.11. *In Vivo Wound Healing Activity on Diabetic Mice and Organ Toxicity Evaluation*

Animals with induced diabetes were confirmed with diabetic symptoms and were subjected to wound healing treatments with the gentamicin-rhEGF-nanofibrous scaffolds and controls. The wound area was measured daily from day 0 to 12 and wounds were monitored qualitatively (Figure 6A), and quantitatively (Figure 6B) for the wound closure to assess the efficacy of therapeutics designed. The results revealed that rhEGF immobilized nanofibrous scaffolds significantly increased the wound closure rates compared to other treatments. The representative images at 1, 4, 8, and 12 days after treatment with rhEGF-PLGA/Gelatin 70:30 nanofibrous scaffold, PLGA/gelatin 70:30 nanofibrous scaffold with gentamicin sulfate, PLGA/gelatin 70:30 nanofibrous scaffold without rhEGF, untreated wound and gentamicin sulfate are shown in Figure 6A. Specifically, the animals with PLGA/Gelatin 70:30 nanofibrous scaffolds with rhEGF and gentamicin sulfate showed 19.13 ± 5.68% open wound area on the 4th day (Figure 6A), 12.99 ± 1.17% open wound area on the 8th day (Figure 6An), and 3.25 ± 2.95% open wound area on the 12th day (Figure 6As), which were much less than other treatments. The data represented the mean ± S.D. for six mice per group.

We also took samples from different organs of mice treated with GS/PLGA/gelatin 50:50 after day 12 and compared with the controls group without any treatment. As shown in Figure 7, histopathological examination results showed that there was no apparent change in different organs morphology and no other abnormal changes in the mice tissue in control versus experimental group. This confirms that the nanofibrous scaffolds, thus, prepared are biocompatible and do not cause any side effects. These results open new opportunities for rapid wound healing in different vascular lesions as advance therapeutics, which is sought as a major challenge in current nanomedicine in vascular biology [51,52].

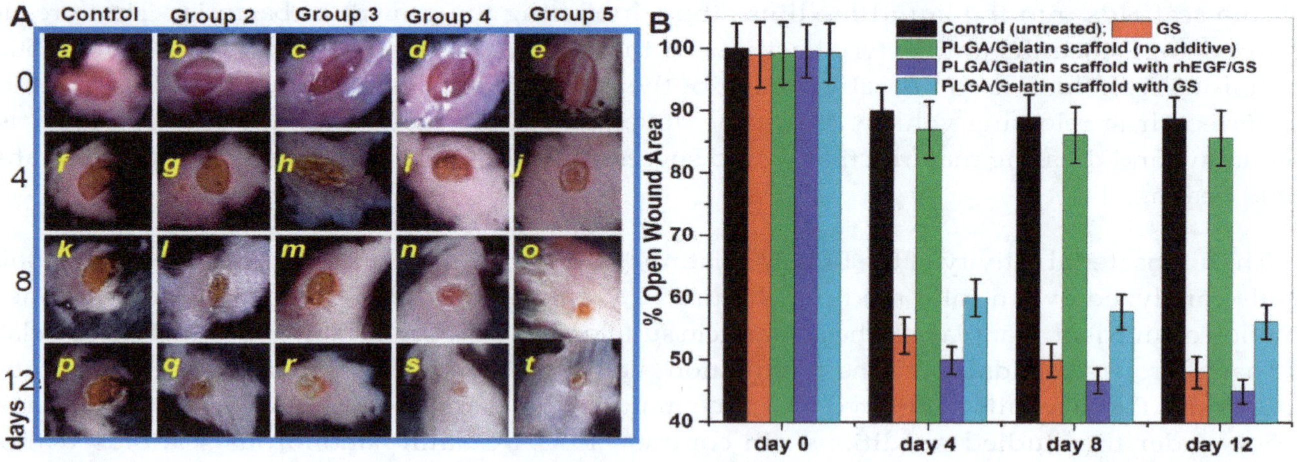

Figure 6. In vivo wound healing assay in mouse model. (**A**) Wound Healing in Diabetic C57/BL6 Mice after Treatment with Various Electrospun Nanofibrous Scaffolds (Batch 1) [a–t represent the extent of wound healing during 12 days period] Group 1—No treatment (negative control); Group 2—0.1% gentamicin sulfate ointment (positive control); Group 3—PLGA/Gelatin 70:30 scaffold without gentamicin sulfate and rhEGF; Group 4—PLGA/Gelatin 70:30 scaffold with gentamicin sulfate and rhEGF; Group 5—PLGA/Gelatin 70:30 scaffold with gentamicin sulfate and without rhEGF. (**B**) Open wound area (% of initial area) over 12 days for each treatment group from control and three experimental groups performed from five different wound healing assays. The results are expressed as the median ± standard deviation from five independent experiments performed in triplicate (n = 5).

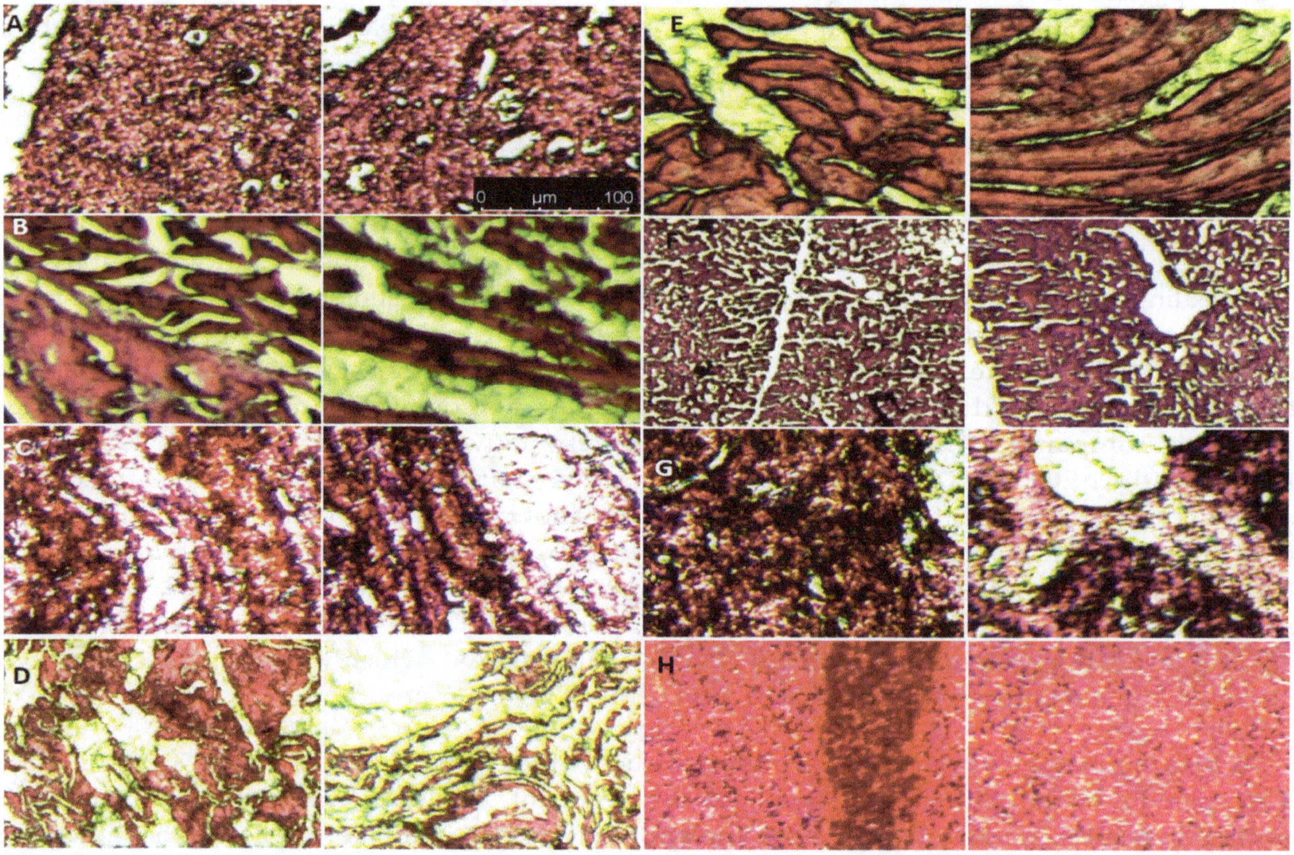

Figure 7. Histological evaluation of In vivo *organ* toxicity with histopathological staining on organ sections. (**A**) Brain (**B**) Heart (**C**) Kidney (**D**) Lung (**E**) Muscle (**F**) Liver (**G**) Pancreases (**H**) Spleen. Each image from **A–H** has control (left panel) and scaffold applied (right panel) sample section with Hematoxylin and Eosin (**H,E**) staining.

4. Conclusions

In summary, a novel nanocomposite carrier device composed of PLGA/Gelatin 70:30 and PLGA/Gelatin 50:50 nanofibrous scaffolds loaded with gentamicin sulfate and immobilized with rhEGF was developed for diabetic wound healing applications. The developed nanofibrous scaffolds resembled the morphology and architecture of the native extracellular matrix (ECM), which makes them useful as a suitable wound-healing scaffold. The gentamicin sulfate stability and bactericidal properties were not affected by the encapsulation process and release. The rhEGF accelerated wound-healing rates at the initial stage of the healing process. The results obtained are promising, since the simultaneous delivery of antibiotic and bioactive molecule from a nanocarrier material to inactivate bacteria in diabetic wounds and hasten the wound healing at the same time was clearly demonstrated. The nanocomposite has the potential to synergistically improve the impaired wound healing in diabetic patients via combined antibacterial activity and rhEGF supply.

Author Contributions: Conceptualization, C.D., A.V.S. and P.W.R.; methodology, C.D., A.V.S., S.P.; software H.P., A.C.P.; validation A.V.S., P.L., A.L., and H.P.; formal analysis, C.D., A.V.S.; investigation, H.P., A.V.S., C.D.; resources, A.C.P., A.L., P.L., P.W.R.; data curation, C.D., A.V.S.; writing—original draft preparation, C.D., A.V.S.; writing—review and editing, A.V.S., C.D., P.W.R., A.L., P.L.; visualization, A.C.P., P.W.R.; supervision, A.V.S., P.W.R.; project administration, P.W.R., A.V.S.; funding acquisition, A.V.S., P.W.R.

Acknowledgments: Charu Dwivedi acknowledges Council of Scientific and Industrial Research (CSIR), Ministry of HRD, Government of India for CSIR-SRF Fellowship support and National Centre of Laboratory Animal Sciences (National Institute of Nutrition-ICMR), Hyderabad, (NCLAS/ASC/2015/B.U./F-278) for providing C57/BL6 mice.

References

1. Xie, Z.; Paras, C.B.; Weng, H.; Punnakitikashem, P.; Su, L.-C.; Vu, K.; Tang, L.; Yang, J.; Nguyen, K.T. Dual growth factor releasing multi-functional nanofibers for wound healing. *Acta Biomater.* **2013**, *9*, 9351–9359. [CrossRef] [PubMed]
2. Singh, A.V.; Subhashree, L.; Milani, P.; Gemmati, D.; Zamboni, P. Interplay of iron metallobiology, metalloproteinases, and fxiii, and role of their gene variants in venous leg ulcer. *Int. J. Low. Extrem. Wounds* **2010**, *9*, 166–179. [CrossRef]
3. Gandhimathi, C.; Venugopal, J.R.; Bhaarathy, V.; Ramakrishna, S.; Kumar, S.D. Biocomposite nanofibrous strategies for the controlled release of biomolecules for skin tissue regeneration. *Int. J. Nanomed.* **2014**, *9*, 4709.
4. Sandhya, S.; Kumar, S.; Vinod, K.; Banji, D.; Kumar, K. Plant as potent anti diabetic and wound healing agent—A review. *Hygeia J. Drugs Med.* **2011**, *3*, 11–19.
5. Tiaka, E.K.; Papanas, N.; Manolakis, A.C.; Maltezos, E. The role of nerve growth factor in the prophylaxis and treatment of diabetic foot ulcers. *Int. J. Burn. Trauma* **2011**, *1*, 68.
6. Djahmi, N.; Messad, N.; Nedjai, S.; Moussaoui, A.; Mazouz, D.; Richard, J.-L.; Sotto, A.; Lavigne, J.-P. Molecular epidemiology of staphylococcus aureus strains isolated from inpatients with infected diabetic foot ulcers in an algerian university hospital. *Clin. Microbiol. Infect.* **2013**, *19*, E398–E404. [CrossRef] [PubMed]
7. Kamtikar, R.; Mitra, N. Clinico microbiological profile of pseudomonas aeruginosa isolated from diabetic foot ulcer. *J. Sci. Innov. Res.* **2014**, *3*, 478–481.
8. Bowen, K. Managing foot infections in patients with diabetes. *Aust. Prescr.* **2007**, *30*, 21–24. [CrossRef]
9. Lipsky, B.A.; Berendt, A.R.; Deery, H.G.; Embil, J.M.; Joseph, W.S.; Karchmer, A.W.; LeFrock, J.L.; Lew, D.P.; Mader, J.T.; Norden, C. Diagnosis and treatment of diabetic foot infections. *Clin. Infect. Dis.* **2004**, *39*, 885–910. [CrossRef] [PubMed]
10. Spichler, A.; Hurwitz, B.L.; Armstrong, D.G.; Lipsky, B.A. Microbiology of diabetic foot infections: From louis pasteur to 'crime scene investigation'. *BMC Med.* **2015**, *13*, 2. [CrossRef]
11. Trivedi, U.; Parameswaran, S.; Armstrong, A.; Burgueno-Vega, D.; Griswold, J.; Dissanaike, S.; Rumbaugh, K.P. Prevalence of multiple antibiotic resistant infections in diabetic versus nondiabetic wounds. *J. Pathog.* **2014**, *2014*, 173053. [CrossRef] [PubMed]
12. Dwivedi, C.; Pandey, H.; Pandey, A.C.; Ramteke, P.W. Nanofiber based smart pharmaceutical scaffolds for wound repair and regenerations. *Curr. Pharm. Des.* **2016**, *22*, 1460–1471. [CrossRef] [PubMed]

13. Choi, J.S.; Leong, K.W.; Yoo, H.S. In vivo wound healing of diabetic ulcers using electrospun nanofibers immobilized with human epidermal growth factor (EGF). *Biomaterials* **2008**, *29*, 587–596. [CrossRef] [PubMed]
14. Herbst, R.S. Review of epidermal growth factor receptor biology. *Int. J. Radiat. Oncol. Biol. Phys.* **2004**, *59*, S21–S26. [CrossRef]
15. Fallon, J.H.; Seroogy, K.B.; Loughlin, S.E.; Morrison, R.S.; Bradshaw, R.A.; Knaver, D.; Cunningham, D.D. Epidermal growth factor immunoreactive material in the central nervous system: Location and development. *Science* **1984**, *224*, 1107–1109. [CrossRef] [PubMed]
16. Vikram Singh, A.; Hasan Dad Ansari, M.; Wang, S.; Laux, P.; Luch, A.; Kumar, A.; Patil, R.; Nussberger, S. The adoption of three-dimensional additive manufacturing from biomedical material design to 3d organ printing. *Appl. Sci.* **2019**, *9*, 811. [CrossRef]
17. Singh, V.; Kashyap, S.; Yadav, U.; Srivastava, A.; Singh, A.V.; Singh, R.K.; Singh, S.K.; Saxena, P.S. Nitrogen doped carbon quantum dots demonstrate no toxicity under in vitro conditions in a cervical cell line and in vivo in swiss albino mice. *Toxicol. Res.* **2019**. [CrossRef]
18. Dwivedi, C.; Pandey, I.; Misra, V.; Giulbudagian, M.; Jungnickel, H.; Laux, P.; Luch, A.; Ramteke, P.W.; Singh, A.V. The prospective role of nanobiotechnology in food and food packaging products. *Integr. Food Nutr. Metab. (IFNM)* **2018**. [CrossRef]
19. Abdel-Wahhab, M.A.; Márquez, F. Nanomaterials in biomedicine. *Soft Nanosci. Lett.* **2015**, *5*, 53–54. [CrossRef]
20. Singh, A.V.; Laux, P.; Luch, A.; Sudrik, C.; Wiehr, S.; Wild, A.-M.; Santomauro, G.; Bill, J.; Sitti, M. Review of emerging concepts in nanotoxicology: Opportunities and challenges for safer nanomaterial design. *Toxicol. Mech. Methods* **2019**, 1–10. [CrossRef]
21. Dwivedi, C.; Pandey, I.; Pandey, H.; Patil, S.; Mishra, S.B.; Pandey, A.C.; Zamboni, P.; Ramteke, P.W.; Singh, A.V. In vivo diabetic wound healing with nanofibrous scaffolds modified with gentamicin and recombinant human epidermal growth factor. *J. Biomed. Mater. Res. Part A* **2018**, *106*, 641–651. [CrossRef] [PubMed]
22. Gupta, K.C.; Haider, A.; Choi, Y.-R.; Kang, I.-K. Nanofibrous scaffolds in biomedical applications. *Biomater. Res.* **2014**, *18*, 5. [CrossRef] [PubMed]
23. Venugopal, J.; Ramakrishna, S. Applications of polymer nanofibers in biomedicine and biotechnology. *Appl. Biochem. Biotechnol.* **2005**, *125*, 147–157. [CrossRef]
24. Wang, S.; Zheng, F.; Huang, Y.; Fang, Y.; Shen, M.; Zhu, M.; Shi, X. Encapsulation of amoxicillin within laponite-doped poly (lactic-co-glycolic acid) nanofibers: Preparation, characterization, and antibacterial activity. *ACS Appl. Mater. Interfaces* **2012**, *4*, 6393–6401. [CrossRef]
25. Hajiali, H.; Shahgasempour, S.; Naimi-Jamal, M.R.; Peirovi, H. Electrospun pga/gelatin nanofibrous scaffolds and their potential application in vascular tissue engineering. *Int. J. Nanomed.* **2011**, *6*, 2133. [CrossRef] [PubMed]
26. Nigam, R.; Mahanta, B. An overview of various biomimetic scaffolds: Challenges and applications in tissue engineering. *J. Tissue Sci. Eng.* **2014**, *5*, 1.
27. Steed, D.L. The role of growth factors in wound healing. *Surg. Clin. N. Am.* **1997**, *77*, 575–586. [CrossRef]
28. Fouad, H.; Elsarnagawy, T.; Almajhdi, F.N.; Khalil, K.A. Preparation and in vitro thermo-mechanical characterization of electrospun plga nanofibers for soft and hard tissue replacement. *Int. J. Electrochem. Sci.* **2013**, *8*, 2293–2304.
29. Ansary, R.H.; Awang, M.B.; Rahman, M.M. Biodegradable poly (D,L-lactic-co-glycolic acid)-based micro/nanoparticles for sustained release of protein drugs-a review. *Trop. J. Pharm. Res.* **2014**, *13*, 1179–1190. [CrossRef]
30. Dwivedi, C.; Pandey, H.; Pandey, A.C.; Ramteke, P.W. Novel gentamicin loaded electrospun nanofibrous scaffolds for wound healing: An in-vitro study. *Int. J. Pharm. Sci. Res.* **2013**, *4*, 2224–2227.
31. Singh, A.V.; Aditi, A.S.; Gade, W.N.; Vats, T.; Lenardi, C.; Milani, P. Nanomaterials: New generation therapeutics in wound healing and tissue repair. *Curr. Nanosci.* **2010**, *6*, 577–586. [CrossRef]
32. Singh, D.; Saraf, S.; Dixit, V.K.; Saraf, S. Formulation optimization of gentamicin loaded eudragit rs100 microspheres using factorial design study. *Biol. Pharm. Bull.* **2008**, *31*, 662–667. [CrossRef]
33. Deng, A.; Yang, Y.; Du, S.; Yang, S. Electrospinning of in situ crosslinked recombinant human collagen peptide/chitosan nanofibers for wound healing. *Biomater. Sci.* **2018**, *6*, 2197–2208. [CrossRef] [PubMed]

34. Kurečič, M.; Maver, T.; Virant, N.; Ojstršek, A.; Gradišnik, L.; Hribernik, S.; Kolar, M.; Maver, U.; Kleinschek, K.S. A multifunctional electrospun and dual nano-carrier biobased system for simultaneous detection of ph in the wound bed and controlled release of benzocaine. *Cellulose* **2018**, *25*, 7277–7297. [CrossRef]
35. Maver, T.; Smrke, D.; Kurečič, M.; Gradišnik, L.; Maver, U.; Kleinschek, K.S. Combining 3d printing and electrospinning for preparation of pain-relieving wound-dressing materials. *J. Sol-Gel Sci. Technol.* **2018**, *88*, 33–48. [CrossRef]
36. Shi, R.; Geng, H.; Gong, M.; Ye, J.; Wu, C.; Hu, X.; Zhang, L. Long-acting and broad-spectrum antimicrobial electrospun poly (ε-caprolactone)/gelatin micro/nanofibers for wound dressing. *J. Colloid Interface Sci.* **2018**, *509*, 275–284. [CrossRef] [PubMed]
37. Dwivedi, C.; Pandey, H.; Pandey, A.C.; Ramteke, P.W. Fabrication and assessment of gentamicin loaded electrospun nanofibrous scaffolds as a quick wound healing dressing material. *Curr. Nanosci.* **2015**, *11*, 222–228. [CrossRef]
38. Gentile, P.; Chiono, V.; Carmagnola, I.; Hatton, P. An overview of poly (lactic-co-glycolic) acid (PLGA)-based biomaterials for bone tissue engineering. *Int. J. Mol. Sci.* **2014**, *15*, 3640–3659. [CrossRef]
39. Singh, A.V.; Mehta, K.K.; Worley, K.; Dordick, J.S.; Kane, R.S.; Wan, L.Q. Carbon nanotube-induced loss of multicellular chirality on micropatterned substrate is mediated by oxidative stress. *ACS Nano* **2014**, *8*, 2196–2205. [CrossRef]
40. Singh, A.V.; Hosseinidoust, Z.; Park, B.-W.; Yasa, O.; Sitti, M. Microemulsion-based soft bacteria-driven microswimmers for active cargo delivery. *ACS Nano* **2017**, *11*, 9759–9769. [CrossRef]
41. Pandey, H.; Parashar, V.; Parashar, R.; Prakash, R.; Ramteke, P.W.; Pandey, A.C. Controlled drug release characteristics and enhanced antibacterial effect of graphene nanosheets containing gentamicin sulfate. *Nanoscale* **2011**, *3*, 4104–4108. [CrossRef] [PubMed]
42. Maver, T.; Gradišnik, L.; Smrke, D.M.; Kleinschek, K.S.; Maver, U. Systematic evaluation of a diclofenac-loaded carboxymethyl cellulose-based wound dressing and its release performance with changing ph and temperature. *AAPS PharmSciTech* **2019**, *20*, 29. [CrossRef] [PubMed]
43. Meng, Z.; Xu, X.; Zheng, W.; Zhou, H.; Li, L.; Zheng, Y.; Lou, X. Preparation and characterization of electrospun plga/gelatin nanofibers as a potential drug delivery system. *Colloids Surf. B Biointerfaces* **2011**, *84*, 97–102. [CrossRef] [PubMed]
44. Meng, Z.; Wang, Y.; Ma, C.; Zheng, W.; Li, L.; Zheng, Y. Electrospinning of plga/gelatin randomly-oriented and aligned nanofibers as potential scaffold in tissue engineering. *Mater. Sci. Eng. C* **2010**, *30*, 1204–1210. [CrossRef]
45. Pal, K.; Banthia, A.K.; Majumdar, D.K. Polyvinyl alcohol–glycine composite membranes: Preparation, characterization, drug release and cytocompatibility studies. *Biomed. Mater.* **2006**, *1*, 49. [CrossRef]
46. Murugan, R.; Ramakrishna, S. Nano-featured scaffolds for tissue engineering: A review of spinning methodologies. *Tissue Eng.* **2006**, *12*, 435–447. [CrossRef]
47. Chong, E.; Phan, T.; Lim, I.; Zhang, Y.; Bay, B.; Ramakrishna, S.; Lim, C. Evaluation of electrospun pcl/gelatin nanofibrous scaffold for wound healing and layered dermal reconstitution. *Acta Biomater.* **2007**, *3*, 321–330. [CrossRef]
48. Gander, B.; Gamazo, C.; Irache, J.M.; Prior, S. Gentamicin-loaded microspheres for treatment of experimental brucella abortus infection in mice. *J. Antimicrob. Chemother.* **2005**, *55*, 1032–1036.
49. Singh, A.V.; Baylan, S.; Park, B.W.; Richter, G.; Sitti, M. Hydrophobic pinning with copper nanowhiskers leads to bactericidal properties. *PLoS ONE* **2017**, *12*, e0175428. [CrossRef]
50. Singh, V.; Kumar, V.; Kashyap, S.; Singh, A.V.; Kishore, V.; Sitti, M.; Saxena, P.S.; Srivastava, A. Graphene oxide synergistically enhances antibiotic efficacy in vancomycin-resistant staphylococcus aureus. *ACS Appl. Bio Mater.* **2019**, *2*, 1148–1157. [CrossRef]
51. Singh, A.V.; Gemmati, D.; Kanase, A.; Pandey, I.; Misra, V.; Kishore, V.; Jahnke, T.; Bill, J. Nanobiomaterials for vascular biology and wound management: A review. *Veins Lymphat.* **2018**, *7*. [CrossRef]
52. Vikram Singh, A. Editorial (thematic issue: Recent trends in nano-biotechnology reinforcing contemporary pharmaceutical design). *Curr. Pharm. Des.* **2016**, *22*, 1415–1417. [CrossRef]

Permissions

All chapters in this book were first published by MDPI; hereby published with permission under the Creative Commons Attribution License or equivalent. Every chapter published in this book has been scrutinized by our experts. Their significance has been extensively debated. The topics covered herein carry significant findings which will fuel the growth of the discipline. They may even be implemented as practical applications or may be referred to as a beginning point for another development.

The contributors of this book come from diverse backgrounds, making this book a truly international effort. This book will bring forth new frontiers with its revolutionizing research information and detailed analysis of the nascent developments around the world.

We would like to thank all the contributing authors for lending their expertise to make the book truly unique. They have played a crucial role in the development of this book. Without their invaluable contributions this book wouldn't have been possible. They have made vital efforts to compile up to date information on the varied aspects of this subject to make this book a valuable addition to the collection of many professionals and students.

This book was conceptualized with the vision of imparting up-to-date information and advanced data in this field. To ensure the same, a matchless editorial board was set up. Every individual on the board went through rigorous rounds of assessment to prove their worth. After which they invested a large part of their time researching and compiling the most relevant data for our readers.

The editorial board has been involved in producing this book since its inception. They have spent rigorous hours researching and exploring the diverse topics which have resulted in the successful publishing of this book. They have passed on their knowledge of decades through this book. To expedite this challenging task, the publisher supported the team at every step. A small team of assistant editors was also appointed to further simplify the editing procedure and attain best results for the readers.

Apart from the editorial board, the designing team has also invested a significant amount of their time in understanding the subject and creating the most relevant covers. They scrutinized every image to scout for the most suitable representation of the subject and create an appropriate cover for the book.

The publishing team has been an ardent support to the editorial, designing and production team. Their endless efforts to recruit the best for this project, has resulted in the accomplishment of this book. They are a veteran in the field of academics and their pool of knowledge is as vast as their experience in printing. Their expertise and guidance has proved useful at every step. Their uncompromising quality standards have made this book an exceptional effort. Their encouragement from time to time has been an inspiration for everyone.

The publisher and the editorial board hope that this book will prove to be a valuable piece of knowledge for researchers, students, practitioners and scholars across the globe.

List of Contributors

Tahereh Fatemian and Ezharul Hoque Chowdhury
Jeffry Cheah School of Medicine and Health Sciences, Monash University Malaysia, Jalan Lagoon Selatan, 46150 Bandar Sunway, Malaysia

Hamid Reza Moghimi
School of Pharmacy, Shahid Beheshti University of Medical Sciences, 19839-63113 Tehran, Iran

Oluwatoyin A. Adeleke
Division of Pharmaceutical Sciences, School of Pharmacy, Sefako Makgatho Health Sciences University, Pretoria 0208, South Africa
Council for Scientific and Industrial Research, Pretoria 0001, South Africa

Rose K. Hayeshi
Council for Scientific and Industrial Research, Pretoria 0001, South Africa
DST/NWU Preclinical Drug Development Platform, Faculty of Health Sciences, North-West University, Potchefstroom 2531, South Africa

Hajierah Davids
Department of Physiology, Nelson Mandela University, Port Elizabeth 6031, South Africa

Verônica da Silva Oliveira, Fernanda Ílary Costa Duarte and Bárbara Cristina Silva Holanda Queiroz
Postgraduate Program in Pharmaceutical Sciences, Health Sciences Center, Federal University of Rio Grande do Norte, Natal-RN 59012-570, Brazil

Ádley Antonini Neves de Lima
Postgraduate Program in Pharmaceutical Sciences, Health Sciences Center, Federal University of Rio Grande do Norte, Natal-RN 59012-570, Brazil
Department of Pharmacy, Universidade Federal do Rio Grande do Norte, Natal-RN 59012-570, Brazil

Amanda Silva de Almeida and Ingrid da Silva Albuquerque
Department of Pharmacy, Universidade Federal do Rio Grande do Norte, Natal-RN 59012-570, Brazil

Attilio Converti
Department of Civil, Chemical and Environmental Engineering, Pole of Chemical Engineering, Genoa University, I-16145 Genoa, Italy

Alexander Ewe, Michael Karimov and Achim Aigner
Rudolf-Boehm-Institute for Pharmacology and Toxicology, Faculty of Medicine, Clinical Pharmacology, Leipzig University, 04107 Leipzig, Germany

Sandra Noske
Rudolf-Boehm-Institute for Pharmacology and Toxicology, Faculty of Medicine, Clinical Pharmacology, Leipzig University, 04107 Leipzig, Germany
Faculty of Chemistry, Technical University Kaiserslautern, 67663 Kaiserslautern, Germany

Špela Zupančič, Petra Kocbek and Julijana Kristl
Faculty of Pharmacy, University of Ljubljana, Aškerčeva 7, SI-1000 Ljubljana, Slovenia

Aleš Berlec
Faculty of Pharmacy, University of Ljubljana, Aškerčeva 7, SI-1000 Ljubljana, Slovenia
Department of Biotechnology, Jožef Stefan Institute, Jamova 39, SI-1000 Ljubljana, Slovenia

Katja Škrlec
Department of Biotechnology, Jožef Stefan Institute, Jamova 39, SI-1000 Ljubljana, Slovenia

Dongwei Wan, Min Zhao and Jingjing Zhang
College of Pharmacy, China Pharmaceutical University, No. 639 Longmian Road, Nanjing 211100, China

Libiao Luan
College of Pharmacy, China Pharmaceutical University, Xuanwumen Campus, No. 24 Tongjiaxiang, Nanjing 210009, China

Silvia Pisani, Enrica Chiesa, Ida Genta and Pietro Grisoli
Department of Drug Sciences, University of Pavia, Viale Taramelli 12/14, 27100 Pavia, Italy

Rossella Dorati, Tiziana Modena and Bice Conti
Department of Drug Sciences, University of Pavia, Viale Taramelli 12/14, 27100 Pavia, Italy
Polymerix S.r.l., Via Taramelli 24, 27100 Pavia, Italy

Giovanna Bruni
Department of Chemistry, University of Pavia, Viale Taramelli 12/14, 27100 Pavia, Italy

Liis Preem, Andres Meos and Karin Kogermann
Institute of Pharmacy, Faculty of Medicine, University of Tartu, Nooruse 1, 50411 Tartu, Estonia

Frederik Bock
Department of Pharmacy, University of Copenhagen, Universitetsparken 2, DK-2100 Copenhagen Ø, Denmark

Mariliis Hinnu, Marta Putrinš, Kadi Sagor and Tanel Tenson
Institute of Technology, Faculty of Natural Sciences, University of Tartu, Nooruse 1, 50411 Tartu, Estonia

Jesper Østergaard
Department of Pharmacy, University of Copenhagen, Universitetsparken 2, DK-2100 Copenhagen Ø, Denmark
LEO Foundation Center for Cutaneous Drug Delivery, Department of Pharmacy, University of Copenhagen, Universitetsparken 2, DK-2100 Copenhagen Ø, Denmark

Ana Paula Dinis Ano Bom, Patrícia Cristina da Costa Neves, Dilson Silva and Sotiris Missailidis
Instituto de Tecnologia em Imunobiológicos (Bio-Manguinhos), Fundação Oswaldo Cruz. Av. Brasil, 4365-Manguinhos, Rio de Janeiro/RJ CEP 21040-900, Brazil

Carlos Eduardo Bonacossa de Almeida
Laboratório de Radiobiologia, Divisão de Física Médica, Instituto de Radioproteção e Dosimetria, Comissão Nacional de Energia Nuclear. Av. Salvador Allende S/N., Rio de Janeiro/RJ CEP 22783-127, Brazil

Inmaculada Mora-Espí, Elena Ibáñez, Jorge Soriano, Carme Nogués and Leonardo Barrios
Unitat de Biologia Cel·lular, Departament de Biologia Cel·lular, Fisiologia i Immunologia, Facultat de Biociències, Universitat Autònoma de Barcelona, Bellaterra, 08193 Barcelona, Spain

Thorarinn Gudjonsson
Biomedical Center, University of Iceland, 101 Reykjavík, Iceland
Department of Anatomy, Faculty of Medicine, and Department of Laboratory Hematology, University Hospital, 101 Reykjavik, Iceland

Urve Paaver, Jyrki Heinämäki and Ivo Laidmäe
Institute of Pharmacy, Faculty of Medicine, University of Tartu, Nooruse 1, 50411 Tartu, Estonia

Ivan Kassamakov, Tuomo Ylitalo and Edward Hæggström
Electronics Laboratory, Department of Physics, (Gustaf Hällströmin katu 2a), University of Helsinki, FI-00014 Helsinki, Finland

Irem Unalan, Stefan J. Endlein, Rainer Detsch and Aldo R. Boccaccini
Institute of Biomaterials, Department of Materials Science and Engineering, Friedrich-Alexander-University Erlangen-Nuremberg, Cauerstraße 6, 91058 Erlangen, Germany

Benedikt Slavik and Andrea Buettner
Chair of Aroma and Smell Research, Department of Chemistry and Pharmacy, Friedrich-Alexander-University Erlangen-Nuremberg, Henkestraße 9, 91054 Erlangen, Germany

Wolfgang H. Goldmann
Institute of Biophysics, Department of Physics, Friedrich-Alexander-University Erlangen-Nuremberg, Henkestraße 91, 91052 Erlangen, Germany

Mónica C. Guadarrama-Acevedo, Raisa A. Mendoza-Flores, Zaida Urbán-Morlán and Gerardo Leyva-Gómez
Departamento de Farmacia, Facultad de Química, Universidad Nacional Autónoma de México, Ciudad Universitaria, Circuito Exterior S/N, Del. Coyoacán, Ciudad de México 04510, México

María L. Del Prado-Audelo
Departamento de Farmacia, Facultad de Química, Universidad Nacional Autónoma de México, Ciudad Universitaria, Circuito Exterior S/N, Del. Coyoacán, Ciudad de México 04510, México
Laboratorio de Posgrado en Tecnología Farmacéutica, FES-Cuautitlán, Universidad Nacional Autónoma de México, Cuautitlán Izcalli 54740, México

David M. Giraldo-Gomez
Departamento de Biología Celular y Tisular, Facultad de Medicina, Universidad Nacional Autónoma de México (UNAM), Edificio "A" 3er piso, Circuito Interior, Avenida Universidad 3000, Ciudad Universitaria, Coyoacán, Ciudad de México 04510, México

Hernán Cortés, Jonathan J. Magaña and Carla D. Florán-Hernández
Laboratorio de Medicina Genómica, Departamento de Genética, Instituto Nacional de Rehabilitación Luis Guillermo Ibarra Ibarra, Ciudad de México 14389, México

Maykel González-Torres
CONACyT-Laboratorio de Biotecnología, Instituto Nacional de Rehabilitación Luis Guillermo Ibarra Ibarra, Ciudad de México 14389, México
Instituto Tecnológico y de Estudios Superiores de Monterrey, Campus Ciudad de México 14380, México

Octavio D. Reyes-Hernández
Laboratorio de Biología Molecular del Cáncer, UMIEZ, Facultad de Estudios Superiores Zaragoza, Universidad Nacional Autónoma de México, Ciudad de México 09230, México

Gabriela Figueroa-González
CONACyT-Laboratorio de Genómica, Dirección de Investigación, Instituto Nacional de Cancerología. Av. San Fernando 22, Tlalpan, Sección XVI, Ciudad de México 14080, México

Benjamín Florán
Departamento de Fisiología, Biofísica & Neurociencias, Centro de Investigación y de Estudios Avanzados del Instituto Politécnico Nacional, Ciudad de México 07360, México

Isaac H. Caballero-Florán
Departamento de Farmacia, Facultad de Química, Universidad Nacional Autónoma de México, Ciudad Universitaria, Circuito Exterior S/N, Del. Coyoacán, Ciudad de México 04510, México
Departamento de Fisiología, Biofísica & Neurociencias, Centro de Investigación y de Estudios Avanzados del Instituto Politécnico Nacional, Ciudad de México 07360, México

Pramod W. Ramteke
Department of Biological Sciences, Sam Higginbottom University of Agriculture, Technology and Sciences, Allahabad 211007, India

Charu Dwivedi
Department of Biological Sciences, Sam Higginbottom University of Agriculture, Technology and Sciences, Allahabad 211007, India
Nanotechnology Application Centre, Faculty of Science, University of Allahabad, Allahabad 211002, India

Avinash C. Pandey
Nanotechnology Application Centre, Faculty of Science, University of Allahabad, Allahabad 211002, India

Himanshu Pandey
Nanotechnology Application Centre, Faculty of Science, University of Allahabad, Allahabad 211002, India
Department of Pharmaceutical Sciences, Faculty of Health Sciences, Sam Higginbottom University of Agriculture, Technology & Sciences, Allahabad 211007, India

Sandip Patil
E-Spin Nanotech Pvt Ltd., Kanpur 208016, India

Peter Laux and Andreas Luch
Department of Chemical and Product Safety, German Federal Institute for Risk Assessment (BfR), Max-Dohrn-Strasse 8-10, 10589 Berlin, Germany

Ajay Vikram Singh
Department of Chemical and Product Safety, German Federal Institute for Risk Assessment (BfR), Max-Dohrn-Strasse 8-10, 10589 Berlin, Germany
Physical Intelligence Department, Max Planck Institute for Intelligent Systems, 70569 Stuttgart, Germany

Index

www.ingramcontent.com/pod-product-compliance
Lightning Source LLC
LaVergne TN
LVHW082140200926
848484LV00008B/2083